OIE/FAO International Scientific Conference on Avian Influenza

Developments in Biologicals

Vol. 124

This series «Developments in Biologicals» begins with Vol. 102 and is the continuation of IABs symposia series «Progress in Immunobiological Standardization», Vols 1-5, «Immunobiological Standardization», Vols 1-22 and «Developments in Biological Standardization», Vols 23-101.

Organized and published by the International Association for Biologicals (IABs)

KARGER

Basel · Freiburg · Paris · London · New York ·
Bangalore · Bangkok · Singapore · Tokyo · Sydney

OIE/FAO International Scientific Conference on Avian Influenza

Paris, France
7-8 April, 2005

Volume editors

Alejandro Schudel
World Organisation for Animal Health – OIE
Paris, France

Michel Lombard
International Association for Biologicals (IABs)
Geneva, Switzerland

Proceedings of a conference organized by the
World Organisation for Animal Health – OIE

42 figures and 27 tables, 2006

KARGER

Basel · Freiburg · Paris · London · New York ·
Bangalore · Bangkok · Singapore · Tokyo · Sydney

Developments in Biologicals

Library of Congress Cataloging-in-Publication Data

OIE/FAO International Scientific Conference on Avian Influenza (2005 : Paris, France)
OIE/FAO International Scientific Conference on Avian Influenza : Paris, France, 7-8 April 2005 / volume editors, Alejandro Schudel, Michel Lombard.
p. ; cm. -- (Developments in biologicals ; v. 124)
"Proceedings of a conference organized by the World Organisation for Animal Health-OIE."
Includes bibliographical references.
ISBN 3-8055-8031-2 (soft cover : alk. paper)
1. Avian influenza--Congresses. I. Schudel, Alejandro. II. Lombard, Michel. III. International Office of Epizootics. IV. Food and Agriculture Organization of the United Nations. V. Title. VI. Series.
[DNLM: 1. Influenza in Birds--epidemiology--Congresses. 2. Influenza A virus--pathogenicity--Congresses. 3. Influenza in Birds--prevention & control--Congresses. 4. Influenza in Birds--transmission--Congresses. 5. Influenza, Human--etiology--Congresses. SF 995.6.I6 O39o 2006]
RA644.I6O34 2006
614.5'18--dc22

2005033508

Bibliographic Indices. This publication is listed in bibliographic services, including Current Contents® and Index Medicus.

Drug dosage. The authors and the publisher have exerted every effort to ensure that drug selection and dosage set forth in this text are in accord with current recommendations and practice at the time of publication. However, in view of ongoing research, changes in government regulations, and the constant flow of information relating to drug therapy and drug reactions, the reader is urged to check the package insert for each drug for any change in indications and dosage and for added warnings and precautions. This is particularly important when the recommended agent is a new and/or infrequently employed drug.

Worldwide distribution by S. Karger AG, Basel (Switzerland).
Printed in Switzerland by Médecine et Hygiène, Genève.
ISBN 3-8055-8031-2

Steering Committee

Dr A. Schudel
Dr J. Domenech
Dr J.-L. Angot
Dr S. Jutzi
Dr D. Wilson

Scientific Programme Committee

Dr I. Capua
Dr D. Alexander
Mr D. Senne
Dr D. Swayne
Dr P. Selleck
Dr S. Marangon
Dr Y. Kida
Dr H. Chen
Dr J. Lubroth
Dr L. Sims

Organization of the Meeting

Opening Session	
Session I	Ecology and Epidemiology Chairperson: *D. Alexander* (VLA, UK) Rapporteur: *D. Swayne* (APHIS, USA)
Session II	Pathogenesis Chairperson: *B. Chantanee* (DLD, Thailand) Rapporteur: *P. Selleck* (AAHL, Australia)
Session III	Human Health Implications of Avian Influenza Chairperson: *F.-X. Meslin* (WHO) Rapporteur: *G. Koch* (CIDC, The Netherlands)
Session IV	Diagnostics Chairperson: *D. Swayne* (APHIS, USA) Rapporteur: *D. Senne* (APHIS, USA)
Session V	Control of Avian Influenza with Focus on Vaccination Chairperson: *I. Capua* (IZS, Italy) Rapporteur: *I. Brown* (VLA, UK)
Session VI	Improvement of Management Tools Chairperson: *P. Vannier* (AFSSA, France) Rapporteur: *D. Suarez* (SEPRL, USA)
Session VII	General Conclusions and Recommendations Chairperson: *B. Vallat* (OIE) Rapporteur: *J. Domenech* (FAO)
Poster Session	

Contents

Opening Session 1

Opening Words on Behalf of WHO 3
F.-X. Meslin
FAO Address 5
S.C. Jutzi
Welcome Speech 11
B. Vallat
Avian Influenza – Past, Present and Future Challenges 15
I. Capua

Session I

Ecology and Epidemiology 21
Chairperson: *D. Alexander* (VLA, UK)
Rapporteur: *D. Swayne* (APHIS, USA)

Epidemiology and Ecology of Highly Pathogenic Avian Influenza with Particular Emphasis on South East Asia 23
V. Martin, I. Sims, J. Lubroth, D. Pfeiffer, J. Slingenbergh, J. Domenech
Ecology and Epidemiology of Avian Influenza in North and South America 37
D.A. Senne, D.L. Suarez, D.E. Stallnecht, J.C. Pedersen, B. Panigrahy
Recent Epidemiology and Ecology of Influenza A Viruses in Avian Species in Europe and the Middle East 45
I.H. Brown, J. Banks, R.J. Manvell, S.C. Essen, W. Shell, M. Slomka, B. Londt, D.J. Alexander
Ecology and Epidemiology of Avian Influenza in Ostriches.... 51
A.J. Olivier

Session II

Pathogenesis 59
Chairperson: *B. Chantanee* (DLD, Thailand)
Rapporteur: *P. Selleck* (AAHL, Australia)

Pathogenicity of Avian Influenza Viruses in Poultry 61
D.E. Swayne, M. Pantin-Jackwood
Library of Influenza Virus Strains for Vaccine and Diagnostic Use Against Highly Pathogenic Avian Influenza and Human Pandemics 69
H. Kida, Y. Sakoda
Swine Influenza in China (Abstract) 73
H. Chen, H. Li, H. Yang, C. Qiao, K. Yu

Session III

Human Health Implications of Avian Influenza 75
Chairperson: *F.-X. Meslin* (WHO)
Rapporteur: *G. Koch* (CIDC, The Netherlands)

Avian Influenza Viruses and Human Health 77
D.J. Alexander
Occupational and Consumer Risks from Avian Influenza Viruses 85
D.E. Swayne

Session IV

Diagnostics 91
Chairperson: *D. Swayne* (APHIS, USA)
Rapporteur: *D. Senne* (APHIS, USA)

Advances in Molecular Diagnostics for Avian Influenza 93
I.H. Brown
Molecular Diagnosis of Avian Influenza during an Outbreak 99
G. Cattoli, I. Capua

Session V

Control of Avian Influenza with Focus on Vaccination 107
Chairperson: *I. Capua* (IZS, Italy)
Rapporteur: *I. Brown* (VLA, UK)

Control of Avian Influenza in Italy: from Stamping out to Emergency and Prophylactic Vaccination 109
S. Marangon, I. Capua
Avian Influenza Vaccination in North America: Strategies and Difficulties 117
D.L. Suarez, C.-W. Lee, D.E. Swayne
Control and Eradication Strategies of Avian Influenza in Mexico 125
C.L. Villareal
Development of a Recombinant Fowlpox Virus Vector-Based Vaccine of H5N1 Subtype Avian Influenza 127
C. Qiao, K. Yu, Y. Jiang, C. Li, G. Tian, X. Wang, H. Chen
Use of Avian Influenza Vaccination in Hong Kong 133
T.M. Ellis, L.D. Sims, H.K.H. Wong, C.W. Wong, K.C. Dyrting, K.W. Chow, C. Leung, J.S.M. Peiris
Use of Strategic Vaccination for the Control of Avian Influenza in Pakistan 145
K. Naeem, N. Siddique
Making Avian Influenza Vaccines Available, an Industry Point of View (IFAH) 151
P. van Aarle

Session VI

Improvement of Management Tools 157
Chairperson: *P. Vannier* (AFSSA, France)
Rapporteur: *D. Suarez* (SEPRL, USA)

OIE Laboratory Standards for Avian Influenza 159
S. Edwards

Surveillance and Compartmentalisation as a Tool to Control Avian Influenza 163
C. Zepeda
Social Economic and Policy Issues in the Long-Term Control of HPAI 171
A. McLeod, E. Guerne-Bleich

General Conclusions and Recommendations 177
Chairperson: *B. Vallat* (OIE)
Rapporteur: *J. Domenech* (FAO)
Panel: *I. Capua* (IZS, Italy), *S. Edwards* (VLA, UK), *K. Sakamoto* (NIAH, Japan), *A. Thiermann* (OIE)

Recommendations 179

Poster Session 187

Phylogenetic Analyses of Genes from South African LPAI Viruses Isolated in 2004 from Wild Aquatic Birds Suggests Introduction by Eurasian Migrants 189
C. Abolnik, E. Cornelius, S.P.R. Bisschop, M. Romito, D. Verwoerd
Ecology and Molecular Epidemiology of H9N2 Avian Influenza Viruses Isolated in Israel during 2000-2004 Epizootic 201
S. Perk, A. Panshin, E. Shihmanter, I. Gissin, S. Pokamunski, M. Pirak, M. Lipkind
HPAI Surveillance Programme in Cambodia: Results and Perspectives 211
S. Desvaux, S. Sorn, D. Holl, D. Chavernac, F. Goutard, J. Thonnat, V. Porphyre, C. Ménard, E. Cardinale, F. Roger
Abstracts 225

Schudel A, Lombard M (eds): OIE/FAO International Scientific Conference on Avian Influenza.
Dev Biol (Basel). Basel, Karger, 2006, vol 124, p 1.

OPENING SESSION

Schudel A, Lombard M (eds): OIE/FAO International Scientific Conference on Avian Influenza.
Dev Biol (Basel). Basel, Karger, 2006, vol 124, pp 3-4.

Opening Words on Behalf of WHO

F.-X. Meslin

World Health Organization, Geneva, Switzerland

Dear Dr. B. Vallat, Dr. S. Jutzi and dear colleagues and friends,

On behalf of Dr. Lee, Director General of the WHO, I want to thank OIE and FAO for their very kind invitation to participate in this important meeting.

According to the programme, Dr. G. Rodier, Director of the Surveillance Response Department, was expected to deliver the WHO address. He is unfortunately unable to, as he is tied up in an emergency meeting on influenza in the USA.

Dr. Lee and Dr. Rodier asked me to convey their best wishes for a very successful meeting.

This is the second international meeting on AI organised by OIE and FAO to which WHO has been invited this year (the first was in Ho Chi Minh City in February) and it is always a pleasure for WHO to be given the opportunity to contribute to the deliberations of the animal health and production sector.

This is not the time to describe the AI situation in any detail as the meeting itself will deal with all aspects including public health, but I would like to mention here that:

- The unprecedented Asian epidemic of HP avian influenza in birds is not yet under control.
- A total of 79 human cases have been reported in three countries with a frightening overall 62 % case fatality rate.
- There are indications of possible changes in human AI clinical presentation and virus pathogenicity.
- The number of reported clusters of human cases is increasing.
- This all seems to indicate that the possibility for a pandemic to emerge is getting closer and WHO is on the alert.

Today, influenza and particularly influenza surveillance and pandemic preparedness are a top priority in WHO, and WHO Member States expect our specialised organisation to do all that is possible to prepare the world for a pandemic. My colleague Klaus Stöhr will tell you more about this during the afternoon session.

WHO fully agrees with FAO and OIE that combating the disease at its source is the best strategy to protect both human and animal health.

We are aware of the large amount of attention paid to the public health implications but that the animal health component should not be forgotten. In relation to this, WHO hopes that FAO and OIE will be able to mobilise the financial and human resources as well as the political support that are needed to control the situation in birds very soon, as the window of opportunity may not last much longer.

From somewhat diverging views at the beginning of the AI crisis in early 2004, I am happy to say that today the three organisations have reached a common understanding of the AI situation: we can see the synergies among our organisations increasing by the day.

For example, our three organisations have decided to:

- Better co-ordinate their AI research and surveillance activities.
- Jointly organise a meeting on reducing the public health risks associated with production, distribution and marketing of live animals in Asia.
- Join forces to detect and contain outbreaks of diseases of common interest more quickly by developing GLEWS.

Once again, I wish to thank the organisers of the meeting for inviting WHO. I am convinced that this event will further strengthen our ability to deal together with the HPAI threat at the international, regional and national level.

I wish you all a very fruitful meeting.

Dr. F.-X. Meslin, World Health Organization, 27, avenue Appia, CH-1211 Geneva 27, Switzerland.
E-mail: meslinf@who.int

Schudel A, Lombard M (eds): OIE/FAO International Scientific Conference on Avian Influenza.
Dev Biol (Basel). Basel, Karger, 2006, vol 124, pp 5-9.

FAO Address

S.C. Jutzi

Animal Production and Health Division, FAO, Rome, Italy

The importance of this scientific conference cannot be overstated. The world's scientific leaders in all aspects related to avian influenza assembled in this room are expected to provide the most up-to-date and effective guidance on how best to handle this very serious threat to animals, human livelihoods and public health. The conclusions and resolutions of this Conference will be instrumental in clarifying all important open questions to be answered when the OIE General Assembly will have to agree next month on the "rules of the game", if I may use this expression.

Avian influenza has had an enormous economic and social impact on affected countries and the risk of this animal disease situation evolving into a global human influenza pandemic is of great public concern. CLSA Asia-Pacific Markets, the Asian investment banking arm of Crédit Agricole of France, estimated in a report released on Monday this week that the disease has already cost Asian nations US$8 to 12 billion. Increasingly, corporate analysts rank highly pathogenic avian influenza as one of the major risks, along with a banking crisis, civil unrest and armed conflict, that could derail the Asian region's current economic expansion.

FAO has recognised the seriousness of this situation and has focused its respective leadership and co-ordination efforts in the Emergency Centre for Control of Transboundary Animal Diseases (ECTAD) under the direction of Dr. Joseph Domenech, Chief Veterinary Officer of FAO. ECTAD was created by the Director General of FAO to enable centralised decision-making on programme management, since it is common practice in Chief Veterinary Offices in the face of epidemic diseases. In partnership with OIE and WHO, FAO has been working closely with affected countries, regional organisations, the international community and donors, to help manage this serious problem.

It is in the interest of all countries, developed or developing, to invest in the containment of avian influenza. The common objective is to protect human health by controlling the disease at source. This means addressing the transmission of the virus where the disease occurs, in poultry, specifically free-range chickens and water fowl, thus curbing disease occurrence in the region before it spreads to other parts of the world. There is a continuing risk of avian influenza spreading that no poultry-keeping country can afford to ignore.

It is likely that avian influenza will persist for many years in some of the countries that had disease outbreaks in 2003 and 2004. The presence of these adaptable viruses in reservoirs such as farmed ducks, wild birds and live-bird markets, means that highly pathogenic avian influenza elimination must be addressed as a long-term goal. In the immediate and short term, the objective, then, is to contain infection in known reservoirs and to minimise the risk of infection spilling over into farmed poultry and humans in villages and farms. In the longer term, FAO and its partners will continue working with affected countries to eliminate infection from as many production systems as possible, using the established, proven tools, and also embracing new technologies and approaches, including vaccination where indicated, based on the relevant scientific research and development efforts. This Conference will help advance decisively the consensus on such technologies and approaches and will thus enhance the effectiveness and efficiency of detection, control and elimination efforts, which the international community is called on to help accelerate.

In the recent FAO/OIE-organised regional avian influenza meeting in Ho Chi Minh City, veterinary service officials and international experts took stock of the experiences with the crisis over the past year and passed a range of resolutions which are considered crucial for the enhanced progress of disease detection, surveillance and control activities set up in the affected countries and the region.

Dr. Domenech will report in detail on this meeting; I therefore highlight only some major elements of the consensus achieved there:

- Regional approaches to problem solution are crucial; regional networks of national laboratories and epidemiology units are essential for enhancing quality, transparency, consistency and reliability of disease information.
- For effective and efficient prevention and control of devastating diseases such as avian influenza, substantially increased investments are required in national veterinary services and surveillance systems at the central, decentralised and local levels, covering farms, villages and markets.
- There are substantial research requirements for filling knowledge gaps in the epidemiology of avian influenza, and in the preparation of vaccines that are more effective and easier to administer than the current ones, both for chicken and ducks.
- Countries, whether or not they are affected by avian influenza, are looking with very high expectations to the conclusion of the on-going updating of OIE's Terrestrial Animal Health Code with respect to this disease.
- International collaboration in support of the affected countries and region is recognised as important. This concerns in particular FAO, OIE and WHO.

In this context, I would like to express my satisfaction with the way in which FAO and OIE have co-ordinated their respective support to the affected countries and region. This was done by implementing the recently renewed and revised FAO/OIE Collaborative Agreement.

This Agreement has enabled a far-reaching initiative which FAO and OIE have recently agreed in setting up the Global Framework for the Progressive Control of Transboundary Animal Diseases or GF-TADs. The goal of this initiative is to help strengthen National Veterinary Services for the application of effective epidemiological knowledge to progressive disease control at source. In addition to the necessary strengthening of the veterinary services at the national level, GF-TADs emphasises regional co-ordination and co-operation as a prerequisite for the effective control of serious, highly contagious diseases that do not respect international borders. The initiative was formally started in Asia last month. Latin America will follow next week.

This initiative, which integrates the complementary roles of FAO and OIE in a synergistic manner, is offered to the international community as an effective instrument for much enhanced transboundary animal disease prevention and control. It is hoped that all countries, regional organisations and donor agencies will resolve to support this global effort for a more effective fight against these devastating animal diseases.

The creation of the OIE/FAO network of avian influenza reference laboratories, which is going to be formally announced during this Conference, is a result of this enhanced inter-agency collaboration. This network will interact closely with the WHO influenza network to achieve common objectives.

As we know, many of the countries currently affected by avian influenza have limited capacity to control these adaptable and highly contagious viruses. They lack effective diagnostic capability and surveillance systems, which are essential for early warning and timely response. Veterinary infrastructures must be strengthened through the provision of scientific and technical advice, equipment and supplies. FAO, in the context of the GF-TADs initiative, continues to place priority on supporting the implementation of more effective systems for diagnosis, surveillance and control. Affected countries still need more help to search actively for infection and conduct detailed epidemiological analysis. This will help to ensure regional sharing of information and international reporting in a timely and transparent manner. Veterinary services also need access to better tools for diagnosis and disease control, including vaccines that are efficient, cost-effective and safe.

FAO allocated US$5.5 m in early 2004 to its avian influenza programme and is running a suite of 19 national, regional and international projects designed to assist the fight against the disease. This complex operation is managed by Dr. Domenech and supported by a multi-disciplinary Task Force, including staff from Headquarters and the Regional Office in Bangkok.

My colleagues will speak during the Conference in some detail on the experiences with this programme; I will limit myself simply to mentioning some major thrusts.

More than 70 expert missions were facilitated to affected countries, expert meetings were called, veterinary systems personnel met on several occasions at regional level; specialised equipment and materials were provided; regional laboratory and epidemiology networks were established and supported; general and country-specific control strategy guidelines were prepared; studies were undertaken on crisis explanation, economic and social impact of the crisis, sector rehabilitation options; and a major effort was undertaken to provide exhaustive and continuous disease intelligence analysis and to maintain communication with all interested parties, including the media. I may mention here the *AIDE News Bulletin* which has been produced on a regular basis, so far in 28 issues. Its 29th issue will appear this week.

I would like to conclude with the major requirements for the support to the affected countries and region: FAO, in agreement with OIE, regional organisations and countries, recommends immediate implementation of the following sets of actions at a national, regional and global level.

At the national level, assistance is required to help governments:

- To strengthen the central animal health and Veterinary Public Health Services to manage national surveillance systems better, to improve early detection and response, define strategies, and monitor their implementation.
- To implement disease prevention and control programmes, including stamping out, biosecurity and vaccination as appropriate.
- To develop better tools (e.g. diagnostic methods, vaccines, antiviral agents) and analyse their effectiveness and costs, under local conditions, to help mitigate risk.

At the regional level, assistance is required to help:

- To support incipient regional diagnostic and surveillance networks, improve the quality of epidemiological information and facilitate transparency, sharing of information and early warning, leading to better prevention and control of avian influenza.
- To strengthen regional co-operation with the goal of helping countries to harmonise surveillance and control strategies, realise economies of scale and scope, and establish sustainable funding and financial instruments for cross-border activities.

At the global level:

- FAO and OIE require sufficient donor support to provide the scientific and technical advice required by countries.
- FAO and OIE are prepared to launch a more formal initiative that would internationally raise and sustain the profile and investment in highly pathogenic avian influenza control with the aim of its ultimate eradication. Various models are feasible, ranging from an International Commission to a Global Programme; it will be part of the GF-TADs initiative mentioned earlier.

FAO, in collaboration with OIE and other partners, has identified a global strategic approach that will require sustained donor support to countries in this region. It is unfortunate that so far the international community has been somewhat slow in responding with such support. FAO is currently in the process of intensive donor contacts so as to revert this situation

Controlling highly pathogenic avian influenza world-wide is our common duty in whatever capacity we are faced with this threat.

Stopping the disease at source is a strategy that fully recognises the importance of sound animal health and veterinary public health infrastructures in dealing with epidemic diseases and promoting food security. It is also the prerequisite for all efforts that countries will undertake in repositioning, rehabilitating or even restructuring their poultry sector. Such repositioning of the poultry sector relies on effective and efficient animal health management capabilities whatever the role of this sector may be.

Finally and importantly, I would like to thank you all for your agreement to participate in this Conference and to contribute your valuable inputs.

Dr. S.C. Jutzi, Animal Production and Health Divison, FAO, Vialle delle Terme di Caracalla, IT-00100 Rome, Italy.
E-mail: Samuel.jutzi@fao.org

Schudel A, Lombard M (eds): OIE/FAO International Scientific Conference on Avian Influenza.
Dev Biol (Basel). Basel, Karger, 2006, vol 124, pp 11-14.

Welcome Speech

B. Vallat

OIE Director General, Paris, France

Dear representatives of international and regional organisations, distinguished delegates of member countries, honourable OIE expert's participants and observers,
Ladies and gentlemen,

It is my great pleasure to welcome you to this International Conference on avian influenza organised by the OIE and the FAO in collaboration with the WHO.

During the past few years, the world has witnessed a global emergence and re-emergence of several infectious animal diseases that have had, and are still having, significant impact on both animal and human health. These infections have not only caused much concern to governments, policy makers and scientists all over the world, but some of them have posed significant threats to the livelihoods of the farming community especially in rural areas. One example is currently being provided by avian influenza (AI), which has presented a crisis unprecedented in scope, geographical distribution and severity. This disease has been, and still is, responsible for disastrous economic losses, especially in Southeast Asia, resulting in millions of people living in poverty. This disease is capable, not only of spreading to other continents, but it has the potential to lead to a human pandemic. This explains our close collaboration with WHO, our main objective being to prevent any pandemic from occurring by eliminating the virus at source, i.e. from animals.

OIE and FAO have already organised, with the support of WHO, a world-wide scientific conference at the beginning of the crisis and then two regional conferences in Southeast Asia to co-ordinate control efforts in the region. In addition to arranging scientific meetings, these two organisations have provided significant technical expertise to countries of the region in terms of capacity building for better surveillance, diagnosis and control of AI. As well as various Technical Cooperation Projects (TCPs) sponsored by FAO, OIE and FAO have solicited, and begun to obtain, further assistance from other regional and international organisations and donors. OIE and FAO are indeed grateful to all those organisations and institutions that have provided assistance, technical or otherwise.

Despite all these efforts though, much remains to be done. According to the latest information, the virus is still circulating in the region, as evidenced by the occurrences of new outbreaks, including human fatalities, both in previously affected countries and in new ones. The potential for the disease to spread to other continents is real and the international scientific community cannot remain insensitive to the challenge of preventing this from happening. The appearance of the disease in previously unaffected countries and its re-emergence in the region demonstrate the difficulties of controlling AI. This also shows the importance of careful, on-going early detection and surveillance strategies and monitoring, together with additional appropriate measures for effective control to achieve the final target, which should be the eradication of the disease.

It is now widely recognised that the current situation in Asia has strong links with traditional animal production and marketing systems, including backyard and subsistence poultry production, multiple animal species farming practices with chickens, ducks and pigs sharing common environments, and live poultry marketing systems. Recent research has also confirmed that aquatic birds, especially ducks, can act as reservoirs of infection with or without clinical signs and are capable of excreting viruses into the environment. It is therefore necessary that more attention be paid to bio-security measures.

The OIE and FAO have thought it wise, and considered it timely, that, following the two regional meetings organised by the two organisations, an international conference be held at the OIE, which has as a main mission the international prevention and control of animal diseases and zoonoses. The main objective of the conference is to review the latest scientific knowledge and to address the different aspects of the control of the disease based on this new knowledge. Presentations will be made on the experience gained in the recent past in the fields of epidemiology, pathogenesis, molecular diagnosis and control and eradication strategies. The conference will also provide an opportunity to evaluate further, and improve, the current standards and guidelines being proposed by the OIE for the better world-wide control of this important disease.

If member countries want to control animal diseases and zoonoses effectively, there is an immediate challenge that lies ahead. Strengthening the capacity of veterinary services for more effective disease control through an effective early detection and response system and follow-up of disease information at national, regional and world-wide level is an absolute necessity. As regards AI, member countries should review poultry marketing systems to obtain a higher level of bio-security, promote more applied research work, including investigations into the possible role of ducks as a reservoir of the disease, and the use of vaccination when relevant as recommended by OIE and FAO. These objectives can only be achieved with a strong and efficient veterinary service. I am happy to state here that, thanks to the persistent efforts of the OIE, strengthening veterinary services to enable better disease early detection, surveillance and response is now accepted by major international organisations as "an international public good".

As outlined earlier, the OIE has been working with its world-wide network of collaborating centres, reference laboratories and scientific experts, international organisations and its member countries. Ad hoc groups comprising the world's most reputed experts have already proposed science-based standards and guidelines on the diagnosis, surveillance and control measures that can be applied safely. These experts have, inter alia, reviewed diagnostic methods and made new recommendations on vaccines and vaccination policies applicable under different epidemiological circumstances. They have also reviewed the existing chapter on AI in the OIE *Terrestrial Animal Health Code* regarding standards to be applied to ensure the safety of the international trade in poultry and poultry products, taking care that, while such trade is being promoted by the removal of unjustified barriers, all reasonable precautions are taken to ensure that the virus is not spread to importing countries. Considerable attention has been given to food safety issues to ensure that the security of consumers is safeguarded and their confidence restored. The OIE has also produced standards related to humane killing of animals during the implementation of stamping-out programmes and the disposal of animal carcasses. All these standards and guidelines have been circulated to member countries for comments and all comments will be duly addressed by the elected experts of OIE specialist commissions and the OIE Central Bureau. After due consideration of comments received, the standards will be submitted for approval by the international committee comprising official representatives of all the 167 OIE member countries during the forthcoming General Session next month.

The OIE is also working in close collaboration with other relevant international and regional organisations including the FAO and WHO to control avian influenza in animals and to prevent a human pandemic. Consultations are on-going and further joint meetings are planned with FAO and WHO.

The OIE has recently proposed a joint OIE/FAO network on AI expertise primarily to promote research on the disease and to provide assistance especially to developing countries in the diagnosis and management of the disease. This OIE/FAO Network which comprises internationally reputed scientists from various parts of the world will have a Steering Committee chaired by the President of the OIE Biological Standards Commission. The Secretariat of the Network will be based in an OIE Reference Laboratory for AI. Another major objective is to set up with WHO a new mechanism allowing the management of the animal human interface through the OIE/FAO animal network and human WHO network. This network will provide the WHO with virus isolates from animals which could be used to produce soon human vaccines in the wake of a potential pandemic.

The official launching of the OIE/FAO Network (OFFLU) will be made during this conference.

Ladies and gentlemen,

The OIE will continue its activities against the disease in 2005 and beyond. It will in this respect continue to work in close collaboration with regional and international organisations. As you aware, the OIE and the FAO have officially agreed to work together in controlling major transboundary animal diseases globally and regionally, within the joint FAO/OIE Global Framework for the Progressive Control of Transboundary Animal Diseases called GF-TADs. The five OIE Regional Representations will serve as permanent secretariats for the five Regional Steering Committees to ensure regional coordination of the clusters of activities, to monitor progress and determine indicators for effective field and laboratory coordination in control efforts. The Regional Steering Committees will be composed of representatives of Chief Veterinary Officers, representatives of the Regional Specialised Organisations involved in animal health, specific donors and representatives of the OIE and the FAO.

The meeting of the Regional Steering Committee for Asia has already been held at the OIE Regional Representation for Asia and the Pacific in Tokyo, Japan. Meetings for the other regions are planned to be held in the near future and as expected, Highly Pathogenic Avian Influenza will be one of the priority issues that will be discussed.

I wish you a successful meeting.

Dr. B. Vallat, World Organization for Animal Health (OIE), 12, rue de Prony, FR-75017 Paris, France.
E-mail: b.vallat@oie.int

Schudel A, Lombard M (eds): OIE/FAO International Scientific Conference on Avian Influenza.
Dev Biol (Basel). Basel, Karger, 2006, vol 124, pp 15-20.

Avian Influenza – Past, Present and Future Challenges

I. Capua

OIE and National Reference Laboratory for Newcastle Disease and Avian Influenza, Istituto Zooprofilattico Sperimentale delle Venezie, Legnaro, Padova, Italy

Abstract: Avian influenza (AI) is an OIE-listed disease that has become of great importance both for animal and for human health. The increased relevance of AI in the fields of animal and human health, has highlighted the lack of scientific information on several aspects of the disease; this has hampered the adequate management of some of the recent crises, thus resulting in millions of dead animals and concern over loss of human lives and over management of the pandemic potential.

The present paper aims to identify areas of knowledge of veterinary competence that need to be explored to generate information to support the global AI crisis.

Given the current situation, it is imperative that close collaboration is sought and achieved by public health officials involved in the veterinary and medical aspects of the disease. In fact, only through the exchange of data, experiences, views and information will it be possible to combat this zoonosis that represents a major threat to public health and animal well-being.

INTRODUCTION

Avian influenza (AI) represents one of the greatest concerns for public health that has emerged in recent times. Over the past five years, there has been a sharp increase in the number of outbreaks of AI, compared to the previous 40 years. It has been calculated that the impact of AI on the poultry industry has increased 100-fold with 23 million birds affected in a 40-year period between 1959 and 1998 and over 200 million from 1999 to 2004 [1]. In fact, from the late 90s, AI infections have assumed a completely different profile both in the veterinary and medical scientific communities. In recent times, some outbreaks have maintained the characteristic of minor relevance while others, such as the Italian 1999-2000, the Dutch 2003, the Canadian 2004 and the ongoing Asian H5N1, have led to devastating consequences for the poultry industry and negative repercussions on public opinion, and in some cases have created significant human health issues, including the risk of generating a new pandemic virus for humans via the avian-human link.

The human health implications of avian influenza infections were revealed during the 1997 Hong-Kong outbreak, in which the H5N1 virus was shown to have infected 18 people, six of whom died. Following this episode, human infection and one death resulted from the H7N7/2003 outbreak in the Netherlands, and the H5N1 virus, which is currently endemic in Asia, has been shown to have caused the death of 49 individuals during 2003-2005 (as of the 4 April 2005). The human health implications of these AI infections are, however, not limited to the consequences of direct infection of human beings with an avian virus. They assume a greater magnitude if the reassortment of an avian virus with a human influenza virus during concurrent infection of a single host occurs. This mechanism could represent the basis for the generation of a new human pandemic virus with inauspicious consequences [2]. The increased relevance of AI in the fields of animal and human health, has highlighted the lack of scientific information on several aspects of the disease; this has hampered the adequate management of some of the recent crises, thus resulting in millions of dead animals and concern over loss of human lives and over management of the pandemic potential.

For this reason and for the devastating effects on the poultry industry, international organisations such as WHO/OIE/FAO have worked together and established a co-ordinated set of guidelines and action plans to combat the on-going Asian epidemic.

It has been recognised that, because of the low profile of AI until 1999, a significant amount of information and specific tools necessary to manage AI epidemics adequately are lacking. This refers both to the EU situation and to the on-going Asian H5N1 crisis. However, in recent years some scientific data has been generated and what is available should represent the initial grounds for an international approach to combat this disease.

The first issue that needs to be resolved encompasses legislative and regulatory aspects, such as the inclusion of low pathogenicity avian influenza (LPAI) viruses in the definition of AI. This proposal logically follows the scientific evidence that LPAI viruses of the H5 and H7 subtype are the progenitors of highly pathogenic avian influenza (HPAI) [3-5]. This represents a crucial aspect for prevention and control of future outbreaks and limiting the circulation of AI viruses, which is among the primary risk factors for the generation of reassortant viruses. It is therefore imperative that official veterinary services identify surveillance for AI as a priority, and manage LPAI outbreaks caused by viruses of the H5 and H7 subtypes in an appropriate manner.

Recent outbreaks in Europe, North and South America, the Republic of South Africa and particularly the on-going Asian H5N1 outbreak have raised the necessity of developing control and management strategies in an unprecedented eco-epidemiological situation. As an example, recent outbreaks of HPAI have affected avian species that exhibit a reduced clinical susceptibility to this virus. There is evidence that birds such as waterfowl and ostriches undergo a completely different pathogenesis from the poultry species (mainly *Galliformes*) that have traditionally been affected by the disease. It would therefore seem reasonable to make cautious assumptions and statements and to develop co-ordinated actions within well-defined research priorities.

The scientific veterinary community has a key role in the adequate management and ultimately in the outcome of the efforts that are being made to combat this global threat. Retrospective analysis of recent outbreaks has permitted the identification of weak points in the management system that represent areas of uncertainty for which improvement is required. On the basis of the eco-epidemiological situation in each country, these areas of uncertainty should be focused on and prioritised to maximise the outcome of the international effort.

Priority Areas of Intervention from a Veterinary Perspective

Limit the extension of the outbreak

Outbreaks that involve significant numbers of animals are characterised by the penetration of infection in the commercial circuit. It is known that biosecurity (encompassing bioexclusion and biocontainment) represents the first and most important means of prevention. It follows that, if biosecurity measures of a high standard are implemented and maintained, these represent a firewall against the penetration and perpetuation in the commercial circuit. However, breaches in biosecurity systems do occur. The occurrence and extent of the breach, on one hand should be evaluated and corrective measures should follow, on the other, indicate the need for the establishment of early warning systems for AI. Some of these are currently being implemented in countries that have identified their densely populated poultry areas (DPPA) as areas at risk, such as The Netherlands and Italy and some states of the USA. These early warning systems include syndrome surveillance programmes and serological monitoring systems [6-8]. However, the early warning systems will have a positive outcome only if an appropriate contingency plan has been developed conjunctly between the official veterinarians and the industry. The firm implementation of the contingency plan is crucial to the reduction of the magnitude of the outbreak.

Impact on the poultry industry and on public veterinary services

Avian influenza has had a devastating impact on the poultry industry in the countries affected by it in recent years. One of the reasons for this lies in the magnitude of the outbreaks, which may have resulted from inappropriate management in the affected countries, at least at the beginning of the outbreak. Until recent times, public and private veterinarians were not adequately trained to diagnose and manage this disease. There has been a great deal of improvement in some countries, but not in others. AI is a transboundary animal disease that has its natural reservoir in migratory waterfowl. No country can consider itself safe from introduction ; therefore specific joint training courses for public and private poultry veterinarians and upgrading of laboratory capacities to face the possible emergency should be considered as national priorities.

Role of waterfowl and other non gallinaceous birds in the epidemiology of AI

Recent outbreaks occurring in areas that have been free historically from HPAI have caused extensive spillover of infection in intensively reared avian species that previously had been affected only sporadically. It should be pointed out that, for example, chickens, ducks and ostriches belong to different families within the class *Aves*, and are therefore phylogenetically quite distinct. Areas of knowledge that are available for gallinaceous birds are therefore not directly applicable to birds belonging to different families. These areas include pathogenesis and evaluation of the carrier state, transmission dynamics and efficacy of vaccination. A co-ordinated set of efforts should be made to develop joint research programmes that complement each other thus avoiding overlap and wasted resources.

Control and prevention

Between December 1999 and April 2003, over 50 million birds died or were depopulated following HPAI infection in the EU alone [1], causing significant economic losses to the private and public sectors. The slaughter and destruction of great numbers of animals is also questionable from an ethical point of view. This would suggest that the strategies and control measures used to combat the disease at the European level require improvement both from a disease control and animal welfare perspective.

Specific recommendations concerning the areas of knowledge that require improvement in the field of AI have been issued by the EU Scientific Committee of Animal Health and Welfare, in the report on "Diagnostic techniques and vaccines for foot-and-mouth disease, classical swine fever, avian influenza and some other important list A diseases" adopted on 24-25 April 2003 [9]. Guidelines on disease prevention and control with particular reference to the Asian crisis have been issued as joint OIE/FAO/WHO recommendations in the recent meetings in Rome (3-4 February 2004), Bangkok (26-28 February 2004) and Ho-Chi Min City (23-25 February 2005).

These recommendations, however, need to be put into practice in a variety of different field situations, and the applicability of one system rather than another in a given situation must be evaluated, bearing in mind the benefits of a successful result but also the drawbacks of a failure.

Vaccination has been shown to be a powerful tool to support eradication programmes in situations in which a stamping-out policy is neither pursuable or desirable. Previous experiences have indicated that, to be successful in controlling and ultimately in eradicating the infection, vaccination programmes must be part of a wider control strategy, which includes monitoring the evolution of infection and biosecurity.

Basic information on the characteristics, efficacy and limitations of currently available products has been generated, and the selection of the product should be carried out on the basis of the eco-epidemiological situation and regulatory position of the given country.

What appears to be lacking in some situations are guidelines that define an appropriate territorial approach. These may be derived from general guidelines on surveillance for epizootic diseases, but must be adapted to the local situations and must be targeted towards a well-defined and pursuable objective.

In addition, because of the recent exposure of a vast variety of avian species to HPAI, it is imperative that specific research programmes are developed to evaluate the efficacy of vaccination in these species and to develop and validate novel vaccination concepts that enable the DIVA (differentiating infected from vaccinated animals) system.

To date, vaccination is not formally regulated under current OIE guidelines. EU Council Directive 92/40/EEC does foresee the use of emergency vaccination, but the consequences on movements of birds and products are not detailed. This regulatory deficiency results in uncertainties in the decision-making process as to whether to vaccinate or not. In the face of an outbreak, exporting countries have not had the legislative support to implement vaccination and continue to trade; this has resulted, for example, in opting for a stamping-out policy, leading to 30,000,000 dead birds in the Netherlands in 2003, with great costs for the industry and the taxpayer. Formal international guidelines and rules on the application of a vaccination programme should be defined.

Human health implications

As a result of the recent cases of human infection caused by AI viruses, and the concern about the generation of a new pandemic virus, AI infections are considered a significant threat to public health.

To limit this occurrence, it appears logical that virus circulation should be reduced and contacts at risk should be avoided. From a superficial point of view, this problem appears to be simple. Instead it is probably the most complex problem to be addressed in developing countries. Most contacts at risk occur between villagers and rural chickens. The nature and entity of these contacts are dependent on social and behavioural practices linked to food security or hobby activities. The modification of these patterns appears to be inapplicable in the short term and, for this reason, pilot vaccination interventions of rural poultry appear to be the only means to achieve a reduction of virus load in the rural environment.

In addition, training courses for farm or other workers potentially exposed to the virus should be developed and applied. They should include outbreak management practices, instructions on how to use protective gear and contingency plans in case of accidental exposure.

Food safety

The zoonotic implications of AI have raised concerns about the safety of food obtained from poultry. AI viruses have been isolated from poultry meat and from commercial eggs [10,11]. The extent of this event is dependent on a series of different factors, including the avian species affected, the viral strain and whether the product is processed or not. Data on the presence of selected AI strains has been generated recently and other studies are in progress [12]. These findings will represent the basis for the assessment of the risk posed by poultry products for human consumption and spread of disease to other animals through swill feeding. The latter event appears to occur rather frequently in some parts of the world and sanitary measures should be taken to prevent it happening.

Given the variety of products originating from poultry that are intended for human consumption, specific tests should be performed to establish whether viable virus can be detected in different commodities. In addition, the evaluation of processing and heat treatment of products should be carried out for different products.

Animal welfare

The occurrence of major outbreaks of epizootic diseases very often results in poor animal welfare. This is related both to the suffering caused to the animal by the disease, and also to movement restrictions imposed on animals that should be slaughtered or relocated. Moreover, particularly for avian species, only recently has there been specific interest in the development of humane, large-scale culling systems. To respect animal welfare, approved culling systems of proven efficacy should be made available or developed on the basis of the requirements and the type of poultry production in the country. Staff destined to culling operations must be trained in times of peace and organised in task forces that are able to work on a 24-hour shift if necessary. In some situations (e.g. if culling capacity is insufficient), vaccination may be seen as a means to preserve animal welfare in the period that precedes culling.

Conclusions

The scientific veterinary community has areas of expertise that can support AI crisis management, however, there are areas in which knowledge needs to improve and the outcome of such effort should be made available to the international scientific community. An enormous effort should be made by national governments and funding bodies to make resources available to develop research programmes based on the priorities that have been identified globally and that appear most relevant to the single country.

It is imperative that transversal research programmes, encompassing veterinary, medical and agricultural science are developed and sustained, to maximise the global effort to combat this disease.

References

1 Capua I, Alexander DJ: Avian influenza: recent developments. Avian Pathol 2004; 33: 393-404.

2 Capua, I, Alexander DJ: Human Health Implications of Avian Influenza Viruses and Paramyxoviruses. Eur J Clin Microbiol Infect Dis 2004; 23:1-6.

3 Garcia M, Crawford JM, Latimer JW, Rivera-Cruz E, Perdue ML: Heterogeneity in the haemagglutinin gene and emergence of the highly pathogenic phenotype among recent H5N2 avian influenza viruses from Mexico. J Gen Virol 1996; 77: 1493-1504.

4 Perdue M, Crawford J, Garcia M, Latimer J, Swayne DE: Occurrence and possible mechanisms of cleavage site insertions in the avian influenza hemagglutinin gene. Proceedings of the 4th International Symposium on Avian Influenza. Athens, Georgia. U.S. Animal Health Association 1998; 182-193.

5 Suarez DL, Senne DA, Banks J, Brown IH, Essen SC, Lee CW, Manvell RJ, Mathieu-Benson C, Mareno V, Pedersen J, Panigrahy B, Rojas H, Spackman E, Alexander DJ: Recombination resulting in virulence shift in avian influenza outbreak, Chile. Emerg Infect Dis 2004; 10:1-13.

6 De Wit JJ, Koch G, Fabri THF, Elbers ARW: A cross sectional serological survey of the Dutch commercial poultry population for the presence of low pathogenic avian influenza infections. Avian Pathol 2004; 33: 565-570

7 Commission Decision 2004/666/CE of 29 September 2004. Official J Eur Commission 2004; L303: 35-44.

8 Akey BL: Low Pathogenicity H7N2 Avian influenza outbreak in Virginia during 2002. Avian Dis 2002; 47: 1099-1103.

9 SCAHAW (Scientific Committee on Animal Health and Animal Welfare): Scientific opinion on recent advances in diagnostic techniques and vaccines for several important OIE List A diseases, including avian influenza. 2003.

10 Tumpey TM, Suarez DL, Perkins LEL, Senne DA, Lee YJ, Mo IP, Sung HW, Swayne DE: Characterization of a highly pathogenic H5N1 avian influenza A virus isolated from duck meat. J Virol 2002; 76: 6344-6355.

11 Cappucci DT, Johnson DC, Brugh M, Smith TM, Jackson CF, Pearson JE, Senne DA: Isolation of avian influenza virus (subtype H5N2) from chicken eggs during a natural outbreak. Avian Dis1985; 29: 1195-1200.

12 Swayne DE, Beck JR: Heat inactivation of avian influenza and Newcastle disease viruses in egg products. Avian Pathol 2004; 33: 512-518.

Dr. I. Capua, OIE and National Reference Laboratory for Newcastle Disease and Avian Influenza, Istituto Zooprofilattico Sperimentale delle Venezie, Viale dell'Università 10, IT-35020 Legnaro, Padova, Italy.
E-mail: icapua@izsvenezie.it

Schudel A, Lombard M (eds): OIE/FAO International Scientific Conference on Avian Influenza.
Dev Biol (Basel). Basel, Karger, 2006, vol 124, p 21.

SESSION I

Ecology and Epidemiology

Chairperson: *D. Alexander* (VLA, UK)
Rapporteur: *D. Swayne* (APHIS, USA)

Schudel A, Lombard M (eds): OIE/FAO International Scientific Conference on Avian Influenza.
Dev Biol (Basel). Basel, Karger, 2006, vol 124, pp 23-36.

Epidemiology and Ecology of Highly Pathogenic Avian Influenza with Particular Emphasis on South East Asia

V. Martin[1], L. Sims[2], J. Lubroth[1], D. Pfeiffer[3], J. Slingenbergh[1], J. Domenech[1]

[1] Animal Health Service, FAO, Rome, Italy

[2] Asia Pacific Veterinary Information Services Pty Ltd, Manunda, Queensland, Australia

[3] Royal Veterinary College, Hatfield, United Kingdom

Abstract: Highly pathogenic avian influenza (HPAI) has been recognised as a serious viral disease of poultry since 1878. The number of recorded outbreaks of HPAI has increased globally in the past 10 years culminating in 2004 with the unprecedented outbreaks of H5N1 HPAI involving at least nine countries in East and South-East Asia. Apart from the geographical extent of these outbreaks and apparent rapid spread, this epidemic has a number of unique features, among which is the role that asymptomatic domestic waterfowl and more particularly free-ranging ducks play in the transmission of highly pathogenic H5N1.

Field epidemiological studies have been conducted by the Food and Agriculture Organization and several collaborative centres to explore the factors that could have led to a change from infection to the emergence of widespread disease in 2003-2004 and 2005. Domestic waterfowl, specific farming practices and agro-ecological environments have been identified to play a key role in the occurrence, maintenance and spread of HPAI.

Although there are some questions that remain unanswered regarding the origins of the 2004 outbreaks, the current understanding of the ecology and epidemiology of the disease should now lead to the development of adapted targeted surveillance studies and control strategies.

INTRODUCTION

Highly pathogenic avian influenza (HPAI), previously known as fowl plague, has been recognised as a serious viral disease of poultry since 1878. The number of recorded outbreaks of HPAI has increased globally in the past 10 years culminating in 2004 with the unprecedented outbreaks of H5N1 HPAI involving at least nine countries in East and South-East Asia. HPAI is a highly contagious disease of domestic fowl whose virus usually finds its origin in water birds. The latter are usually not affected by the disease and serve as the entry point of infection into domestic poultry. Many of the strains that circulate in wild birds are either non-pathogenic or low pathogenic for poultry. However, a virulent strain may emerge either by genetic mutation or by reassortment of less virulent strains.

Once introduced into domestic flocks, wild birds are probably not essential for the maintenance of an outbreak which spreads through other methods, involving movement of infected poultry, contaminated equipment, vehicles, personnel and other means.

Recent serious epidemics have occurred in Hong Kong in 1997-1998 and 2003, Chile in 2002, The Netherlands in 2003 and South Korea in 2003. In addition, since the outbreak in Hong Kong where 18 people were infected and six people died of an avian influenza strain, directly contracted from infected birds, the role of the avian species in the epidemiology of human influenza had to be reconsidered as well as the importance of the disease as a public health issue.

The magnitude of the 2004 epidemic highlights HPAI as a major epidemic transboundary disease with the potential to generate a dramatic situation, threatening the livelihood of millions of people who depend on poultry for their subsistence.

The seriousness of the problem was initially brought to international attention in December 2003 when the high rate of mortalities in poultry were reported in Vietnam. However, the situation was probably dormant for some months or more, underestimated or simply not recognised due to deficient disease surveillance systems.

When the extent of this disease became internationally known, with the almost simultaneous declarations in a number of Asian countries for the first time, there was considerable concern among both veterinary and public health authorities – especially as the virus also caused fatal disease in humans.

Apart from the geographical extent of these outbreaks and apparent rapid spread, this epidemic has a number of unique features, among which is the role that asymptomatic domestic waterfowl and more particularly free-ranging ducks play in the transmission of highly pathogenic H5N1.

This study presents the results of field epidemiological and ecological studies that have been conducted by the Food and Agriculture Organization and several collaborative centres to explore the factors that could have led to a change from infection to emergence of widespread disease in 2003-2004 and 2005. Domestic waterfowl, specific farming practices and the agro-ecological environment were identified as playing a key role in the occurrence, maintenance and spread of HPAI. Targeted surveillance activities and the control of infection at source is now urgently needed to prevent the emergence of a new pandemic strain that would threaten the world.

Materials and Method

Epidemiological data and information were collected and derived from a number of sources including published scientific papers, official government disease reports, Genbank accessions, reports from FAO and other consultants and news articles from reliable sources. The quality of the data was not always optimal for the purpose of disease and epidemiological analysis, and what has been reported did not always reflect what actually occurred. The absence of population-at-risk data in most countries visited represented a major constraint for disease analysis which was difficult to overcome.

When possible, spatio-temporal analytical studies using logistic regression techniques have been attempted to explore the contribution of identified risk factors further in the occurrence of avian influenza. These analyses have been jointly carried out with the National Veterinary Services of affected countries. The results of these studies, such as the ones carried out in Vietnam and Thailand, have been instrumental in understanding the epidemiology and ecology of HPAI in the region.

Results

The exploration of risk factors on a regional scale, recognised as playing an important role in the genesis of HPAI outbreaks in the past, enabled a preliminary understanding of the ecology of the 2004 epidemic. Various maps representing poultry density, water bodies, land cover and irrigated lands were inserted into a geographical information system together with reported AI outbreaks, in an attempt to identify possible relationships with environmental risk factors (maps 1 to 3). Due to serious data limitations and the absence of population-at-risk data, these relationships could not be explored using statistical methods.

However, this exploratory approach gave early indications of possible relationships existing between outbreaks, irrigated lands and areas of low to medium poultry population densities.

These relationships were further investigated through the implementation of national studies that were carried out in Thailand and Vietnam using logistic regression techniques. Both studies highlighted the importance of farming management practices and more particularly the role of free-ranging ducks in the occurrence and maintenance of the infection.

In Thailand, a preliminary indication of the involvement of ducks raised in free-ranging systems was provided through the mapping of chicken outbreaks in combination with free-ranging duck populations (maps 4 to 6). These relationships, including a broader range of risk factors, were further explored through regression logistic models (Slingenbergh et al. – work in progress).

In Vietnam, two main clusters of infections were detected in the South and the North of the country (maps 7, 8 and 9) and were related to the main river systems, namely the Mekong delta in the South and the Red River in the North. During the second wave of outbreaks, most outbreaks occurred in the South of the country where duck production is predominant.

Logistic regression was used to investigate the role of various risk indicators including waterfowl distribution, terrestrial poultry density, type of farming systems and crop production. Interestingly, a strong correlation between outbreak locations and rice field production as well as the increase in the percentage of irrigated lands was identified. An outbreak probability map showing high risk areas of disease occurrence was produced (map 10).

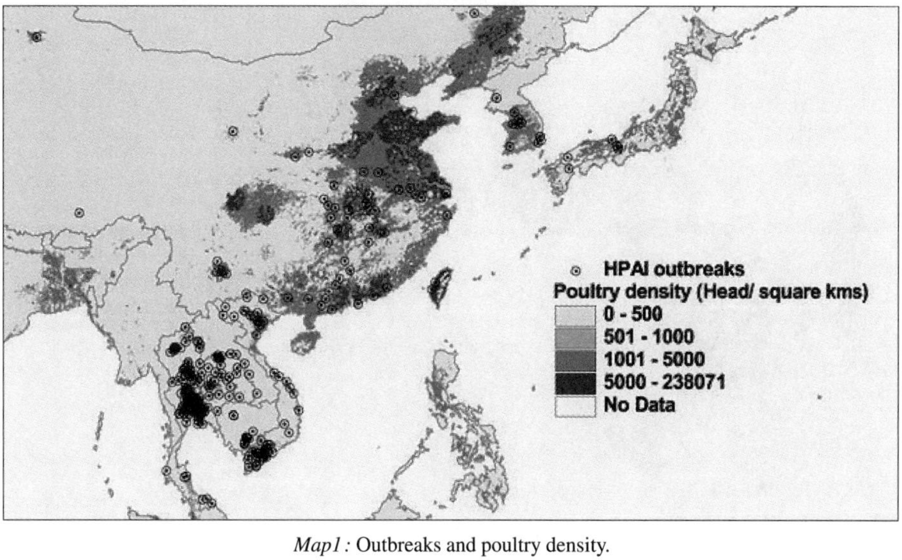

Map1 : Outbreaks and poultry density.

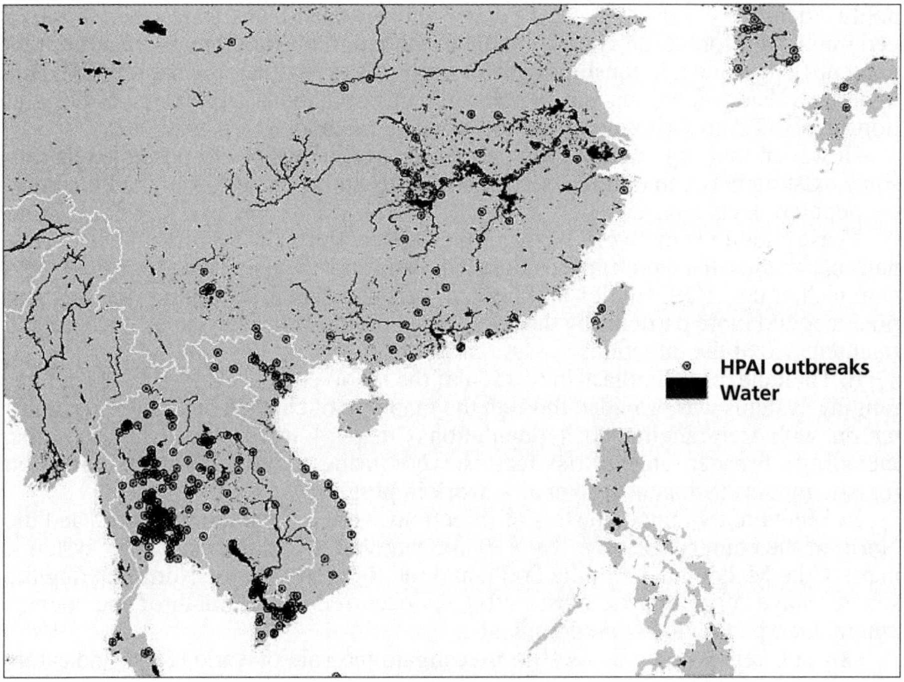

Map 2: Water bodies and outbreaks.

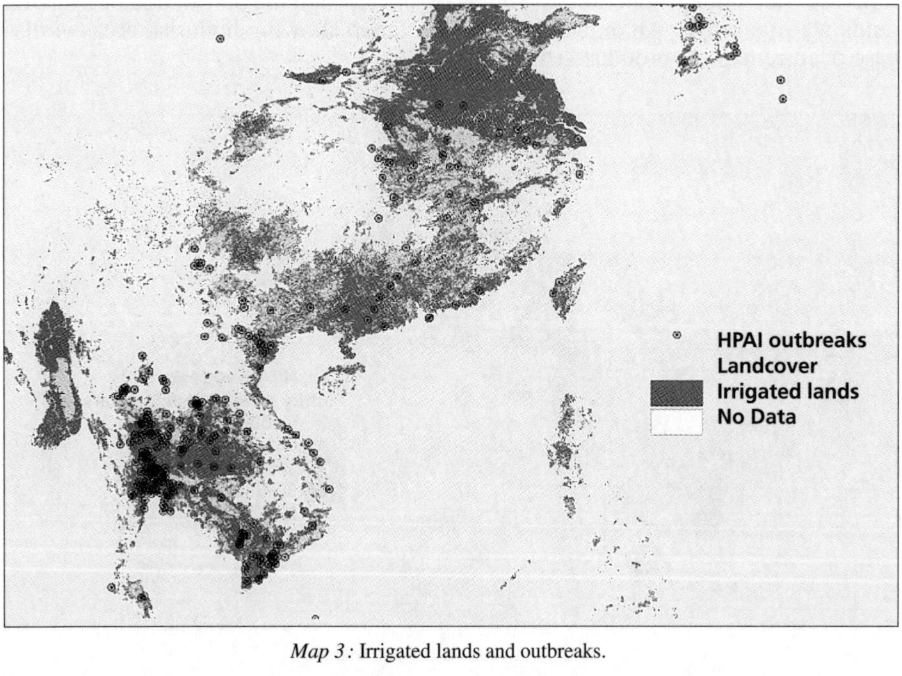

Map 3: Irrigated lands and outbreaks.

Maps 4 to 6: Thailand.

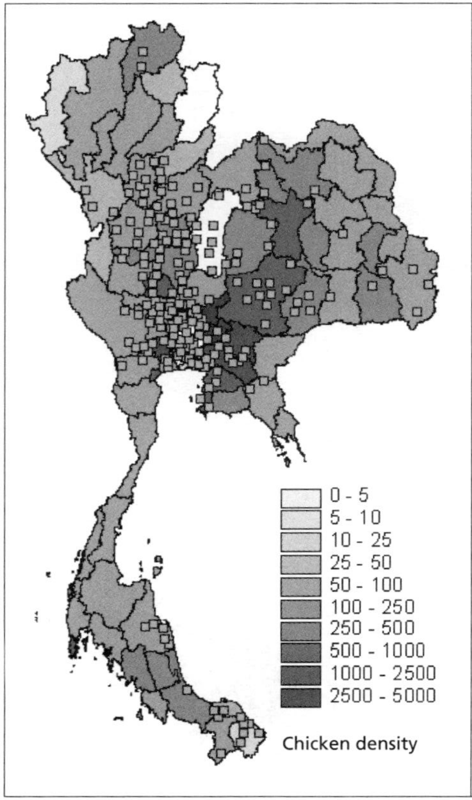

Map 4: Chicken outbreaks in Thailand and chicken distribution.
(Slingenbergh et al. work in progress.)

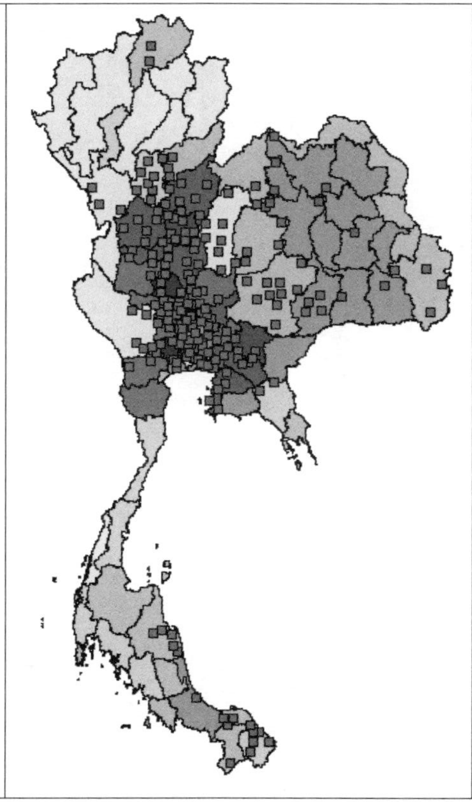

Map 5: Chicken outbreaks in Thailand and duck distribution.
(Slingenbergh et al. – work in progress.)

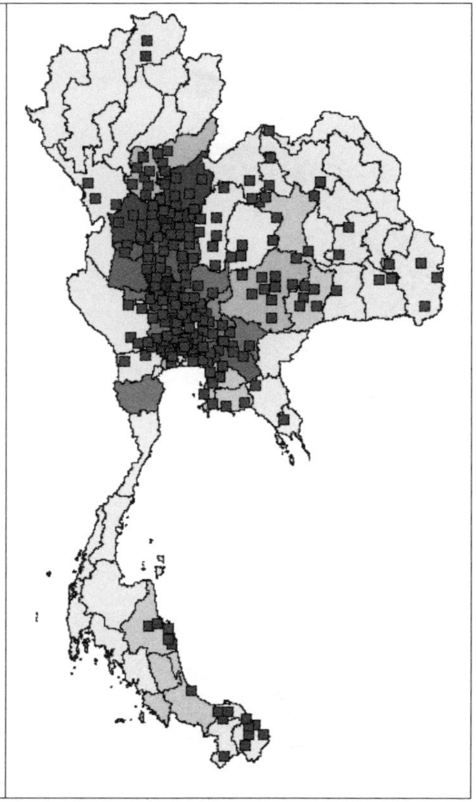

Map 6: Chicken outbreaks in Thailand and free-ranging duck distribution.
(Slingenbergh et al. – work in progress.)

Maps 7-9: Cluster of infection in Vietnam.

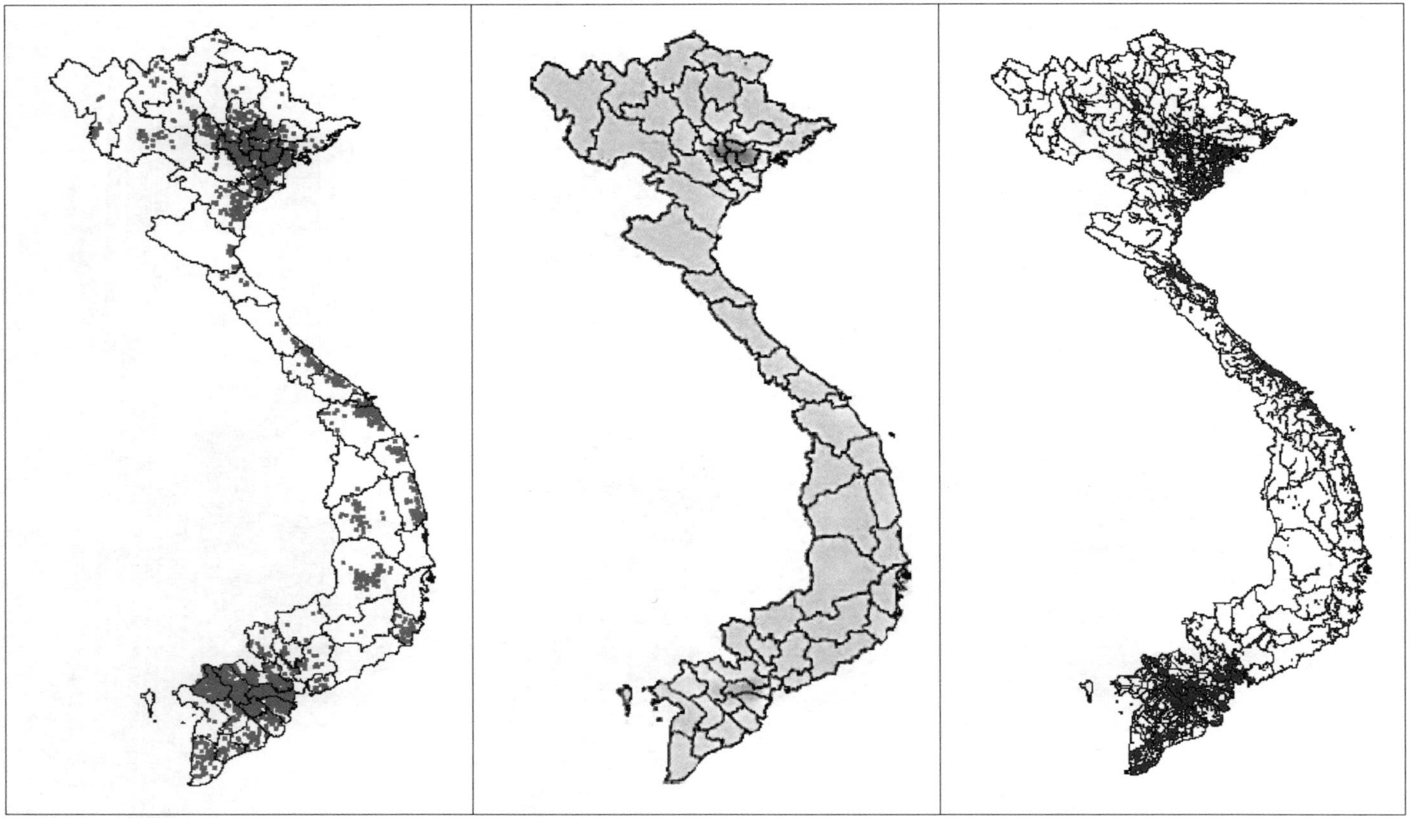

Map 7: Outbreak data (2004) – Source of data: Department of Animal Health.

Map 8: Main cluster of infection (dark spots).

Map 9: Main river systems in Vietnam.

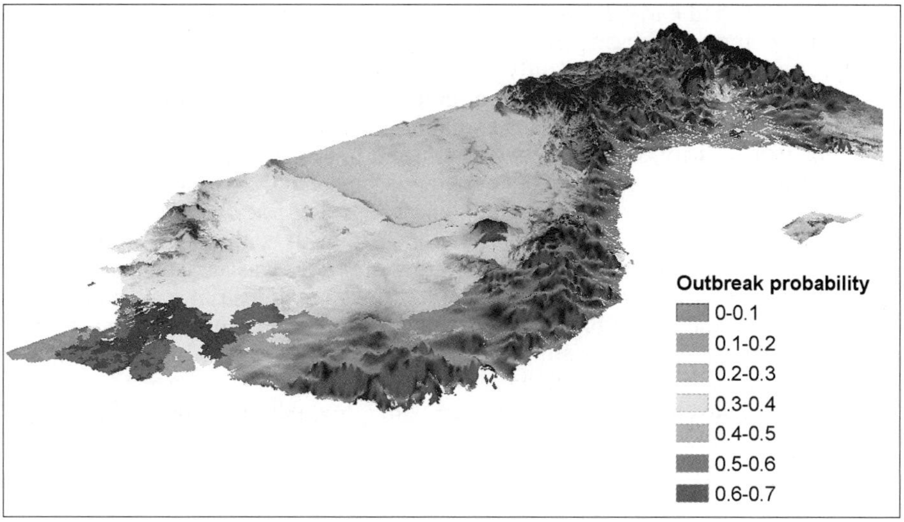

Map 10: Outbreak probability in Vietnam – risk map.

Increases in Poultry Populations

FAO livestock statistics demonstrate the marked increase in the number of poultry being raised in Asia over the past seven years. The figures for Viet Nam provide a clear example of the extent and rapidity of this increase (Fig. 1). In some countries, smallholders have markedly increased the size of their flocks in response to market signals but have not concurrently increased biosecurity levels to match this investment. In addition there has been little or no government intervention to ensure that this was done. This factor probably played a role in the emergence of HPAI in Asia.

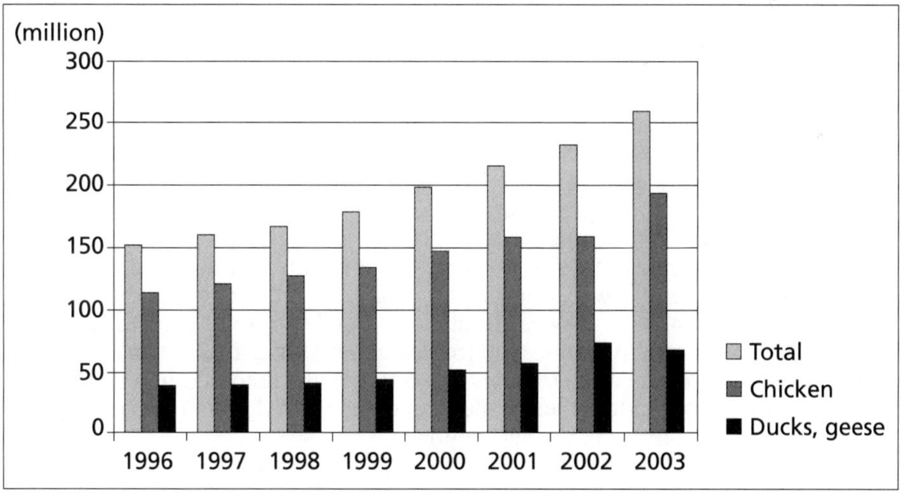

Fig. 1: Increase in poultry population in Vietnam.

In late 2003 and early 2004 a significant number of cases of H5N1 HPAI were reported in commercial farms. However, results from Thailand on confirmed cases of infection in the period from 3 July to 30 September 2004 demonstrated that more than 64 % of infected farms/premises or holdings contained 1000 or fewer poultry. This trend towards involvement of the smallholder and village sector has continued into 2005. Biosecurity is effectively non-existent in this sector.

A preliminary analysis carried out of outbreaks in China, based on the numbers of poultry culled in the 3 km zone, around 44 outbreak sites for which data were available indicated that 50 % of cases were reported in areas with a poultry density of fewer than 2000 per sq km (Table 1). The largest category was areas with fewer than 1000 poultry per sq km, which are those with little if any industrial scale production.

The distribution of outbreaks according to poultry density in China is also shown in Figure 2. This diagram shows that most cases occurred in areas with an average density < 5000 poultry/km^2.

Cases in Malaysia involved a province with a low poultry density. The largest infected village flock contained only 500 birds.

Table 1 : Density of poultry around sites of disease reported in China in 2004.

0-999/sq km	1000-1999	2000-2999	3000-3999	4000-4999	5000-5999	6000-6999	7000 +
16	5	6	5	3	2	2	5

Discussion

Overview of the situation

Although the disease has been known for over a century, the HPAI epidemic in 2004 has been unsurpassed historically by its magnitude and the scale of its geographical distribution, forcing countries to react promptly by ordering massive stamping out exercises and in some cases vaccination campaigns. International trade was disrupted and international organisations joined efforts to respond as fast as possible to this emergency situation. Some of the main features of this outbreak are summarized below:

- *Unprecedent regional scale :* the disease was reported in several countries at the same time which was an unusual characteristic, creating some degree of panic in national veterinary services and in the scientific community, fearing a possible reassortment of the virus with human influenza viruses and opening the way to a wider human pandemic [1]. H5N1 was not suspected in the first instance since it is not always included in the differential diagnosis of national veterinary services. Indeed, poultry deaths are seasonal and particularly frequent at the time the disease occurred. In some countries, significant mortalities are annually anticipated before the wet season, particularly in the months of February to April. Diseases such as Newcastle disease, Gumboro, fowl cholera and duck plague are usually held responsible for heavy mortalities in chicken and ducks. However, the abnormal magnitude of poultry deaths recorded in Vietnam this year triggered the alert and led to the suspicion of HPAI which was then discovered in other countries of the sub-region.
- *High virulence :* as observed for the first time in Hong-Kong in 1997, the virus was found to be highly pathogenic for humans and directly linked with human

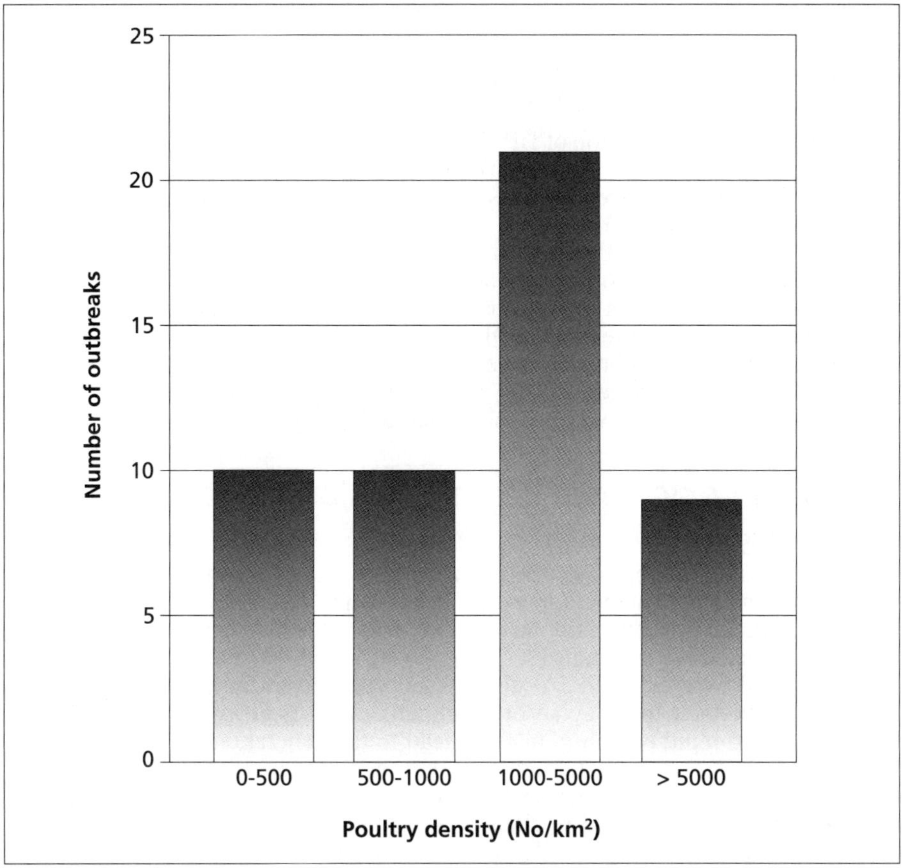

Fig. 2: Poultry density at outbreak sites in China.

infection and deaths. The H5N1 strain involved in the current epidemic was also found to be highly virulent and responsible for the deaths of many species of poultry as well as wild birds. Zoo animals (tiger and clouded leopard) as well as domestic cats were also affected.

- *Clinical signs and species affected:* the most common signs observed in terrestrial poultry were depression, ruffled feathers, cyanosis of wattles and combs, and diarrhoea. Specific respiratory signs were generally not seen. Death was documented one to three hours after initial clinical signs were observed. In some occasions, the H5N1 strain also affected domestic ducks with a certain degree of variability [2]. Examination of H5N1 isolates of the Z genotype for pathogenicity in ducks revealed that these isolates could be divided into three broad groups:
  - (i) those that kill all inoculated ducks with neurological signs of disease;
  - (ii) those that kill a percentage of ducks without neurological signs of disease;
  - (iii) those that replicate but cause no signs of disease.
    (K. M Sturm-Ramirez et al. Unpublished findings)

- *Multiple sources of infection.* Molecular epidemiological studies have shown that multiple strains of H5N1 were circulating in the region, complicating the understanding of the epidemiology of the disease and discarding the possibility of having a unique source of infection.

After the initial declaration of HPAI in Vietnam, the disease was rapidly notified in neighbouring countries (Vietnam, Thailand, Lao PDR, China, Cambodia, Japan) while the disease reappeared in the Republic of Korea where it had already been reported in December 2003.

At the end of January 2004, almost all provinces of Thailand and Vietnam were affected and 16 provinces out of 53 notified the disease in China (map 11).

The crisis had taken an international dimension and developed beyond South East Asian countries to threaten the whole region, if not the world.

A second wave of outbreaks started in June 2004 and peaked at the end of the year in Thailand and in early 2005 in Vietnam (Fig. 3). Malaysia also became infected during the second wave of the epidemic in August 2004.

Epidemiological and Ecological Considerations

Virus cycle

Understanding the ecology of influenza viruses, i.e. the interrelationships of the virus and its environment, including the mechanism of spread to spillover and dead-end host is crucial if we wish to find ways to prevent the repeated occurrence of the disease in affected Asian countries.

Influenza A viruses of all 16 subtypes are perpetuated in aquatic birds of the world. After transfer to an avian or mammalian host (spill-over host), influenza viruses undergo rapid evolution that can lead to the generation of new and highly pathogenic strains [2]. Genetic and antigenic analyses of H9N2 viruses isolated from domestic ducks in Southern China during 2000-2001 has provided evidence that these viruses established in chicken and quail have been transmitted back to domestic ducks, generating double or triple reassortants with viruses already resident in ducks [3]. The same mechanism may apply to H5N1 viruses with a two-way transmission between terrestrial and aquatic birds, increasing the opportunity to generate influenza viruses with pandemic potential (Fig. 4).

Live bird markets are likely to act as a reservoir of avian influenza viruses and to play a significant role in the maintenance of infection, and contribute to the secondary spread of the disease through animal movements. Indeed, live poultry markets where duck, geese, quail, pheasants and chickens are raised or housed together provide optimal conditions for the reassortment and evolution of influenza viruses.

Virus evolution

H5N1 viruses have been isolated from free-ranging wildlife at several intervals throughout the years. HPAI (H5N1) has certainly been present in the region since the first detection of the infection in geese in 1996 (Guangdong province of China).

After its first detection in 1996 in Guangdong province, the disease broke out in Hong Kong in 1997. A Goose/GD/96-like virus was later considered to be the origin of the H5 component of the 1997 Hong Kong H5N1 virus. The disturbing event of the 1997 epidemic was the transmission of the disease to humans (confirmed in 18 people), leading to the deaths of six. The same year, the virus was also detected in geese in Guangdong province.

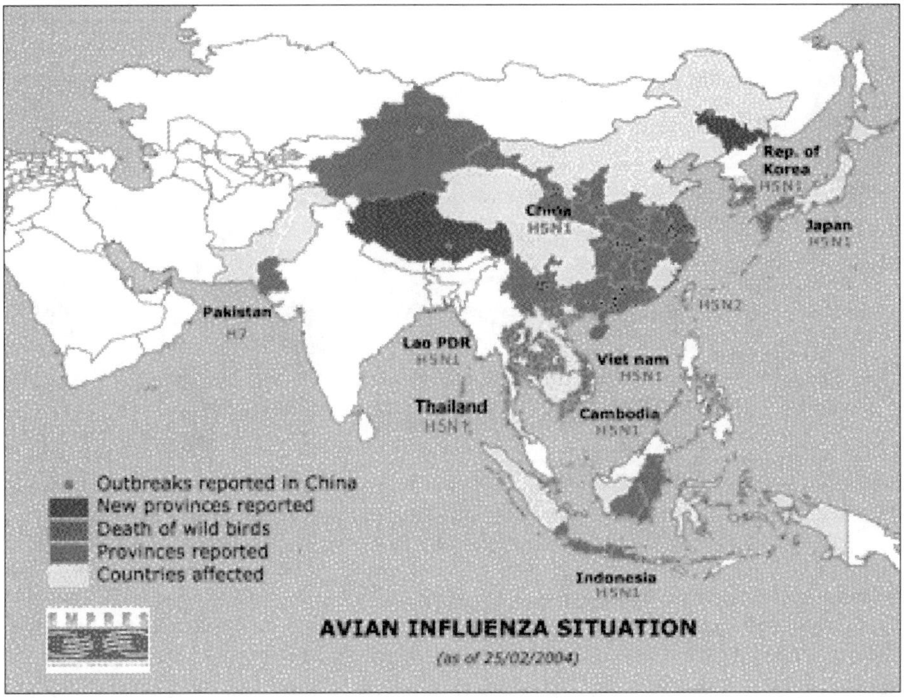

Map 11 : Situation on the 25 February 2004.

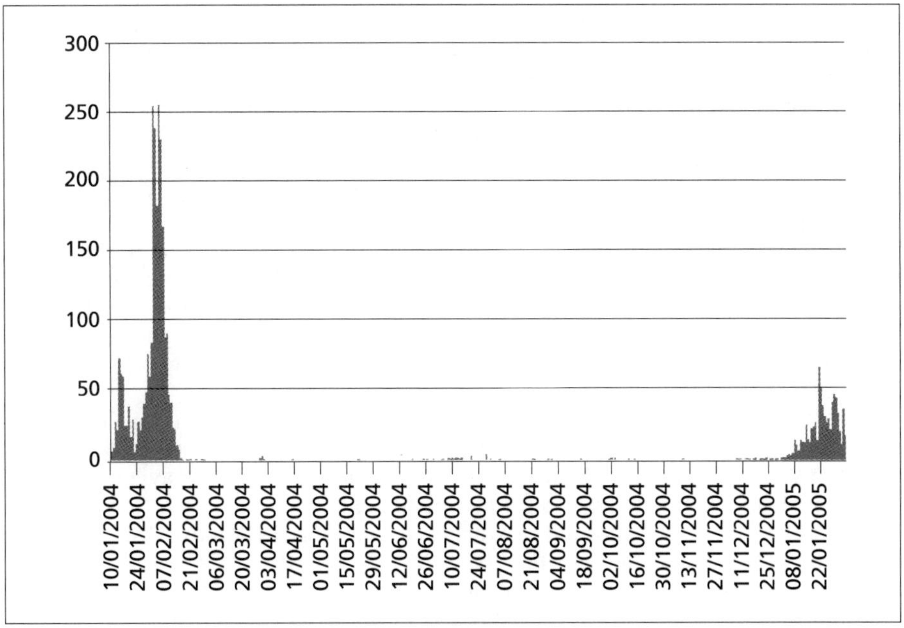

Fig. 3 : Outbreaks of HPAI in Vietnam (January 2004 – January 2005).

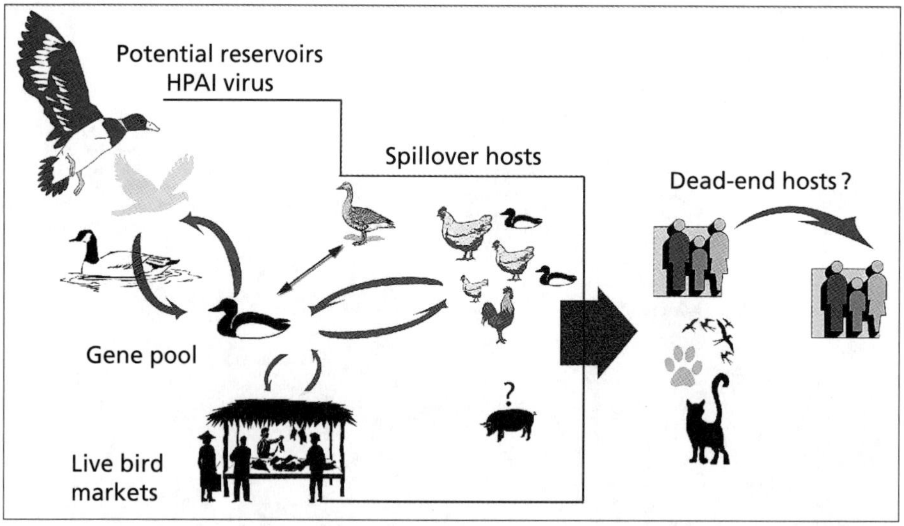

Fig. 4: Current understanding of the ecology of HPAI virus in Asia.

From 1999 onwards, virus circulation was detected in Hong Kong in avian species through blood testing, swabbing of cages and testing of faecal samples. It appeared that the number of H5N1 virus isolations from ducks and geese increased from 1999 to 2001.

In late 2000, the virus changed genetically, incorporating new genes from other influenza viruses. These genes were believed to be from influenza viruses derived from other aquatic birds. Further, viruses isolated from a goose and a duck in December 2000 have acquired NS, PA, M, and PB2 genes from the aquatic avian influenza gene pool through reassortment. For pandemic preparedness, it is important to monitor whether these reassortant viruses have the capacity for interspecies transmission to terrestrial poultry or mammals [4]. In May 2001, an avian H5N1 influenza virus was isolated from duck meat that had been imported to the Republic of Korea from China [5].

Two H5N1 HPAI viruses were also detected in geese in markets in one small surveillance study in live poultry markets in Vietnam [6]. Genetic characterisation of these viruses is continuing but the haemagglutinin of these viruses differs considerably from that found in viruses in Vietnam in 2004. Based on the HA gene it appears to be similar to other viruses found in domestic waterfowl elsewhere in Asia in 2001-02 [6].

In 2002, mortalities of wild birds due to HPAI were reported in Hong Kong. This was the first report of deaths in wild birds in Asia. An H5N3 virus was isolated from dead terns in 1961 in South Africa but, in other parts of the world, avian influenza viruses isolated from wild birds have low pathogenicity.

In January 2003, the mortality extended to waterfowl (flamingo) in Kowloon Park, Hong Kong and later in the year (May 2003) the H5N1 virus was also detected in Japan in imported duck meat.

Samples collected from live bird markets in Southern China from 2002 to 2004 confirmed that "Z" genotype viruses persisted in domestic waterfowl throughout this period. This "Z" genotype has been evolving for several years in terrestrial and aquatic poultry before the widespread outbreaks of disease in 2004.

The Role of the Farming System in Asia and Domestic Waterfowl in the Maintenance and Spread of H5N1 HPAI

Various studies have shown that AI was affecting areas of medium concentration (< 5000 birds per square kilometre) and by extension, medium-scale farming systems, compared to areas with very high or very low poultry density.

The level of biosecurity in semi-commercial farming systems, lower than that practised in large scale commercial enterprises, could have played a major role in the introduction and spread of the disease, offering an entry point for the virus through close contact with waterfowl and migrating wild birds.

In addition, there is increased evidence that domestic waterfowl have played a key role in the genesis of the 2003-04 outbreak. Much of this can be ascribed to the ability of asymptomatic ducks to carry H5N1 HPAI viruses. Significant genetic changes occurring in these viruses in late 2000 to early 2001, leading to the carriage of these viruses by healthy ducks, appears to be a unique feature of the H5N1 avian influenza viruses circulating in Asia. Those isolated elsewhere from domestic ducks have been LPAI viruses.

The precise extent of infection in domestic ducks in Asia is still not known, although it appears that it is not occurring in all parts of Asia. H5N1 HPAI was detected in some flocks of ducks in the Republic of Korea in early 2004 but continuing surveillance since the virus was eradicated has so far only detected one flock with a low pathogenicity H5N2 virus. This has a markedly different HA genome from the goose GD/96 lineage.

However, H5N1 HPAI virus is still present in domestic waterfowl in a number of Asian countries. In Viet Nam and Thailand they are believed to be playing a key role in the maintenance of infection, especially free-grazing ducks. Domestic ducks in China were known to be infected in the past with viruses becoming progressively more pathogenic for mammals [7] but many of these are now vaccinated, which should reduce their contribution to the virus load in the environment.

Countries with significant duck populations will need to assess the levels of infection in these birds through serological and viral surveillance studies. They will also have to devise appropriate management strategies for these ducks. Changing of management practices so that ducks are raised in confined premises is one possible option but would have major socio-economic and environmental consequences (ducks are a form of biological pest control, removing snails from paddies and providing natural fertiliser). If this is not feasible, vaccination would be another possible strategy. Initial laboratory studies indicate that vaccination of ducks can reduce the excretion of virus in experimentally infected ducks but until more field studies are available there is no way of predicting the extent of reduction that would be obtained.

If control measures including animal culling, vaccination and movement management have been instrumental in reducing the incidence of the disease and bringing it under control in many places, the disease seems to be established in some ecosystems and tends to reoccur at regular intervals. Stopping the cycle of infection between reservoir and spillover species is of critical importance and should involve the use of adapted control strategies including vaccine in identified reservoir populations.

CONCLUSION

The recent epidemiological findings on HPAI in Asia provide reasons to believe that the disease has been smouldering for some time in domestic and wild birds, waiting for determinant factors to emerge. Indeed, the presence of H5N1 infection was first encountered in 1996 and various reports provide evidence that the disease was present long before it was detected and reported through official channels, allowing the virus to recombine and become more virulent over the years. The regional scale of the problem can certainly be linked to a lack of emergency preparedness, especially when it deals with the emergence of new and more virulent strains of viruses, such as AI.

Intensive farming practices and inadequate disease reporting, early warning mechanisms and monitoring programmes have also played a major role in the development of the 2004 epidemic and its international dimension. Waterbirds and live bird markets have also been recognised as playing a major role in the cycle of infection. Targeted surveillance and control activities have to be implemented at these places.

Changing farming, trading and veterinary practices should be encouraged to mitigate the effect of such crises which have the potential to set back economic development progress for long periods of time because of the need to divert funds away from development to emergency, disaster, and reconstruction activities.

REFERENCES

1 Li KS, et al: Genesis of a highly pathogenic and potentially pandemic H5N1 influenza virus in eastern Asia. Nature 2004; 430 (6996): 209-213.

2 Webster RG: Microbiological adaptation and change: avian influenza. Revue Scientifique et technique de l'Office international des epizooties 2004; 23 (2): 453-465.

3 Li KS, et al: Characterization of H9 subtype influenza viruses from the ducks of southern China: a candidate for the next influenza pandemic in humans? J Virol 2003; 77 (12): 6988-6994.

4 Guan Y, et al: H5N1 influenza viruses isolated from geese in Southeastern China: evidence for genetic reassortment and interspecies transmission to ducks. Virology 2002; 292 (1): 16-23.

5 Tumpey TM, et al: Evaluation of a high-pathogenicity H5N1 avian influenza A virus isolated from duck meat. Avian Dis 2003; 47 (3 Suppl): 951-955.

6 Nguyen DC, et al: Isolation and characterization of avian influenza viruses, including highly pathogenic H5N1, from poultry in live bird markets in Hanoi, Vietnam, in 2001. J Virol 2005; 79 (7): 4201-4212.

7 Chen H, et al: The evolution of H5N1 influenza viruses in ducks in Southern China. Proc Natl Acad Sci U S A 2004; 101 (28): 10452-10457.

Dr. V. Martin, Animal Health Service, FAO, Viale delle Terme di Caracalla, IT-00100 Rome, Italy.
E-mail: vincent.martin@fao.org

Schudel A, Lombard M (eds): OIE/FAO International Scientific Conference on Avian Influenza.
Dev Biol (Basel). Basel, Karger, 2006, vol 124, pp 37-44.

Ecology and Epidemiology of Avian Influenza in North and South America

D.A. Senne[1], D.L. Suarez[2], D.E. Stallnecht[3], J.C. Pedersen[1], B. Panigrahy[1]

1 U.S. Department of Agriculture, APHIS, National Veterinary Services Laboratories, Ames, IA, USA

2 U.S. Department of Agriculture, Agriculture Research Service, Southeast Poultry Research Laboratory, Athens, GA, USA

3 University of Georgia, College of Veterinary Medicine, Southeastern Cooperative Wildlife Disease Study, Athens, GA, USA

Key words: Avian influenza, ecology, epidemiology, highly pathogenic avian influenza, low pathogenicity avian influenza, poultry, surveillance, live-bird markets, wild aquatic birds, ducks, swine influenza, avian influenza infections in humans.

Abstract: Wild waterfowl and shorebirds are known to be the natural reservoir for influenza A viruses. Surveillance studies in waterfowl and shorebirds in North America show that influenza A viruses are repeatedly recovered from these birds. However, the virus recovery is influenced by geography, season, age and species of birds. In addition to the natural reservoir, the live-bird marketing system (LBMS) in certain regions of the United States has been recognized as a man-made reservoir of influenza viruses and has been linked to several outbreaks of low pathogenicity avian influenza (LPAI) in poultry. Outbreaks of LPAI in commercial poultry is attributed to movement of infected birds, dirty or improperly cleaned crates, and contaminated vehicles from the LBMS to poultry farms. However, in the majority of outbreaks in poultry, the source of infection is suspected to be wild aquatic birds or the source is unknown. Since 2002, three outbreaks of highly pathogenic avian influenza (HPAI) have occurred in the Americas; one each in Chile (H7N3), United States (H5N2), and Canada (H7N3). In each of these outbreaks, a precursor virus of low pathogenicity mutated to become highly pathogenic after circulating in poultry. The HPAI viruses recovered from the three outbreaks had unique molecular and phenotypic characteristics that do not conform to other known HPAI viruses. These findings emphasize the need for monitoring wild and domestic bird species for presence of influenza A viruses.

Introduction

Avian influenza (AI) is caused by influenza A viruses of the Family *Orthomyxoviridae* and is distributed worldwide. The genome of influenza A viruses is single-stranded negative-sense RNA that occurs in eight distinct segments. The virus is enveloped; on the envelope are two major surface proteins: the haemagglutinin (H), and neuraminidase (N). Based on antigenic differences in H and N proteins, the avian influenza virus is divided into subtypes. Sixteen H and nine N subtypes are recognized. An avian influenza virus (AIV) carries only one of 16 H and one of nine N on its surface. Wild birds, especially waterfowl and shorebirds of the Orders Anseriformes and Charadriiformes are the natural reservoir for influenza A viruses [1,2] and represent the original source of all avian influenza viruses (AIV) that infect domestic birds and mammals, including humans [3]. Worldwide, all 16 H and nine N subtypes, in 144 possible combinations, have been detected in one or the other of these orders of birds.

In poultry, disease caused by AIV varies from an inapparent to a systemic disease with high mortality [4]. Highly pathogenic avian influenza (HPAI) has only been associated with H5 and H7 subtypes; however, an overwhelming majority of H5 and H7 subtypes have low pathogenicity for domestic poultry. Influenza A viruses usually do not produce disease in the natural reservoir species and are shown to be genetically stable [3]. When introduced into a new and unnatural host such as domestic poultry, the viruses, particularly some strains of H5 or H7 subtype, may undergo molecular changes leading to the emergence of a highly pathogenic virus [3]. Since 1983, there have been five recorded outbreaks of highly pathogenic avian influenza (HPAI) in the Americas; four in North America and one in South America. In each of these outbreaks, a precursor virus of low pathogenicity was detected in poultry before the emergence of the HPAI virus [5-9, Suarez, personal communication].

The intent of this paper is to provide a general overview of the ecology of influenza in the Americas and to highlight some of the significant epidemiological findings regarding AIV infections in domestic poultry and humans. A more detailed account of infections in poultry and caged birds in the Western Hemisphere can be found in the proceedings of the 5th International Symposium on Avian Influenza [10].

Surveillance Studies in Wild Aquatic Birds in North and South America

Isolations of AIV have been reported from over 100 species of wild birds worldwide [11]. Surveillance of wild bird populations in North America began in the early 1970s and has continued, although efforts have decreased in recent years. Limited surveillance of wild bird populations in South America has yielded at least one AIV isolate from a wild bird [Suarez, personal communication].

Species within two orders of birds are important in the epidemiology of influenza A viruses. These are Anseriformes (duck, geese, and swans) and Charadriiformes (gulls, terns, and shorebirds). Within the Anseriformes, mallards (*Anas platyrhynchos*) have accounted for most of the reported isolations, although infection is common in most duck species. Prevalence of infection reported from mallards can exceed 30 %, but varies greatly depending on season and location. Seasonal variation is driven by migratory behaviour with peak prevalence occurring in late summer and early autumn related to the pre-migration staging of juvenile (susceptible) birds. Such staging occurs in more northern latitudes and prevalence decreases as birds move south to wintering areas. The prevalence often drops to less than 1 % when the birds are on their wintering grounds. The epidemiology of influenza A viruses in species within the Charadriiformes is not so clear. Although AI viruses have been isolated from many species in this order, prevalence is generally low. One exception is the ruddy turnstone *(Arenaria interpres)* where high infection rates have been observed. The high prevalence rates, however, have only been observed at Delaware Bay locations during the spring. In the case of turnstones, the infection probably relates to the congregation of shorebirds during spring migration due to seasonal and local availability of eggs from spawning horseshoe crabs. Besides this case involving this single species, little is known about seasonal or spatial relationships associated with influenza A virus infection in other species in the order Charadriiformes.

It is important to emphasize that all influenza A virus subtypes are not equally represented in wild bird populations. In ducks, the H3, H4, and H6 subtypes predominate as reported in independent studies in North America and other parts of the world since 1970. In gulls and shorebirds, the H9 and H13 subtypes predominate [12]; additional work is needed to understand subtype diversity within these populations fully. Regarding wild bird reservoirs for the H5 and H7 influenza A viruses, two observations are important. First, no isolations of HPAI virus have been made from wild bird populations in North or South America. Second, H5 and H7 viruses are not common in any of the recognized wild avian reservoirs. Based on 3,109 isolates from ducks in Alberta [12], New York [13], Pennsylvania [14], Germany [15], Canada [16], Ohio [17], and Louisiana [18], H5 and H7 viruses respectively represented only 0.25 % and 0.61 % of total isolates. In more recent work in shorebirds at Delaware Bay [Stallknecht, unpublished data] the H5 and H7 viruses respectively represented only 2 % and 1 % of 150 isolates. Regional variation in H5 and H7 prevalence can occur but, in general, these subtypes are not commonly isolated from wild birds.

Emergence of HPAI from LPAI Precursor Viruses in North and South America

Highly pathogenic avian influenza (HPAI) is a disease that is reportable to the World Organization for Animal Health (OIE) because of the seriousness of the disease and high potential for spread through international movement of poultry and poultry products. Viruses characterized as HPAI must fulfil a criterion of virulence for chickens: intravenous pathogenicity index of ≥ 1.2 or 75 % mortality in eight experimentally inoculated chickens; or a multiple dibasic amino acid motif at the haemagglutinin cleavage site compatible with known HPAI viruses.

Since 1983, five outbreaks of HPAI have occurred in the Americas, three caused by H5N2 subtype and two by the H7N3 subtype viruses: (i) H5N2 in the USA, 1983-84; (ii) H5N2 in Mexico, 1994-95; (iii) H7N3 in Chile, 2002; (iv) H5N2 in the USA, 2004, and (v) H7N3, Canada, 2004. In each of these outbreaks, a precursor virus of low pathogenicity was detected in poultry before the emergence of the HPAI virus. However, the length of time the LPAI virus circulated in poultry before becoming highly pathogenic varied from 11 days to more than two years. The nature of the mutations near the haemagglutinin cleavage site was also different. For example, in the U.S. outbreak of 1983-84, the LPAI virus circulated for six months before mutating to HP through the loss of a carbohydrate side chain located near the haemagglutinin cleavage site [5]. In Mexico (1994-95), a LPAI H5N2 virus was widely disseminated in 11 states before it was isolated. It was estimated that the

LPAI virus circulated for approximately 14 months before mutating to the HP form; the mutation occurred by insertion of multiple basic amino acids at the haemagglutinin cleavage [6]. In Chile, (2002), a LPAI H7N3 virus was detected in a broiler breeder flock. Within four weeks the virus mutated to become HP. The mutation involved the insertion of a 30 nucleotide insert from the nucleoprotein gene by non-homologous recombination [7]. In the 2004 U.S. outbreak, the progenitor of the HP H5N2 virus was most probably a LP H5N3 virus that was isolated in 2002 and continued to circulate undetected in an unknown reservoir for approximately two years. The emergence of the HP H5N2 virus involved a reassortment of genes from the H5N3 virus and the substitution of a non-basic amino acid for a basic one [Suarez, personal communication]. Finally, in the 2004 outbreak in Canada, a LP H7N3 virus was isolated from a 56 week-old broiler breeder flock. The virus mutated to HP in 11 days after infecting a younger flock of broiler breeders on the same farm. Like the Chile H7N3 virus, the Canadian H7N3 virus also mutated by non-homologous recombination; the mutation occurred by the insertion of a 21-nucleotide insert from the matrix gene instead of the nucleoprotein gene [8,9].

Historically, all HPAI viruses isolated before 2002 were not only highly virulent for chickens but also had the molecular marker for high virulence (multiple dibasic amino acids at the haemagglutinin cleavage site). However, in the three outbreaks of HPAI in North and South America since 2002, the virus recovered was either not virulent for chickens or lacked the typical molecular marker associated with high virulence. The 2002 Chile HPAI virus was virulent for chickens but did not have a multiple basic amino acid motif at the cleavage site of the haemagglutinin. The event in Chile prompted the OIE to create an ad hoc committee to revise the Terrestrial Animal Health Code Chapter on HPAI to reflect the inconsistency of the Chile isolate with the current definition. Since the Chile outbreak, two additional outbreaks of HPAI have occurred, one in the United States (H5N2) and the other in Canada (H7N3), where the viruses responsible for the outbreaks also were inconsistent with the current OIE definition for HPAI viruses. In the case of the 2004 outbreak in the USA, the H5N2 virus met the molecular definition but was not pathogenic for chickens, whereas the Canadian H7N3 virus met the virulence criterion, but like the Chile virus, did not meet the molecular criterion for HPAI. The unusual properties of these HPAI viruses combined with the fact that all three viruses appeared to have evolved from a LP precursor, the ad hoc committee has recommended that all infections with H5 and H7 AIV be notified to the OIE. Justification for this recommendation can be supported by the fact that, given the current understanding of virulence, it is not possible to predict which LPAI viruses have the potential to become HPAI viruses; therefore, all H5 and H7 infections in poultry are notifiable.

Role of Live-Bird Markets in the Ecology of Avian Influenza in North America

Live-bird markets (LBMs), or wet markets as they are sometimes called, are common in many regions of the world and serve as a source of poultry meat for local patrons who choose to buy fresh poultry for consumption. Awareness of these markets as a potential reservoir of AI virus has dramatically increased since 1997 when infections in poultry and humans with HPAI H5N1 were linked to markets in Hong Kong as the source of the virus. In the USA, LBMs have been recognized as a significant reservoir of AI viruses for poultry since 1986, when an epidemiological link was made between LPAI H5N2 influenza virus infections in commercial poultry in Pennsylvania and the presence of the same lineage of H5N2 virus in the LBM system in the northeastern USA [19]. Since that time, the markets have been routinely monitored for the presence of AI virus.

The LBM system in the northeast USA consists of approximately 120 markets that sell about 25 million birds annually. The majority of poultry entering the system come from large and small flocks in nearby states that are monitored for AI, but a significant number of birds enter the system through a complex network of dealers, wholesalers, and poultry auctions that buy and sell birds to the LBMs from sources that are not monitored for AIV. The complex marketing activities and a mixed population of susceptible and infected birds make the markets an ideal environment for transmission, adaptation and evolution of AIVs. Surveillance studies show that a variety of subtypes of AIV are routinely isolated each year from birds and the environment within the markets [20]. In some cases certain subtypes of AIV are shown to persist in the market system for several years [Senne, unpublished data].

In 1994, a LPAI H7N2 virus was introduced into the northeast LBM system; the virus has persisted in the markets despite the efforts by the states to eradicate the virus from the market system. Sequence analysis of isolates recovered over time show that the H7N2 virus is accumulating mutations (additional basic amino acids near the cleavage site of the H protein) that favour the emergence of a highly pathogenic virus [21]. In addition, since 1996, the lineage of LPAI H7N2 virus found in the LBMS has been linked to eight LPAI outbreaks in commercial poultry, resulting in the destruction of millions of birds and an economic loss of millions of dollars to the poultry industry, including costs of eradication and loss of export markets.

Subtypes of AIV Found in Domestic Poultry and Methods of Spread

The source of AI virus for domestic poultry and the mode of introduction into a flock in most cases are unknown. However, circumstantial evidence indicates that infections in chickens and turkeys are most probably transmitted from wild bird species by direct or indirect contact. In North America, subtypes of AIV detected in domestic poultry correlates closely with subtypes found in natural reservoir species. For example, from 1996 to 2001, subtypes H1-12 and N1-4, N6-9 were detected in domestic poultry, either by detection of specific antibodies or isolation of the virus [10]. The H14 through H16 subtypes have not been detected in poultry or wild birds in the Americas. Once AIV is introduced into poultry from the natural reservoir species, the virus can spread to other poultry by a variety of methods including movement of infected birds, contaminated vehicles, bird crates, equipment, and by maintenance, utility, vaccination and artificial insemination crews. Backyard flocks, range-reared poultry, and organically grown poultry play a particularly important role in the epidemiology of AI; these birds can acquire infection by direct contact or by sharing common water sources with wild birds or AIV-contaminated environments. For example, in Minnesota during the 1980s and early 1990s, many infections were detected each year in range-reared commercial turkeys. In the early 1990s producers stopped the practice of range-rearing turkeys in favour of confinement rearing; as a result, AIV infection in turkeys in the state is under control.

In the United States the live-bird markets that are common in some of the large metropolitan areas can serve as a man-made reservoir of influenza virus and the markets have been linked to several outbreaks of LPAI infections in poultry. Also, swine have been shown to be a source of H1 and H3 influenza virus infections in turkey breeders and market turkeys when these birds are raised in close proximity to swine [22].

Human Infections with Avian Influenza Viruses in North America

Direct transmission of avian H5N1 and H9N2 influenza viruses from poultry to humans in Hong Kong in 1997 and 1999 respectively, has kindled a renewed interest in the role of AIVs as zoonotic agents. Although there have been several outbreaks of AIV in poultry in North America during the past 30 years, there are only three documented cases of human infections with avian influenza virus; all involved subtype H7. The three documented cases have occurred since 2002 and all resulted in mild infections. Two of the cases involved people culling poultry to control outbreaks of AI. The first case was confirmed by the Centers for Disease Control (CDC) in 2002 when antibodies to H7N2 were detected in an individual experiencing a respiratory illness; however, no virus was isolated. Before the illness, the affected individual had been helping with the culling of infected flocks experiencing an outbreak of LPAI (H7N2) in chickens and turkeys in the Shenandoah Valley, Virginia, USA. The individual recovered without complications [CDC, unpublished data, <http://www.cdc.gov/flu/avian/outbreaks/us.htm>].

The second case, also confirmed by the CDC [CDC unpublished data, <http://www.cdc.gov/flu/avian/outbreaks/us.htm>], occurred in 2003 in a patient with a serious underlying medical condition. The person was admitted to a New York hospital with respiratory symptoms. Preliminary laboratory tests showed that respiratory secretions were positive for influenza A virus, presumed to be H1 or H3. The patient recovered and went home after a few weeks. Subsequent confirmatory tests showed that the patient was infected with an H7N2 avian influenza virus. Molecular studies on the isolate performed at the Southeast Poultry Research Laboratory, Athens, Georgia, showed the H7N2 virus to be similar to the LPAI H7N2 viruses associated with the LBMS in the Northeast United States [Spackman, personal communication]. However, the affected individual denied having contact with poultry.

The third case was reported by Health Canada in 2004 [23]. In this case, two individuals were infected with H7N3 virus after assisting with culling operations associated with an outbreak of HPAI H7N3 in poultry in the Frazer Valley, British Columbia, Canada. Both persons developed conjunctivitis and other influenza-like symptoms The illness in both individuals resolved after treatment with oseltamivir.

Conclusions

Domestic poultry can be exposed to a variety of subtypes of AIV that can originate from a number of sources, including wild aquatic birds, LBMs, and backyard poultry. Swine can also be an important source of the H1 and H3 subtypes of influenza virus for turkeys in North America. Since there are no control measures that can be used to control infection in wild birds, prevention of influenza infection in poultry from wild birds must rely upon good husbandry and biosecurity programmes. The development of effective surveillance programmes for AI virus infections in poultry, with particular emphasis on detection of H5 and H7 subtypes, is essential to identify infected flocks quickly and prevent the emergence of HPAI viruses in domestic poultry.

References

1 Slemons RD, Johnson DC, Osborn JS, Hayes F: Type-A influenza viruses isolated from wild free-flying ducks in California. Avian Diseases 1974; 18: 119-124.

2 Kawaoka Y, Chambers TM, Sladen WL, Webster RG: Is the gene pool of influenza viruses in shorebirds and gulls different from that in wild ducks? Virology 1988; 3: 247-250.

3 Webster RG: Influenza: an emerging disease. Emerging Infectious Diseases 1998; 4 (3): 436-41.

4 Swayne DE, Halvorson DA: Influenza, in Saif YM, Barnes J, Glisson JR, Fadley AM, McDougald LR, Swayne DE (eds): Diseases of Poultry, 11th ed. Ames, Iowa, Iowa State Press, Blackwell Publishing, 2003, pp 135-160.

5 Kawaoka Y, Naeve CW, Webster RG: Is virulence of H5N2 influenza viruses in chickens associated with loss of carbohydrate from the hemagglutinin? Virology 1984; 139 (2): 303-316.

6 Horimoto T, Rivera E, Pearson J, Senne, D, Krauss S, Kawaoka Y, Webster RG: Origin and molecular changes associated with emergence of a highly pathogenic H5N2 influenza virus in Mexico. Virology 1995; 213 (1): 223-230.

7 Suarez DL, Senne DA, Banks J, Brown IH, Essen SC, Lee CW, Manvell RJ, Mathieu-Benson C, Moreno V, Pedersen JC, Panigrahy B, Rojas H, Spackman E, Alexander DJ: Recombination resulting in virulence shift in avian influenza outbreak, Chile. Emerging Infectious Diseases 2004; 10 (4): 693-699.

8 Bowes VA, Ritchie SJ, Byrne S, Sojonky K, Bidulka JJ, Robinson JH: Virus characterization, Clinical presentation, and pathology associated with H7N3 avian influenza in British Columbia broiler breeder chickens in 2004. Avian Diseases 2004; 48 (4): 928-934.

9 Hirst M, Astell CR, Griffith M, Coughlin SM, Moksa M, Zeng T, Smailus DE, Holt RA, Jones S, Marra MA, Petric M, Krajden M, Lawrence D, Mak A, Chow R, Skowronski DM, Tweed SA, Goh S, Brunham RC, Robinson J, Bowes V, Sojonky K, Byrne SK, Li Y, Kobasa D, Booth T, Paetzel M: Novel avian influenza H7N3 strain outbreak, British Columbia. Emerging Infectious Diseases 2004; 10 (12): 2192-2195.

10 Senne DA: Avian influenza in the Western Hemisphere including the Pacific Islands and Australia. Avian Diseases 2003; 47 (special issue): 798-805.

11 Stallknecht DE, Shane SM: Host range of avian influenza virus in free-living birds. Veterinary Research Communications 1988; 12: 125-141.

12 Kawaoka Y, Chambers TM, Sladen WL, Webster RG: Is the gene pool of influenza viruses in shore birds and gulls different from that in wild ducks? Virology 1988; 163: 247-250.

13 Diebel R, Emord DE, Dukelow W, Hinshaw VS, Wood JM: Influenza viruses and paramyxoviruses in duck in the Atlantic Flyway, 1977-1983, including an H5N2 isolate related to the virulent chicken virus. Avian Diseases 1985; 29: 970-985.

14 Hinshaw VS, Nettles VF, Schorr LW, Wood JM, Webster RG: Influenza virus surveillance in waterfowl in Pennsylvania after H5N2 avian outbreak. Avian Diseases 1986; 30: 207-212.

15 Ottis K, Bachman PA: Isolation and characterization of ortho- and paramyxoviruses from feral birds in Europe. Zbl Vet Med B1983; 30: 22-35.

16 Boudreault A, Lecomte J, Hinshaw VS: Antigenic characterization of influenza A viruses isolated from avian species in Ontario, Quebec and Maritimes during the 1977 season. Revue Canadienne De Biologie 1980; 39: 107-114.

17 Slemons RD, Shieldcastle MC, Heyman LD, Bednarik KE, Senne DA: Type A influenza viruses in waterfowl in Ohio and implications for domestic turkeys. Avian Diseases 1991; 35: 165-173.

18 Stallknecht DE, Shane SM, Zwank PJ, Senne DA, Kearney MT: Avian influenza viruses from migratory and resident ducks of coastal Louisiana. Avian Diseases 1990; 34: 398-405.

19 Senne DA, Pearson JE, Panigrahy B: Live poultry markets: a missing link in the epidemiology of avian influenza. In Proceedings of the 3rd International Symposium on Avian Influenza 27-29 March 1992, The Wisconsin Center, The University of Wisconsin, Madison, Wisconsin 2004, pp 50-80.

20 Panigrahy B, Senne DA, Pedersen JC: Avian influenza virus subtypes inside and outside the live bird markets, 1993-2000: a spatial and temporal relationship. Avian Diseases 2002; 46 (2): 298-307.

21 Senne DA, Suarez DL, Pedersen JC, Panigrahy B: Molecular and biological characteristics of H5 and H7 avian influenza viruses in live-bird markets of the northeastern United States, 1994-2001. Avian Diseases 2003; 47 (3 Suppl): 898-904.

22 Choi YK, Lee JH, Erickson G, Goyal SM, Joo HS, Webster RG, Webby RJ: H3N2 influenza virus transmission from swine to turkeys, United States. Emerging Infectious Diseases 2004; 10 (12): 2156-2160.

23 Tweed SA, Skowroski DM, David ST, Larder A, Petric M, Lees W, Li Y, Katz J, Krajden M, Tellier R, Halpert C, Hirst M, Astell C, Lawrence D, Mak A: Human illness from avian influenza H7N3, British Columbia. Emerging Infectious Diseases 2004; 10 (12): 2196-2199.

D.A. Senne, Avian Section, National Veterinary Services Laboratories, 1800 Dayton Avenue, Ames, IA 10050, U.S.A.
E-mail: dennis.a.senne@aphis.usda.gov

Schudel A, Lombard M (eds): OIE/FAO International Scientific Conference on Avian Influenza.
Dev Biol (Basel). Basel, Karger, 2006, vol 124, pp 45-50.

Recent Epidemiology and Ecology of Influenza A Viruses in Avian Species in Europe and the Middle East

I.H. Brown, J. Banks, R.J. Manvell, S.C. Essen, W. Shell, M. Slomka, B. Londt, D.J. Alexander

Veterinary Laboratories Agency (Weybridge), Addlestone, Surrey, United Kingdom

Abstract: There have been at least ten distinct outbreaks of LPAI or HPAI in poultry caused by H5 or H7 viruses in the last eight years in Europe and the Middle East. There appears to be an increased occurrence of such episodes consistent with global trends. As a result, surveillance systems have been enhanced to facilitate early detection of infection in poultry, together with active surveillance of wild bird populations.

These complementary activities have resulted in the detection of a number of viruses in wild bird populations, including some with high genetic similarity to newly detected viruses in poultry, for example, H7N3 in Italy and H7N7 in the Netherlands. Furthermore, there is evidence for continued circulation of H5 and H7 viruses in wild *Anseriformes*, thereby presenting a real and current threat for the introduction of viruses to domestic poultry, especially those reared in outdoor production systems. Viruses of H9N2 subtype continue to circulate widely in the Middle East and are associated with significant disease problems in poultry.

The epidemiology has the potential to be complicated further by introduction of novel viruses through illegal importation of captive birds, such as was detected with H5N1 in Belgium in 2004. Continual genetic exchange in the avian virus gene pool and independent evolution of all gene segments either within an individual host species or among wild bird hosts suggests that these viruses are not in evolutionary stasis in the natural reservoir.

INTRODUCTION

The genetic pool of all avian influenza (AI) viruses is primarily in aquatic birds, which are responsible for the perpetuation of these viruses in nature [1]. The range of influenza virus subtypes infecting poultry is more limited, with some haemagglutinin (HA) subtypes predominating, including H5, H6, H7 and H9. Influenza A viruses infecting poultry can be divided into two distinct groups on the basis of their ability to cause disease. The highly pathogenic avian influenza (HPAI) viruses can cause up to 100 % flock mortality; these viruses are restricted to the H5 and H7 subtypes, although not all viruses of these subtypes can cause HPAI. All other viruses cause a much milder disease, consisting of mild respiratory disease, depression and reduction in egg production in layers. In some circumstances, more serious disease can occur if infection is exacerbated by other factors, such as presence of other pathogens or influence by environmental conditions.

The social and economic impact of HPAI can be immense, typified by the current on-going veterinary and public health crises in eastern Asia as a result of H5N1. The last outbreak of HPAI in Europe was in the Netherlands in 2003 resulting from infection with H7N7 [2]. This outbreak led to the death or culling of 30 million birds; the economic costs are estimated at 270 million Euros in direct compensation and > 1 billion Euros in indirect costs.

Since 1959, approximately 24 primary outbreaks of HPAI in poultry have been reported [3], of which ten (38 %) have been in Europe and one (on-going) in the Middle East. There appears to have been an upward trend in the incidence of these episodes world-wide, with six (25 %) occurring since 2002. Although some of this may be because of better reporting and recognition, there appears to be an underlying trend that may be consistent with intensification of poultry production and recent impetus in some regions towards outdoor production.

There is an on-going background risk of introduction of AI into poultry populations from infected wild birds that may come into contact directly or indirectly with domestic poultry. As a result, surveillance systems have been enhanced in many areas both in wild birds and poultry to understand virus epidemiology better and provide improved early warning systems for detection of virus in poultry populations.

In this paper, we review and report on the epidemiology of AI viruses primarily of H5, H7 and H9 subtypes based on viruses isolated recently in Europe and the Middle East and submitted to the International Reference Laboratory at VLA-Weybridge, UK.

Epidemiology of H5 in Europe

Although there have been no outbreaks of HPAI from H5 viruses in Europe since 1998, there is current evidence for circulation of these subtypes (summarised in Table 1) in the wild bird population and there are occasional incidents of subsequent detection in poultry, principally, but not exclusively, in ducks that are reared outdoors, thereby presenting greater risk of introduction. There appears to be an increasing trend, but it is unclear whether this is because of enhanced surveillance in some countries or as a result of increased prevalence in bird populations, including "spikes" of circulation in wild aquatic species, especially ducks.

Surveys of wild birds in northern Europe in 1999 to 2000 identified one H5 virus from a total of 8500 birds sampled [4]. This would appear to be lower than the perceived prevalence in 2003-2004 in

Table 1: Influenza A viruses of H5 and H7 subtype isolated from avian species in European countries 2003-2004.

Subtype	Poultry	Wild birds
LPAI		
H5N2	1*	2
H5N3	2	1
H5N7	1	0
H7N1	0	1
H7N3	2	1
H7N4	0	1
H7N7	1	2
HPAI		
H5N1	0	1**
H7N7	3 (253)	0

* Number of countries isolating virus.

** Imported captive birds.

() Number of outbreaks.

wild bird populations, when fewer birds were sampled but from across a more diverse region of Europe. The detection of H5N1 in smuggled eagles from the Far East in Belgium in 2004 demonstrates the potential risk of virus introduction. Fortunately, these birds were seized at the port of entry and, despite being healthy, were shown to be infected with H5N1 virus very similar to those strains associated with current epidemics in eastern Asia and therefore distinct from other H5 viruses detected in Europe [5].

Broadly, recent European viruses are antigenically homogeneous, however, there is some heterogeneity and some strains exhibit high levels of antigenic similarity with most viruses analysed including historical strains. Evaluation of antigenic properties of avian viruses is becoming an increasing requirement for defining and selecting the most appropriate strains for use in serosurveillance for LPAI and vaccine banks. The recent European H5 viruses could be clearly distinguished in haemagglutinin inhibition (HI) tests from their counterparts in Asia and North America.

Genetic analyses of the HA gene revealed significant heterogeneity. Viruses isolated in Europe during the last seven years form several distinct groups indicating some genetic diversity in the prevailing gene pool. Viruses isolated in 2002 could be clearly distinguished from selected viruses detected in 2003 and 2004, which all clustered closely together. All the viruses examined were distinct from the Italian HPAI viruses of H5N2 that are known to be more closely related to Hong Kong strains from 1997 [6]. This is consistent with the reported similarity of 95 % between an H5N7 virus isolated from mallards in Denmark in 2003 and H5N2 Chicken/Italy/312/97 [7].

Epidemiology of H7 in Europe and the Middle East

As with H5 viruses, there is continued evidence for widespread circulation in Europe of H7 viruses, principally in wild birds. This is supported by the continual introduction of LPAI viruses to poultry populations in northern Italy presumably from wild birds [3,8]. It has been postulated that backyard flocks of poultry, particularly those that contain domesticated ducks and geese, may act as a link between wild birds and the commercial poultry sector [9]. The detection of several H7 subtypes (Table 1) from more than one country, mainly in wild ducks, indicates a continuing, real and perhaps increasing threat of introduction to poultry. It has been postulated that the outbreak virus responsible for the H7N7 epidemic in northern Europe in 2003 was derived from a progenitor virus whose gene segments were very similar to those from viruses isolated from wild birds within the previous few years [Koch, personal communication]. Nevertheless, as for H5, only a single H7 virus was isolated from an extensive survey of wild bird populations [4].

In Pakistan, outbreaks of HPAI resulting from H7N3 began in 1995 and initiated a vaccination campaign using vaccines with homologous HA. Further outbreaks occurred in 2001, involving similar viruses but of both LPAI and HPAI forms. Continuing epidemics in poultry were confirmed in 2003 and 2004.

Genetically, the Eurasian viruses form a distinct lineage and can be clearly separated from prevailing viruses in the Americas and Australasia. The recent viruses from outbreaks in Europe have similar topologies consistent with similarities in the circulating H7 gene pool in wild birds in the region, but are clearly distinguishable from viruses circulating ten years earlier. Interestingly, viruses from eastern Europe in 1995 form a distinct sublineage. The H7N3 viruses from Pakistan group together in a distinct sublineage of the Eurasian lineage. Virus from the recent outbreaks, whilst closely related to, can be clearly differentiated from, the 1995 isolates, suggesting some drift in the HA of these viruses.

Epidemiology of Other Influenza Virus Subtypes in Europe and the Middle East

Subsequent to the first reports of H9N2 viruses in poultry in the Middle East in the late 1990s, these viruses have continued to persist and spread, often in association with significant disease problems, occasionally with high mortality even though the viruses are classified as LPAI. The disease presentation is often complicated by the presence of other pathogens and adverse environmental factors. During 2004, the reference laboratory at VLA-Weybridge continued to receive numerous virus isolates from a total of eight countries in the Middle East. Genetic analyses of the HA of a limited number of these viruses indicates that they are quite distinct from the earlier isolates, forming a unique sublineage. It is possible that the widespread use of autogenous vaccines may contribute to the continued evolution of these viruses in poultry.

In Europe, programmes of enhanced and focused surveillance since 2003 for influenza A viruses in avian species have resulted in the isolation of other subtypes. In poultry species, viruses were isolated from ducks (H6N1, H6N2, H3N8), turkeys (H6N2, H9N9), geese (H1N1, H6N2) and ostriches (H2N3). In wild birds, the surveillance was largely focused on **anseriformes** and led to the isolation of H1N1, H2N3, H3N2, H3N8, H4N6, H6N1, H6N2, H6N5, H6N6, H6N8, H9N9, H10N4, H10N5, H10N6, H10N7, H11N9 virus subtypes. In addition, surveillance of various other wild bird species resulted in the isolation of H9N9, H10N4, H13N6 and H16N3 virus subtypes.

Evolution of AI Viruses in Avian Species

Broadly, viral gene lineages are segregated according to host grouping and geographical location but there are exceptions through migratory bird movements or trade in live birds and animals. Examination of a relatively small number of viruses derived from wild birds and poultry in Europe and Africa indicated considerable genetic heterogeneity in the internal protein genes of viruses co-circulating in bird populations in the same geographical region.

It would appear that there is continual genetic exchange in the avian virus gene pool among contemporary viruses in bird populations that contributes to the extensive genetic diversity within the genes encoding the internal proteins. Viruses in the east hemisphere avian lineage did not show consistent topologies in relation to their position within the lineage for each gene segment, suggesting some genetic variability in the genome resulting from genetic exchange among co-circulating avian viruses. The Eurasian avian viruses contain different genetic "imprints" amongst the internal protein genes, with individual viruses located in heterologous sublineages between gene segments.

This indicates independent evolution of all gene segments either within an individual host species or, perhaps more likely, between wild bird hosts. Transmission to poultry from wild birds results in a rapid evolution in the gene's encoding internal proteins [10] as the virus adapts to the new host group. The high efficiency of virus replication in wild bird hosts provides significant opportunity for generation of genetic variants and suggests that these viruses are not in evolutionary stasis in the natural reservoir.

Future Perspectives

Recent history dictates that influenza is an increasing problem for poultry production that is probably linked to changes in agricultural practices. The epidemiology of the viruses appears to be increasing in complexity and may be directly influenced by modern production systems together with alternative control strategies. In addition, recent evidence supports the emergence of viruses directly from avian species that may present threats to human health.

To gain a better understanding of the epidemiology of AI and how it is changing, together with early detection of viruses that have the potential to produce devastating consequences for the farming community, enhanced and improved surveillance is vital. In the European Union, new initiatives to improve surveillance for influenza viruses of H5 and H7 subtypes have been formally implemented in all member states. Active surveillance based on serological detection of infection is conducted on a statistical basis to detect defined prevalence with appropriate confidence in all poultry populations, with particular focus on higher risk categories and those more susceptible to infection. In addition, the programmes provide an opportunity to enhance and conduct surveillance in wild bird populations in the region.

Summary Conclusions

There is growing evidence for increased incidence and prevalence of H5 and H7 viruses in poultry populations world-wide. This apparent increase needs to be balanced against improved surveillance, which is often targeted on higher risk groups, thereby resulting in better detection. Nevertheless, the frequent introduction of viruses to poultry, presumably from wild birds, either directly or through farmed species that are raised outdoors, does raise the possibility that the epidemiology is changing consistent with changes in poultry production and management.

Surveillance has identified co-circulation of multiple H5 and H7 viruses with distinct genetic characteristics in Europe both in wild birds and poultry. These viruses can exhibit some antigenic differences that may have implications for future surveillance and control through vaccination. In Pakistan, recent HPAI of H7N3 subtype appears to have evolved compared with earlier viruses and emphasises the importance of good surveillance in vaccinated populations. Influenza viruses of H9N2 subtype continue to change genetically and present significant problems in the Middle East. The genetic pool in wild birds is very diverse and is subject to continual exchange among different host species thereby providing an evolving gene pool of influenza viruses.

Acknowledgements

The authors would like to highlight the invaluable contribution made by all laboratories and other institutes in submitting viruses to the AI reference laboratory at VLA-Weybridge.

References

1 Alexander DJ: A review of avian influenza. In Proceedings of the ESVV Symposium on influenza viruses of wild and domestic animals, Ghent, 16-18 May 1999. Vet Micro 2000; 74: 3-13.

2 Elbers ARW, Fabri THF, Vries TS, de Wit JJ, Pijpers A, Koch G: The highly pathogenic avian influenza A virus (H7N7) epidemic in The Netherlands in 2003: lessons learned from the first five outbreaks. Av Dis 2005, in press.

3 Capua I, Alexander DJ: Avian influenza: recent developments. Av Path 2004; 33 (4): 393-404.

4 Fouchier RAM, Olsen B, Bestebroer TM, Herfst S, van der Kemp L, Rimmelzwaan GF, Osterhaus ADME: Influenza A virus surveillance in wild birds in Northern Europe in 1999 and 2000. Av Dis 2003; 47: 857-860.

5 van Borm S, Lambrecht B, Boschmans M, Decaestecker M, Morales D, Gonze M, Vandenbroeck M, van den Berg T: Isolation and characterisation of a highly pathogenic H5N1 influenza virus from eagles smuggled from Thailand into Europe. In Proceedings of the OIE/FAO International Conference on Avian Influenza, Paris, 7-8 April 2005; 65.

6 Donatelli I, Campitelli L, Di Trani L, Puzelli S, Selli L, Fioretti A, Alexander DJ, Tollis M, Krauss S, Webster RG: Characterization of H5N2 influenza viruses from Italian poultry. J Gen Viro 2001; 82: 623-630.

7 Bragstad K, JorGensen PH, Handberg KJ, Mellergaard S, Corbet S, Fomsgaard A: New avian influenza A virus subtype combination H5N7 identified in Danish mallard ducks. Virus Res 2005; in press.

8 Campitelli L, Mogavero E, Alessandra de Marco M, Delogu M, Puzelli S, Frezz F, Facchini M, Chiapponi C, Foni E, Cordioli P, Webby R, Barigazzi G, Webster RG, Donatelli I: Interspecies transmission of an H7N3 influenza virus from wild birds to intensively reared domestic poultry in Italy. Virol 2004; 323: 24-36.

9 Terregino C, Cattoli G, De Nardi R, Beato MS, Capua I: Isolation of influenza A viruses subtype H7N7 and H7N4 from waterfowl in Italy. Vet Rec 2005; 156 (9); 292.

10 Zhou NN, Shortridge KF, Claas ECJ, Krauss SL, Webster RG: Rapid evolution of H5N1 influenza viruses in chickens in Hong Kong. J Virol 1999; 73; 3366-3374.

Dr. I.H. Brown, Veterinary Laboratories Agency-Weybridge, New Haw, Addlestone, Surrey KT15 3NB, U.K.
E-mail: i.h.brown@vla.defra.gsi.gov.uk

Schudel A, Lombard M (eds): OIE/FAO International Scientific Conference on Avian Influenza.
Dev Biol (Basel). Basel, Karger, 2006, vol 124, pp 51-57.

Ecology and Epidemiology of Avian Influenza in Ostriches

A.J. Olivier

Klein Karoo Group, Research and Development: Ostrich Laboratory, PO Box 241, Oudtshoorn, 6620, South Africa

Abstract: Avian influenza is important because of its potential devastating effect on poultry health and trade. The ostrich industry of South Africa has not escaped the consequences of control and export restrictions resulting from notifiable virus infections.

Ostrich farmers first observed a syndrome of green urine in the early and mid 1980s. An H7N1 subtype, causing high mortality in young ostriches but with a low pathogenicity index for chickens, was first isolated in 1991. The first highly pathogenic subtype affecting ratites was reported during the 2000 epidemic of H7N1 in Italy. Low pathogenic subtypes were isolated in South Africa from 1991 to 2004, with one HPAI isolated in 2004.

International research work on ostriches with both H5 and H7 subtypes, in both low and high pathogenic pathotypes, found the severity of clinical disease was not directly correlated to the pathotype.

The ecology and epidemiology of infections in ostriches is not well understood. Surveys suggest local migratory water birds may play an important role. They have direct contact with ostrich flocks through the free-range production systems. Seasonal occurrence is seen, with the wet colder months more favourable for virus survival and detection. Management, population density, immune status and age are other important determinants of the severity of disease.

Surveillance and monitoring must be implemented to understand the ecology and epidemiology, which extends to the validation and standardisation of diagnostic and serological methods for ostriches. Serious consideration should be given to vaccination, education and the use of separate production zones as part of a control programme.

INTRODUCTION

Ostrich farming in South Africa is focused on export of leather and fresh ostrich meat products to trade partners, (in USA, Japan, and Europe respectively). The world market share of the South African industry is around 60 %. Main production systems, export slaughter and processing facilities are located within a limited semi-arid region (Klein Karoo) within the Western Cape province (WC) representing 70-80 % of the South African industry. The Eastern Cape (EC) and Northern Cape (NC) are the other provinces raising slaughter ostriches, mainly by contract growers for larger producers in the Western Cape.

The production system is unique, since it is based on extensive farming production systems. In August 2004, an isolation was made of an avian influenza (AI) virus in a feedlot farm in the EC, which was sequenced and classified as a high pathogenic (HPAI) pathotype. This resulted in the implementation of control measures, mass destruction and burial to eradicate the disease from the province. The South African Government suspended all export, and international trade partners placed a ban on importation of all fresh ostrich products to their countries.

The summary of AI isolations from ostriches in Table 1, reflects the limited knowledge the poultry industry had before the 1980s on this virus. It was only in the early 1990s, after the first ostrich influenza outbreak, that more regular isolations were recorded. This first virus isolation, was an H7N1 subtype with a low pathogenicity for chickens [1]. This was made during an epizootic in 1991, which saw high mortality in young ostriches. Factors contributing to increased mortality were other infectious agents and stressors, such as high population densities, inadequate ventilation and bad hygiene resulting from poor management practices [1,2].

Table 1 : Isolations of avian influenza viruses in Southern Africa.

Year	Pathotype	Species	Area
1961	LP H5N3	"Tern"	South Africa
1991	LP H7N1	Ostrich	Klein Karoo district*/**
1994	LP H5N9	Ostrich	RSA
1995	LP H9N2	Ostrich	RSA
1995	LP H5N2	Ostrich	Zimbabwe
1996	LP H5N2	Ostrich	Zimbabwe
1998	LP H10N2	Wild water birds	Klein Karoo district**
1998	LP H6N8	Egyptian geese	Oudtshoorn (serology)
1998	LP H6N8	Ostrich	Oudtshoorn
2001	LP H10N1	Ostrich	Dr Rust/Oudtshoorn*
2002/3	LP H6N2	Chickens	KZN, Gauteng, North West & Western Cape provinces
2004	H5N2	Egyptian geese	Oudtshoorn**
2004	H5N2	Ostrich	Eastern Cape **
2004	H5N3/H5N1	Wild water birds	Gauteng Province**

* Isolated at the Klein Karoo Group Research Laboratory.
** Isolated at a provincial veterinary laboratory (Stellenbosch or OVI).

An H6N8 virus was isolated from ostriches showing signs of disease in 1998, shortly after an AI survey identified wild birds with positive titres, by the Onderstepoort Veterinary Institute (OVI) in the Klein Karoo area [3]. During 2001, an H10N1 isolate was made from ostrich chicks showing signs of depression and "green urine". Since 2002, a low pathogenic H6N2 virus has been circulating among chickens in South Africa. Fortunately, this isolate has so far not been found in ostriches.

An investigation in the winter of 2004 into increased mortality on a feedlot farm in the EC, some 500 km from the Klein Karoo region, isolated an H5N2 virus. It was classified as an HPAI type based on the nucleotide sequence of the haemagglutinin, although the intravenous pathogenicity index (IVPI) was that of a low pathotype (LPAI) [4,5]. No further isolations were made on other farms in the area, but a number of healthy flocks showed sero-conversion, without any signs of infection.

Ecology

Our practical experience during outbreaks of low pathogenic types and the more recent highly pathogenic subtype in the EC show that the epidemiology, pathogenesis, and diagnosis are not always straightforward.

Ostrich farmers in the area first observed a syndrome, which they described as "green urine" with respiratory signs, in the early 1980s [1, personal observation]. This syndrome was not confirmed as AI since these signs are not pathogenomic and various differential diagnoses exist. There was a seasonal pattern to the occurrence, with the autumn and winter months being the most common times for the green urine to be observed. This is the main rainfall season and is when producers plant various small grains for grazing or harvest. It was also associated with drought conditions.

Clinical disease

The H7N1 outbreak of 1991 affected young ostriches, but adults showed no symptoms. Signs were the classical green urine, depression, poor appetite and mortality after two to three days or slow recovery over two to three weeks. Worst affected were young birds (< 8 months) kept at high stock densities, suffering from poor body condition or kept in conditions of poor hygiene. Birds were treated with hepatic stimulants and multivitamins. An experimental vaccine was used to control the outbreak with very good success [1,2].

With the 2004 H5N2 outbreak on the feedlot farm in the EC, similar signs were observed, with acute hepatitis, peritonitis and respiratory pathology the primary lesions. Various management and environmental factors contributed to the severity of clinical disease, such as very high population density, introduction of various age groups from a number of grower farms, adaptation stress associated with new rations and environment, and very cold weather. The roles of secondary infections were highlighted, with good response after veterinary intervention with antibiotic treatment and vitamins. This was shortly before final diagnosis and mass destruction. Mortality rate was around 18 % and limited to a few camps.

Diagnosis

Diagnosis of infections can be very difficult. This may be because of the nature of low pathogenicity infections in ostriches with non-specific clinical signs. Low morbidity and lower mortality, slow infection rate and secondary infections mask a possible viral aetiology among a flock. Serological responses after antigen exposure are another factor that may reduce excretion, severity of clinical signs and consequent detection.

Current situation

The control measures implemented during the EC outbreak resulted in over 30,000 ostriches being culled and destroyed. This was devastating to the industry since these birds represent almost 40 % of the EC ostrich population. The culling of chicks, slaughter ostriches and irreplaceable breeding stock will have a long-term negative effect on the industry.

An investigation into the historical results of cases at the ostrich laboratory of the Klein Karoo Group during 2004 indicated no live virus isolation through conventional embryonated specific-pathogen-free (SPF) eggs or antigen detection by polymerase chain reaction (PCR) methods. These cases were part of routine diagnostic investigation and post-mortem examinations from mortalities in the area.

Initial serological and antigen detection (by RT-PCR) of all registered export ostrich farms in the WC revealed 11.7 % serological positive slaughter ostriches on 10 % of farms. Initial epidemiological investigations revealed the prevalence of some clusters. These findings may be slightly biased towards farms along rivers. It must be noted that none of the farms in the WC experienced abnormal mortality rates during the period of the H5N2 outbreak in the EC.

Of importance is the finding in other poultry species (chickens). No virus activity was found, serologically or clinically in the EC or during the WC surveillance. This was despite some rural chickens being present on the affected farms. This is very significant, since commercial poultry production areas are distinctly separated from ostrich production areas because of climatic and economic factors.

Epidemiology

Wild waterfowl dynamics

In 1998, the Ostrich Division of the OVI identified AI as one of the potential threats to the ostrich industry and its trade. A survey was initiated and wild bird samples were collected in the Klein Karoo region during the winter of 1998 [3]. In total, 262 aquatic wild birds, comprising 14 species were sampled. From eight samples, avian influenza virus serotype H10N9 was isolated, with one bird serologically positive for H6.

A second survey was performed by the Klein Karoo Group in conjunction with the OVI and University of Pretoria Faculty of Veterinary Science, during the early winter of 2004. An H5N2 virus was isolated from an Egyptian goose sampled from a farm in the region. This was similar to the virus later isolated in the EC, differing in its pathotype being a low pathogenic strain. There are indications that this virus may have originated from strains found in Europe and Siberia. Although the Egyptian goose from which the isolate was made is locally nomadic, it does have contact with migratory species at lagoons and rivers along the southern coast of South Africa.

Ostrich production management systems

Ostrich farming is a free-range production system, making use of flood-irrigated lucerne pastures for younger chicks and open grazing pastures for slaughter birds [2]. The Klein Karoo area is a semi-arid region with a very low non-seasonal rainfall pattern with rain occurring mainly in autumn and winter. This results in farms being concentrated along rivers and irrigation schemes. Open water-storage systems, such as farm dams are important sources of water for livestock. Farmers also produce wheat and barley for the ostriches to graze in the winter. Unfortunately, both these practices create ideal environments for the attraction of various wild bird species, notably waterfowl.

Because of the low rainfall, drought situations and planted pastures, wild birds are attracted to food and water provided for ostriches (personal observation). This close connection between wild avian species and ostriches may have resulted in a number of AI outbreaks over the years, as can be seen from isolation first in wild bird species followed closely by the occurrence of an outbreak or isolation in ostriches [3].

Trade Implications

Avian influenza epidemics result in trade bans, of poultry and poultry products including ostriches, between influenza-free and -infected trade partners [2,5-7].

Agriculture is the cornerstone of economic activities in the WC, so the ostrich industry is of strategic importance. The socio-economic impact of the disease and the resulting control strategies can be enormous in the WC. Almost 18,000 jobs depend directly on the ostrich industry. Each of these jobs supports a further five dependants.

The core of a control strategy must be to ensure a sustainable poultry and ostrich industry in South Africa, while at the same time maintaining food safety and security.

Research

Limited international work with both H5 and H7 subtypes, in both low and high pathogenic pathotypes found the clinical disease was not associated with the pathotype [8-13]. Ostriches infected with high pathogenic types showed slight depression, ruffled feathers and a heamorrhagic diarrhoea. In the case with the H7 pathotypes, depression, ruffled feathers, anorexia, and younger birds with sneezing and open mouth breathing were observed in one trial.

Another trial had no clinical disease in ostriches challenged with an H5 pathotype. The virus was transmitted to in-contact sentinel birds a few days post-infection. Virus could be recovered from tracheal and cloacal swabs from infected ostriches and their sentinel controls. Recovery of viruses was from three days up to 11-14 days post-infection. Tracheal swabs were the recommended samples to take, but cloacal swabs should be included for the few birds that show shedding in this way. Significant antibody responses were detected with the H7 trial, but low serological responses in an H5 trial. Sero-conversion was rapid within a week after challenge with other H5 viruses.

Prevention, Control and Eradication

Strategies for control of AI vary from no action in low pathogenic infections to the extreme of stamping out or depopulation programmes for eradication of high pathogenic strains [13]. These strategies are strongly influenced by international trade agreements, domestic expectations, sanitary and health requirements and also pathogenicity, species affected, risk assessments, geographical distribution and economic implications. With HPAI, an approach of precludement of introduction, and exposure to poultry is followed. If HPAI does occur, eradication by depopulation with or without vaccination may be considered. Both high and low pathogenic control strategies require a comprehensive, integrated national surveillance and monitoring programme; practical biosecurity measures, education of all producers involved, movement control, depopulation programmes with all high pathogenic and some H5 and H7 strains and vaccination as part of a programme of national Government control [5-7,14-16].

The South African Veterinary Authority's disease-control policies must ensure the above to the citizens of South Africa and to trading partners. This can be achieved through increased veterinary involvement in controlling a disease like AI, by establishing a technical advisory group comprising veterinarians of both sectors (poultry and ostrich), the Department of Agriculture, epidemiologists, virologists and international experts.

AI is an important emerging disease threatening the unique ostrich industry, which is under constant exposure and risk because of the free-range or extensive production systems it employs.

The ostrich industry could be crucial in being an early warning system to the South African AI surveillance and monitoring programme. This surveillance system must be transparent, developed and implemented by both industries. A well founded contingency plan needs to be in place to deal with the unique ostrich and poultry situation, and with the effect of control measures on irreplaceable breeding flocks concentrated in a small geographical area. The ostrich industry must consider seriously the use of vaccination, increased biosecurity and AI education as part of the control strategy, because of the constant exposure to virus. Research is urgently needed to understand the behaviour of the AI virus in ostriches since they are not just big chickens.

References

1 Allwright DM, Burger WP, Geyer A and Terblanche AW: Isolation of an influenza A virus from ostriches (*Struthio camelus*). Avian Pathology 1993; 22:59-65.

2 Huchermeyer FW: Diseases of ostriches and other ratites. Agricultural Research Council, Promedia, Pretoria, pp154-155.

3 Pfitzer S, Verwoerd DJ, Gerdes GH, Labuschagne AE, Erasmus A, Manvell RJ, Grund Ch: Newcastle disease and avian influenza A virus in wild waterfowl in South Africa. Avian Dis 2002; 44: 655-660.

4 Alexander DJ: A review of avian influenza in different bird species. Veterinary Microbiology 2000; 74: 3-13

5 Swayne DE, Suarez DL: Highly pathogenic avian influenza. Rev Sci Tech 2000; 19 (2): 463-482.

6 Capua I, Alexander DJ: Review article – Avian Influenza: recent developments. 2004; Avian Pathology 33 (4), 393-404.

7 CEC, Council Directive 92/40/EEC of 19th May 1992. Introducing Community measures for the control of avian influenza. Official Journal of the European Communities 1992; L167: 1-15.

8 Capua I, Cattoli G, Manvell RJ, Burlini F: Highly pathogenic avian influenza (H7N1) in ostriches farmed in Italy. Vet Rec 2000; 356.

9 Capua I, Mutinelli F, Bozza MD, Terregino, Cattoli G: Highly pathogenic avian influenza (H7N1) in ostriches (*Struthio camelus*). Avian Pathology 2000; 29: 643-646.

10 Clavijo A, Riva J, Pasick J: Pathogenicity of a Ratite origin influenza A H5 virus in ostriches (*Struthio camelus*). Avian Dis 2003; 47 (3 Suppl): 1203-1207.

11 Manvell RJ, English C, Jørgensen PH, Brown IH: Pathogenesis of H7 influenza A viruses isolated from ostriches in the homologous host infected experimentally. Avian Dis 2003; 47 (3 Suppl): 1150-1153.

12 Manvell RJ, Jørgensen PH, Nielson OL, Alexander DJ: Experimental assessment of the pathogenicity of two avian influenza A H5 viruses in ostrich chicks (*Struthio camelus*) and chickens. Avian Dis 1998; 27: 400-404.

13 Swayne DE, Beck JR, Perdue ML, Brugh M, Slemons RD: Assessment of the ability of ratite origin influenza viruses to infect and produce disease in rheas and chickens. Avian Dis 1996; 2: 438-447.

14 Halvorson DA: The control of H5 or H7 Mildly pathogenic avian influenza: a role for inactivated vaccine. Avian Pathology 2002; 31: 5-12.

15 Zampaglione M: Joint OIE/FAO press release. Update on highly pathogenic avian influenza control methods in Asia including use of vaccination. Promed 27 Sept 2004 (edited) <http://www.isid.org>.

16 Avian Influenza, poultry vaccines (16). Promed, 20 Oct 2004, <http://www.isid.org>.

Dr. A.J. Olivier, Klein Karoo Group, Research and Development: Ostrich Laboratory, PO Box 241, Oudtshoorn, 6620, South Africa.
E-mail: aolivier@kleinkaroo.com

Schudel A, Lombard M (eds): OIE/FAO International Scientific Conference on Avian Influenza.
Dev Biol (Basel). Basel, Karger, 2006, vol 124, p 59.

SESSION II

Pathogenesis

Chairperson: *B. Chantanee* (DLD, Thailand)
Rapporteur: *P. Selleck* (AAHL, Australia)

Schudel A, Lombard M (eds): OIE/FAO International Scientific Conference on Avian Influenza.
Dev Biol (Basel). Basel, Karger, 2006, vol 124, pp 61-67.

Pathogenicity of Avian Influenza Viruses in Poultry

D.E. Swayne, M. Pantin-Jackwood

Southeast Poultry Research Laboratory, Agricultural Research Service,
U.S. Department of Agriculture, Athens, GA, USA

Abstract: Historically, the pathogenicity of avian influenza (AI) viruses has been based on lethality for the major domesticated poultry species, the chicken. All AI viruses are categorised as either low (LP) and high pathogenicity (HP), but, within each category, pathobiological changes vary with host species and virus strain. Typically, AI viruses that are HP produce a similar severe, systemic disease with high mortality in chickens and a similar pathobiology in other galliforme birds, but usually either produce no infection or mild disease in ducks. The newer H5 and the H7 HPAI viruses have shifted to increased virulence for chickens as evidenced by shorter mean death times (MDT). Furthermore, the Asia H5N1 HPAI viruses have changed from producing inconsistent respiratory infections in ducks to some strains being HP (Hong Kong 2002 viruses) with virus in internal organs and brain, and excretion of large virus quantities from respiratory, and to a lesser extent, intestinal tracts. However, the quantities of virus shed per bird are still 1 % of that produced in chickens. With 2003-2004 Asian H5N1 AI viruses, the isolates have been highly lethal for young ducks but this virulence is age dependent. Across all bird species, the ability to produce severe disease and death is associated with high virus replication titres in the host, especially in specific tissues such as brain and heart.

INTRODUCTION

Avian influenza (AI) viruses vary in their ability to infect and cause disease in a host species [1]. All AI viruses are classified into two pathotypes (low (LP) and high pathogenicity (HP)) based on the existing World Organisation for Animal Health (OIE) criteria. For AI viruses to be HP, they must meet one of two criteria: (i) any AI virus that has intravenous pathogenicity index (IVPI) > 1.2 or is lethal for 75 % or more of intravenously inoculated susceptible chickens *(Gallus gallus domesticus)*; or (ii) any AI virus of H5 or H7 subtypes that has amino acid sequence at the haemagglutinin proteolytic cleavage site compatible with HPAI virus. All other AI viruses are categorised as LP. The pathogenicity designations are based on the ability to produce disease and/or death in the major poultry species, i.e. chickens. However, similar lethality and pathobiological changes have occurred in other birds of the family, *Galliformes*.

LPAI virus infections in galliformes are usually subclinical, but can produce clinical problems, such as drops in feed and water consumption, respiratory signs, egg production drops, ruptured egg yolks in the coelomic cavity and, rarely, renal disease with visceral urate deposition. Mortality rates are low unless complicated by secondary viral or bacterial infections. By contrast, HPAI virus infections in galliformes produce a multi-organ systemic disease with high mortality rates and do not require the presence of secondary pathogens. The high lethality for galliformes is evident regardless of the bird's age.

Critical Factors

The host, virus and environment all impact the outcome of exposure. Several concepts must be recognised in order to understand the pathobiology of AI viruses. First, the AI virus must have the ability to replicate in respiratory and/or intestinal epithelial cells of the host following exposure; i.e. infectivity. This infectivity depends on several virus features including: (i) binding of the haemagglutinin surface glycoprotein to host cellular sialoligosaccharide receptors to initiate formation and internalisation of phagocytic endosomes; (ii) cleavage of the whole haemagglutinin protein (HA0) into the HA1 and HA2 fragments, which results in fusion of the virus envelope with the endosome membrane to release the nucleocapsid into the cell cytoplasm; and (iii) the replication of the viral genome via the polymerase complex utilising the cell's metabolic machinery [2]. Second, the pathogenicity (i.e. ability to produce lesions, disease and/or death) is a multi-genic trait, but the cleavability of the haemagglutinin protein has the major impact in determining HP for galliforme birds. Third, the expression of pathogenicity is directly associated with the quantity of virus produced during replication. Finally, infectivity is dependent on how well the virus is adapted to the specific host species.

In general, HPAI viruses, as defined by high lethality in intravenous-inoculated chickens, also express high lethality in other galliforme hosts with an intravenous lethality test. In addition, the production of mortality by natural route of exposure, such as intranasal inoculation, also produces high lethality in chickens but the mean death times (MDT) are lengthened and vary with individual virus strains (Table 1). In an intranasal experimental study using H5 HPAI viruses isolated between 1959 and 1984, the viruses most consistently produced high mortality rates in turkeys (*Meleagris gallopavo*) and chickens, and fewer were highly lethal for Japanese quail (*Coturnix coturnix japonicus*) (Table 1) [3]. The viruses grew to high titres in the respiratory and intestinal tracts of chickens and turkeys. By contrast, none of these six viruses caused clinical signs or mortality for domestic ducks (*Anas platyrhyncos*) and with most viruses, no virus replication occurred.

By contrast, the Asian H5N1 HPAI viruses have emerged to be unique in their ability to cause disease and death in a variety of poultry species, and this pathogenicity varies with individual virus strains [4-15]. The first outbreaks in chickens were reported in Hong Kong during March 1997; this initial virus isolate (A/chicken/Hong Kong/220/1997 [H5N1]) was considered an early prototype for the pathobiology potential of Asian H5N1 AI viruses in various bird species.

In a pathogenesis study using standard 10^6 mean embryo infectious doses (EID_{50}) given intranasally in 20 different animal species, the animal species could be placed into four different pathobiological groups based on virus replication, pathology, morbidity and mortality [9]. There was an association between the quantity of virus isolated and the ability to produce disease, lesions and death. The first group (Group 1)

Table 1 : Mortality patterns (dead/total challenged) and mean death times (days) in 2 week old chickens, turkeys and ducks, and 4-8 week old Japanese quail inoculated intranasally with approximately 10^6 mean embryo infectious doses of individual highly pathogenic avian influenza virus strains.

Virus	Chickens	Turkeys	J. Quail	Ducks
A/chicken/Scot/59 (H5N1)	5/10 (4.6)	2/10 (6.5)	0/10	0/10
A/Tern (South Africa/61 (H5N3)	10/10 (5.0)	10/10 (5.5)	2/10 (7)	0/10
A/turkey/Ontario/7732/66 (H5N9)	5/10 (3.8)	10/10 (6.3)	0/10	0/10
A/chicken/Pennsylvania/1370/83 (H5N2)	9/10 (5.0)	10/10 (4.8)	1/10 (7)	0/10
A/turkey/Ireland/1378/83 (H5N8)	9/10 (4.3)	10/10 (5.5)	10/10 (5.1)	0/10
A/duck/Ireland/113/84 (H5N8)	10/10 (2.7)	10/10 (3.8)	10/10 (5.1)	0/10

developed severe disease with greater than 75 % mortality, and they had exudative, necrotic, haemorrhagic and/or suppurative lesions in multiple visceral organs. This group includes all the galliformes (chickens, turkeys, Japanese quail, Bobwhite quail [*Colinus virginianus*], pheasants [*Phasianus colchicus*], chukkar partridges [*Alectoris chukar*], and Pearl guineafowl [*Numida meleagris*]) and zebra finches *(Taeniopygia guttata)*.

Group 1 was subdivided into two subgroups based on the primary site of virus replication and lesions. Subgroup A had primary replication in vascular endothelium and phagocytic leucocytes throughout the body. Subgroup B had primary replication in parenchymal cells of visceral organs principally cardiac myocytes, adrenal corticotrophic cells, pancreatic acinar cells, and neurons and glial cells of the brain. For birds that died early, the virus replication and lesions fit subgroup A, while birds that survived a few days typically fit into subgroup B.

The second group (Group 2) had delayed morbidity, mortality between 0 % and 75 % and presented with neurological signs. The pathobiological changes focused primarily on the nervous system tissues, and less so on the heart and pancreas. The brain had the most severe lesions and greatest concentration of influenza-specific antigen. Animals within this group included geese *(Anser anser domesticus)*, emus *(Dramaius novaehollandiae)*, house finches *(Carpodacus mexicanus)* and budgerigars *(Melopsittacus undulatus)*.

The third group (Group 3) had minimal morbidity, no mortality and mild respiratory lesions. Affected animals included domestic ducks, house sparrows (*Passer domesticus*) and laughing gulls *(Larus atricilla)*. Pathobiological changes centred on the respiratory system (ducks and gulls) or heart and gonad (sparrows). Virus detection was minimal and in low titres.

The fourth group (Group 4) lacked morbidity, mortality, pathology and virus replication except a single isolation from a starling. This group included pigeons *(Columba livia)*, starlings *(Sturnus vulgaris)*, rats *(Rattus norvegicus)* and rabbits *(Lepus oryctolagus)*.

The virulence of the Asian H5N1 AI viruses for chickens has varied with individual virus strains (Table 2) [4-6,11-13,16]. In the regulatory intravenous pathogenicity test, all viruses were uniformly lethal, causing death in 100 % of the chickens, but varied in MDT, which ranged from 1 to 4.1 days. The shortest MDT

Table 2: Mortality rates and mean death times in chickens intravenously inoculated with different Asian H5N1 HPAI viruses isolated between 1997-2003.

Virus	% mortality	Mean death time (days)
A/chicken/Hong Kong/220/97	100	1.0, 1.0
A/Hong Kong/156/97	100	2.0, 2.0, 2.0
A/environment/Hong Kong/437-4/99	100	3.4
A/environment/Hong Kong/437-6/99	100	3.0
A/environment/Hong Kong/437-8/99	100	3.3
A/environment/Hong Kong/437-10/99	100	4.1
A/duck/Anyang/ES/01	100	3.0
A/goose/Vietnam/113/01	100	1.1
A/goose/Vietnam/324/01	100	1.0
A/chicken/Korea/ES/03	100	1.0

were produced by viruses isolated from chickens and geese, and the longest by viruses isolated from humans, ducks and environmental samples from the western wholesale market of Hong Kong. However, complicating the interpretation was the usage of varying inoculum doses with each virus strain as mandated by the testing protocol to use 1:10 dilution of the virus-containing infectious allantoic fluid.

In another series of studies using a natural route of exposure (i.e. intranasal pathogenicity tests), the virus dose was controlled (10^6 EID_{50}) in order to compare the virus pathogenesis among virus isolates in chickens. All the Asian H5N1 AI viruses produced 100 % mortality in chickens, but the MDT were longer than in the intravenous test, and varied by virus strain ranging from 1.5 to 5.5 days for isolates from birds and 1.5 to 2.4 days for isolates from humans (Table 3) [4-6,11-13,16] (unpublished data). The longest MDT were for the isolate obtained from the wholesale market environment; this virus also had the lowest peak replication titre from the oropharynx, suggesting poor adaptation to the chicken. The other isolates replicated and were shed from the oropharynx and cloaca, but the cloacal titres were lower than oropharyngeal titres except for the A/duck/Anyang/01 isolate. The brain had high titres of virus, but the heart had the highest tissue titres, suggesting that lethality was associated with high titre replication and damage to vital organs.

By contrast, the pathobiology of the Asian H5N1 viruses for domestic ducks has varied more widely than in chickens, with mortality rates ranging from 0 % to 100 % (Table 4) [4,5,8,13,16] (unpublished data). Only two of the viruses were HP in ducks and these were isolated from captive or wild birds in Hong Kong during 2002. In all situations, the virus replication titres were lower for the oropharynx and cloaca of the ducks than the chickens. Unlike chickens, where the high lethality was uniform regardless of age, the high lethality was seen only with young ducks and was not present in older ones (Table 5) (unpublished data). This age dependence of the lethality explains the lack of, or low, mortality reported for infected ducks in the field. In ducks, AI virus replication is predominantly respiratory and not intestinal, with moderate titres in brain and heart for 2001-2004 isolates.

Table 3: Data from 3-6 week old chickens intranasally inoculated with 10^6 EID_{50} of Asian H5N1 HPAI viruses isolated from birds and humans.

Virus	Age (wks)	MDT (days)	Virus titres (log10 EID_{50}/ml or g) Oral	Cloacal	Brain	Heart
A/chicken/Hong Kong/220/97	4	1.5	4.7	4.2	6	–
A/Hong Kong/156/97	4	2.4	6	3.7	–	–
A/Hong Kong/491/97	4	1.6	6.4	5.8	6.3	9.8
A/environment/Hong Kong/437-6/99	4	5.5	1.7	–	–	–
A/duck/Anyang/AVL-1/01	4	2.9	3.1	6.7	–	–
A/goose/Vietnam/113/01	4	2.6	–	–	–	–
A/goose/Vietnam/324/01	4	2.4	–	–	–	–
A/chicken/Korea/ES/03	3-6	2	6.2	6	7.2	9.3
A/chicken//Indonesia/7/03	4-6	2.1	6.4	5.6	7.6	–
A/Hong Kong/213/03	4	2.1	7.4	4.5	7.4	10
A/Vietnam/1203/04	4	1.5	6.3	5.9	7.7	10
A/chicken/Supranburi/2(1)/04	3	1.8	4.7	–	–	–

Table 4: Mortality (%), mean death times (days) and virus isolation (no. positive/total tested) and titration (log10 EID_{50}/ml or g) data from 2 week old ducks intranasally inoculated with 10^6 EID_{50} of Asian H5N1 HPAI viruses isolated from birds and humans.

Virus	Mort %	MDT (days)	Virus titres (log10 EID_{50}/ml or g) Oral	Cloacal	Brain	Heart
A/chicken/Hong Kong/220/97	0	0	4/4(2.0)	2/4(1.2)	0/4	–
A/environment/Hong Kong/437-6/99	38	5.3	3/4(1.7)	1/4(1.2)	0/4	0/4
A/environment/Hong Kong/437-6/99	0	0	4/4(2.1)	4/4(2.5)	0/4	0/4
A/chicken/Hong Kong/317.5/00	0	0	4/4(1.9)	4/4(2.5)	0/4	–
A/duck/Anyang/AVL-1/01	0	0	4/4(2.6)	4/4(1.3)	4/4(3.1)	–
A/goose/Vietnam/113/01	0	0	1.8	–	1.5	–
A/goose/Hong Kong/739.2/02	88	4.7	3.8	–	–	–
A/Egret/Hong Kong/757.2/02	100	5.3	2.7	–	5.5	–
A/Hong Kong/213/03	0	0	2.7	–	–	–
A/chicken/Korea/ES/03	25	4	3/4(1.7)	1/4(1.6)	1/4(2.1)	2/4 (2.7)

Table 5: Mortality (%), mean death times (days) and virus isolation (no. positive/total tested) and titration (log10 EID_{50}/ml or g) data from 2 and 4 week-old ducks intranasally inoculated with 10^6 EID_{50} of A/chicken/Indonesia/7/2003 H5N1 HPAI viruses.

Age	Mortality (%)	Virus titres (EID_{50}/ml or gm) Oropharynx	Cloacal	Brain	Heart
2	50(7)	3/4(2.5)	0/4	4/4(3.7)	4/4(4.6)
4	0	3/4(3.0)	2/4(1.3)	–	–
4	0	–	–	–	–

Likewise, the lesions produced in ducks varied to a greater extent than in chickens with the individual virus strains. The 1997-2001 Hong Kong H5N1 HPAI viruses either produced no lesions or occasionally mild respiratory infection with associated lesions in ducks, i.e. pathobiology groups 3 or 4. However, beginning in 2001, the pathobiology of H5N1 HPAI viruses in ducks began to change and show wide variations in lesions and lethality. For example, the A/duck meat/Anyang/ES/01 H5N1 HPAI virus isolate produced predominantly respiratory (rhinitis, sinusitis, laryngitis, tracheitis and pneumonia) lesions without clinical signs or lethality, but it also produced mild lesions and had low titre virus replication in skeletal muscle and brain. The A/goose/Vietnam/113/01, A/human/Hong Kong/213/03 and A/chicken/S. Korea/ES/03 virus isolates produced respiratory lesions (air sacs and lungs) and mild myocarditis or myocardial necrosis (Group 3). The greatest change in pathobiology occurred with A/Egret/Hong Kong/757.2/02 and A/goose/Hong Kong/739.2/02, which produced systemic infection with associated lesions of non-suppurative meningoencephalitis, autonomic neuritis, pancreatic necrosis, hepatic necrosis, myocardial necrosis and myocarditis (10-80 % myocytes had virus infection), adrenal gland necrosis, skeletal muscle degeneration and necrosis, and respiratory tract inflammation (Group 1). Finally, A/chicken/Indonesia/7/03 isolate produced autonomic ganglioneuritis, encephalitis, myocarditis, and sinusitis (Group 2). These data indicate that the H5N1 HPAI viruses vary greatly in their ability to infect and cause disease in ducks.

Conclusions

- All AI viruses are categorised into one of two pathotypes based on intravenous chicken pathogenicity — low (LP) and high pathogenicity (HP) viruses.
- The pathobiology of HPAI viruses in chickens varies with the strain and they express similar pathogenicity for other birds in the order *Galliformes.*
- Historically, ducks have been resistant to HPAI virus infections or, if infections were produced, only minor respiratory lesions occurred. This is also true for the early Asian H5N1 HPAI viruses.
- Since 2001, H5N1 HPAI viruses have shown great variations in virulence for domestic ducks, changing from respiratory only to infections producing lesions in a few internal organs to some recent isolates producing severe systemic infection and lesions.

Acknowledgements

The author appreciates the assistance given in conducting studies and receiving virus isolates from Southeast Poultry Research Laboratory (Laura Perkins, Chang-Won Lee, David Suarez, Mike Perdue, Terry Tumpey and Joan Beck), Centres for Disease Control (Terry Tumpey, Jackie Katz, Nancy Cox, Alexander Klimov, Yumi Matsuoka and Doan Nguyen), National Institutes of Health (Kanta Subbarao), Hong Kong Department of Fisheries, Agriculture and Conservation (Les Sims, Trevor Ellis and Howard Wong), Thailand Department of Livestock Development (Chantanee Buranthai, Sudurat Damwatanapokin and Arunee Chaisingh) and South Korean National Veterinary Research and Quarantine Service (Inpil Mo, Jae-Hong Kim and Yong-Kuk Kwon).

References

1 Swayne DE, Halvorson DA: Influenza, in Saif YM, Barnes HJ, Fadly AM, Glisson JR, McDougald LR, Swayne DE (eds): Diseases of Poultry. Ames, IA, Iowa State University Press, 2003, pp 135-160.

2 Palese P, Garcia-Sastre A: Influenza Viruses (Orthomyxoviruses): Molecular Biology, in Granoff A, Webster RG (eds): Encylopedia of Virology. San Diego, Academic Press, 1999, vol 2, pp 830-836.

3 Alexander DJ, Parsons G, Manvell RJ: Experimental assessment of the pathogenicity of eight influenza A viruses of H5 subtype for chickens, turkeys, ducks and quail. Avian Pathol 1986; 15: 647-662.

4 Cauthen AN, Swayne DE, Schultz-Cherry S, Perdue ML, Suarez DL: Continued circulation in China of highly pathogenic avian influenza viruses encoding the hemagglutinin gene associated with the 1997 H5N1 outbreak in poultry and humans. J Virol 2000; 74: 6592-6599.

5 Nguyen DC, Uyeki TM, Jadhao S, Maines T, Shaw M, Matsuoka Y, Smith C, Rowe T, Lu X, Hall H, Xu X, Balish A, Klimov A, Tumpey TM, Swayne DE, Huynh Lien PT, Nghiem HK, Nguyen Hanh HT, Hoang LT, Cox NJ, Katz JM: Isolation and characterization of avian influenza viruses, including highly pathogenic H5N1, from poultry in live bird markets in Hanoi, Vietnam, in 2001. J Virol 2005; 79: 4201-4212.

6 Perkins LEL, Swayne DE: Pathobiology of A/chicken/Hong Kong/220/97 (H5N1) avian influenza virus in seven gallinaceous species. Vet Pathol 2001; 38: 149-164.

7 Perkins LEL, Swayne DE: Susceptibility of laughing gulls (Larus atricilla) to H5N1 and H5N3 highly pathogenic avian influenza viruses. Avian Dis 2002; 46: 877-885.

8 Perkins LEL, Swayne DE: Pathogenicity of a Hong Kong-origin H5N1 highly pathogenic avian influenza virus for emus, geese, ducks, and pigeons. Avian Dis 2002; 46: 53-63.

9 Perkins LEL, Swayne DE: Comparative susceptibility of selected avian and mammalian species to a Hong Kong-origin H5N1 high-pathogenicity avian influenza virus. Avian Dis 2003; 47: 956-967.

10 Perkins LEL, Swayne DE: Varied pathogenicity of a Hong Kong-origin H5N1 avian influenza virus in four passerine species and budgerigars. Vet Pathol 2003; 40: 14-24.

11 Suarez DL, Perdue ML, Cox N, Rowe T, Bender C, Huang J, Swayne DE: Comparison of highly virulent H5N1 influenza A viruses isolated from humans and chickens from Hong Kong. J Virol 1998; 72: 6678-6688.

12 Subbarao K, Klimov A, Katz J, Regnery H, Lim W, Hall H, Perdue M, Swayne D, Bender C, Huang J, Hemphill M, Rowe T, Shaw M, Xu X, Fukuda K, Cox N: Characterization of an avian influenza A (H5N1) virus isolated from a child with a fatal respiratory illness. Science 1998; 276: 393-396.

13 Tumpey TM, Suarez DL, Perkins LEL, Senne DA, Lee JG, Lee YJ, Mo IP, Sung HW, Swayne DE: Characterization of a highly pathogenic H5N1 avian influenza a virus isolated from duck meat. J Virol 2002; 76: 6344-6355.

14 Chen H, Deng G, Li Z, Tian G, Li Y, Jiao P, Zhang L, Liu Z, Webster RG, Yu K: The evolution of H5N1 influenza viruses in ducks in southern China. Proceedings of the National Academy of Sciences of the United States of America 2004; 101: 10452-10457.

15 Sturm-Ramirez KM, Ellis T, Bousfield B, Bissett L, Dyrting K, Rehg JE, Poon L, Guan Y, Peiris M, Webster RG: Reemerging H5N1 influenza viruses in Hong Kong in 2002 are highly pathogenic to ducks. J Virol 2004; 78: 4892-4901.

16 Lee C, Suarez DL, Tumpey TM, Sung H, Kwon Y, Lee Y, Choi J, Joh S, Kim M, Lee E, Park J, Lu X, Katz JM, Spackman E, Swayne DE, Kim J: Characterization of Highly Pathogenic H5N1 Avian Influenza A Viruses Isolated from South Korea. J Virol 2005; 79: 3692-3702.

Dr. D.E. Swayne, Southeast Poultry Research Laboratory, Agricultural Research Service, U.S. Department of Agriculture, 934 College Station Rd, Athens, GA 30605, USA.
E-mail: dswayne@seprl.usda.gov

Schudel A, Lombard M (eds): OIE/FAO International Scientific Conference on Avian Influenza.
Dev Biol (Basel). Basel, Karger, 2006, vol 124, pp 69-72.

Library of Influenza Virus Strains for Vaccine and Diagnostic Use Against Highly Pathogenic Avian Influenza and Human Pandemics

H. Kida, Y. Sakoda

Department of Disease Control, Hokkaido University Graduate School of Veterinary Medicine, Sapporo, Japan

Abstract: To prepare for the emergence of pandemic influenza in birds and mammals including humans, we have carried out global surveillance of avian influenza. Influenza A viruses of 48 combinations of 15 HA and 9 NA subtypes out of 135 theoretical combinations have been isolated from faecal samples of ducks in Alaska, Siberia, Mongolia, Taiwan, China and Japan. So far, viruses of 73 other combinations have been generated by genetic reassortment in chicken embryos. Thus, avian influenza viruses of 121 combinations of HA and NA subtypes have been stocked for use in vaccine and diagnosis. Their pathogenicity, antigenicity, genetic information, and yield in chicken embryo have been analysed and registered in the database.

Background

Although many infectious diseases have been eradicated or controlled in the last century, influenza remains to be overcome, since influenza A viruses cause occasional catastrophic pandemics in humans, poultry and mammals. In addition, recent outbreaks of highly pathogenic avian influenza (HPAI) in the world have sent alarm signals as we realise that there is no border for infections. These outbreaks have given rise to concern for human health as well as the livestock industry. H5N1 avian influenza viruses have jumped the species barrier and caused severe disease with high mortality in humans in Hong Kong in 1997, and Vietnam, Thailand and Cambodia in 2004-2005; eight deaths of 18 cases, and 29 of 37, 11 of 16, and one of one, respectively. It is now obvious that live-bird markets play an important role in the generation of highly pathogenic strains.

To elucidate the origin and evolution of pandemic influenza viruses, we have conducted global surveillance of influenza in birds, animals and humans. On the basis of antigenic and genetic analyses of influenza virus isolates from migratory ducks, domestic ducks, pigs and humans, and experimental infection studies of birds and animals with those viruses, we proposed that the haemagglutinin (HA) gene of A/Hong Kong/68 (H3N2) strain was introduced into the precedent human H2N2 Asian influenza virus by genetic reassortment in pigs through domestic ducks from an H3 influenza virus circulating in migratory ducks in southern China [2-5].

Ecological studies have revealed that a vast influenza virus gene pool for avian and mammalian influenza exists in migratory ducks. Each of the known subtypes of influenza A virus perpetuates among migratory ducks and their nesting lake water in nature [6,9]. Experimental infection studies established that influenza viruses preferentially replicate in the columnar epithelial cells in the colon, causing no disease signs and are excreted in high concentration in ducks [1]. Influenza viruses have been isolated from freshly deposited faecal materials and from lake water, indicating that migratory ducks have an efficient way to transmit viruses, i.e. via faecal material in the water supply.

In comparison with influenza viruses of humans, those in ducks are in evolutionary stasis [2]. The remarkable lack of amino acid changes among influenza viruses isolated from migratory ducks suggests that the virus genes in this host are subject to stringent stabilising selection. The genetic and antigenic conservation of influenza viruses in ducks suggests that the virus and host have reached a long established adaptive optimum. Such a stasis in migratory ducks is further evidence that the duck population is the natural reservoir of influenza viruses.

In experimental infection of pigs, most tested strains of each of the known HA subtypes of avian influenza virus replicated in the upper respiratory tract of the animals. Co-infection of pigs with a swine virus and with an avian virus unable to replicate in this animal generated reassortants, whose polymerase and HA genes were entirely of avian origin; these could be passaged in pigs [5]. The results indicate that avian viruses of any subtype can contribute genes in the generation of reassortants, so that none of the 15 HA and nine neuraminidase (NA) subtypes can be ruled out as potential candidates for future pandemics in humans and poultry. The direct transmission of H5N1 influenza viruses from domestic poultry to humans in Asia and Europe in recent years further emphasised the need to have information on all influenza A subtypes circulating in avian species in the world.

To provide information on the ecology of influenza viruses in the natural host, virological surveillance of avian influenza was carried out in Alaska and Siberia during the breeding season in summer. Influenza viruses of different subtypes were isolated from faecal samples of ducks and water samples of the lakes where they nest. Even in autumn, when the ducks had left for migration to the south, viruses were still isolated from the lake water. This indicated that influenza viruses are maintained in the duck population by water-borne transmission in nature and revealed the mechanism of year-by-year perpetuation of the viruses in the frozen lake water while ducks are absent. Phylogenetic analysis of the isolates from Alaska indicates that ducks carrying these viruses migrate to the south through the continent of North America and not to Asia [6].

Influenza virus isolates from faecal samples of ducks in their nesting areas in Siberia phylogenetically belonged to Eurasian lineage and were closely related to those from birds, pigs and horses in Asia. It was noted that these isolates closely correlated to the H5N1 influenza virus isolates from chickens and humans [9]. Antigenic and phylogenetic analysis of the HA of H5 influenza virus isolates from ducks in Japan revealed a close relationship with those of H5N1 influenza viruses from Hong Kong, southern China, Thailand, Vietnam and Japan, indicating that the

H5HA of these viruses originates from influenza viruses maintained in migratory ducks nesting in Siberia. These results indicate that the precursor genes of pandemic influenza viruses are perpetuated in water in the lakes where ducks nest in their northern territory.

Vaccine strains should be antigenically closely related to the pandemic strain, avirulent for humans and chicken embryos, of high yield in chicken embryos, and immediately prepared when the causative virus is characterised. We tested immunogenicity in mice to inactivated avirulent H5N4 influenza viruses isolated from reservoir host ducks. The results showed that they were potent enough to protect animals from challenge with a lethal dose of the highly pathogenic H5N1 virus [8].

Results

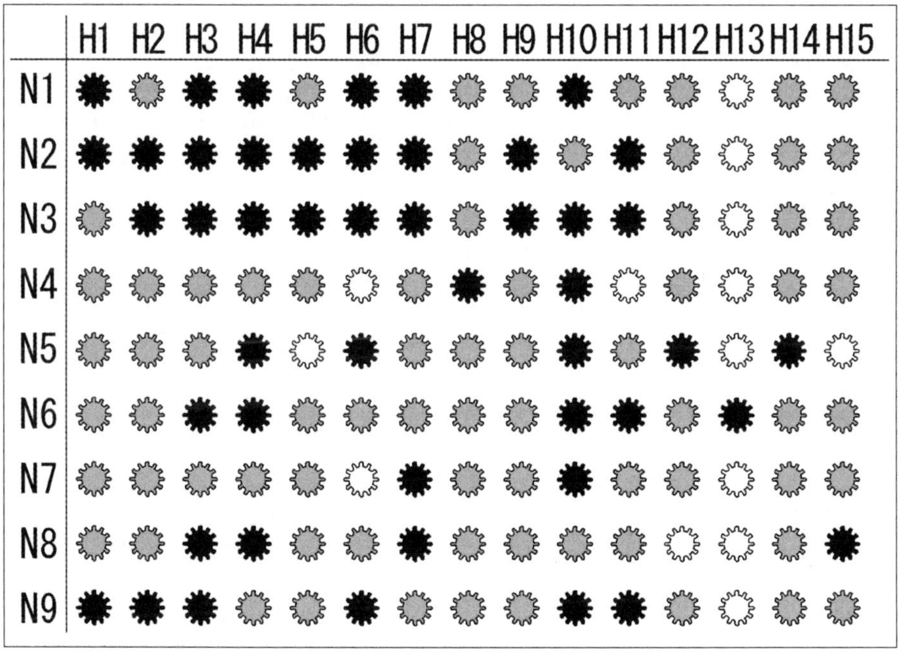

Fig. 1: Present status of the library of influenza virus strains for vaccine and diagnostic use. Influenza viruses of 48 combinations of HA and NA subtypes have been isolated from faecal samples of ducks in Alaska, Siberia, Mongolia, Taiwan, China and Japan (shown in black). So far, 73 other combinations have been generated by genetic reassortment procedure in the laboratory (shown in grey). Thus, avian influenza viruses of 121 combinations of HA and NA subtypes have been stocked as vaccine strain candidates. Their pathogenicity, antigenicity, genetic information and yield in chicken embryo have been analysed.

For the prediction of possible HA and NA subtypes of pandemic strains emerging in poultry and humans, the surveillance study of avian influenza has been carried out since 1976. Influenza virus isolates of 48 combinations of HA and NA subtypes have been isolated from faecal samples of ducks in Alaska, Siberia, Mongolia, Taiwan, China and Japan. So far, viruses of more than 73 other combinations have been generated by genetic reassortment in chicken embryos. Thus, avian influenza viruses of 121 combinations of HA and NA subtypes have been stocked as vaccine strain candidates and diagnostic use (Fig. 1). Their pathogenicity, antigenicity, genetic information and yield in chicken embryo have been analysed and registered in the database.

Discussion

Since influenza A viruses of all the known subtypes are perpetuated among migratory ducks and their nesting lakes, we must accept that influenza is not an eradicable disease. At present, prevention and control should be the only realistic goals. Since it is now clear that humans, pigs, poultry and migratory ducks are associated with the interspecies transmission of influenza virus and the emergence of pandemics in birds and mammals including humans, it is essential to expand global surveillance in these species. Live-poultry markets provide a critical environment for genetic mixing and spreading of influenza viruses. Continued surveillance and epidemiological monitoring and analysis should serve to reduce the possibility of the emergence of highly pathogenic avian influenza virus strains in these markets.

References

1 Kida H, Yanagawa R and Matsuoka Y: Duck influenza lacking evidence of disease signs and immune response. Infect Immun 1980; 30: 547-553.

2 Kida H, Kawaoka Y, Neave CW and Webster RG: Antigenic and genetic conservation of H3 influenza virus in wild ducks. Virology 1987; 159: 109-119.

3 Kida H, Shortridge KF and Webster RG: Origin of the hemagglutinin gene of H3N2 influenza viruses from pigs in China. Virology 1988; 162: 160-166.

4 Yasuda J, Shortridge KF, Shimizu Y and Kida H: Molecular evidence for a role of domestic ducks in the introduction of avian H3 influenza viruses to pigs in southern China, where the A/Hong Kong/68 (H3N2) strain emerged. J Gen Virol 1991; 72: 2007-2010.

5 Kida H, Ito T, Yasuda J, Shimizu Y, Itakura C et al: Potential for transmission of avian influenza viruses to pigs. J Gen Virol 1994; 75: 2183-2188.

6 Ito T, Okazaki K, Kawaoka Y, Takada A, Kida H et al: Perpetuation of influenza A viruses in Alaskan waterfowl reservoirs. Arch Virol 1995; 140: 1163-1172.

7 Ito T, Couceiro NJSS, Kelm S, Baum LG, Krauss S, Castrucci MR, Donatelli I, Kida H et al: Molecular basis for the generation in pigs of influenza A viruses with pandemic potential. J Virol 1998; 72: 7367-7373.

8 Takada A, Kuboki N, Okazaki K, Ninomiya A, Kida H et al: An avirulent avian influenza virus as a vaccine strain against a potential human pandemic. J Virol 1999; 73: 8303-8307.

9 Okazaki K, Takada A, Ito T, Imai M, Kida H et al: Precursor genes of future pandemic influenza viruses are perpetuated in ducks nesting in Siberia. Arch Virol 2000; 145: 885-893.

Dr. H. Kida, Research Center for Zoonosis Control, Department of Disease Control, Hokkaido University Graduate School of Veterinary Medicine, Kita 18, Nishi-9, Kita-ku, Sapporo, 060-0818 Japan.
E-mail: kida@vetmed.hokudai.ac.jp

Schudel A, Lombard M (eds): OIE/FAO International Scientific Conference on Avian Influenza.
Dev Biol (Basel). Basel, Karger, 2006, vol 124, p 73.

Swine Influenza in China

H. Chen, H. Li, H. Yang, C. Qiao, K. Yu

Harbin Veterinary Research Institute, Chinese Academy of Agriculture Sciences, Harbin, P. R. China

Abstract: Swine influenza is a common infectious respiratory disease of pigs that caused by influenza A viruses, and H1N1 and H3N2 are currently the most popular subtypes of influenza viruses circulated in pig population in China. H9N2 virus was detected from pigs that imported from Mainland China in Hong Kong in 1998, and extensive viral surveillance conduced since then indicated that H9N2 viruses are widely distributed in pig population in China. Phylogenetic analysis indicated that H9N2 viruses from pigs are highly related, implying they may establish a stable lineage in pigs in China. During the routine surveillance, we also isolated 2 H5N1 viruses from pigs in Fujian province in 2001 and 2003, respectively. Molecular analysis indicated that the two viruses are origin from duck H5N1 viruses. Their replication in chickens, mice and pigs has also been investigated.

Schudel A, Lombard M (eds): OIE/FAO International Scientific Conference on Avian Influenza.
Dev Biol (Basel). Basel, Karger, 2006, vol 124, p 75.

SESSION III

Human Health Implications of Avian Influenza

Chairperson: *F.-X. Meslin* (WHO)
Rapporteur: *G. Koch* (CIDC, The Netherlands)

Schudel A, Lombard M (eds): OIE/FAO International Scientific Conference on Avian Influenza. Dev Biol (Basel). Basel, Karger, 2006, vol 124, pp 77-84.

Avian Influenza Viruses and Human Health

D.J. Alexander

Virology Department, Veterinary Laboratories Agency Weybridge, Addlestone, Surrey, United Kingdom

Abstract: Influenza A viruses cause natural infections of humans, some other mammals and birds. Few of the 16 haemagglutinin and nine neuraminidase subtype combinations have been isolated from mammals, but all subtypes have been isolated from birds.

In the 20th century, there were four pandemics of influenza as a result of the emergence of antigenically different strains in humans: 1918 (H1N1), 1957 (H2N2), 1968 (H3N2) and 1977 (H1N1). Influenza A viruses contain eight distinct RNA genes and reassortment of these can occur in mixed infections with different viruses. The 1957 and 1968 pandemic viruses differed from the preceding viruses in humans by the substitution of genes that came from avian viruses, suggesting they arose by genetic reassortment of viruses of human and avian origin.

Up to 1995, there had been only three reports of avian influenza viruses infecting humans, in 1959, 1977 and 1981 (all H7N7), but, since 1996, there have been regular reports of natural infections of humans with avian influenza viruses: in England in 1996 (H7N7), Hong Kong 1997 (H5N1), 1999 (H9N2), and 2003 (H5N1), in The Netherlands 2003 (H7N7), Canada 2004 (H7N3), Vietnam 2004 (H5N1) and Thailand 2004 (H5N1). The H5N1 virus is alarming because 51 (64 %) of the 80 people confirmed as infected since 1997 have died.

INTRODUCTION

Influenza viruses have negative sense RNA genomes and are placed in the *Orthomyxoviridae* family in three genera or types, A, B and C, which were originally differentiated on the basis of the antigenic nature of the internal nucleocapsid or the matrix protein. Influenza C viruses are restricted mainly to humans and cause a fairly mild respiratory infection. Influenza B virus infections are also mainly restricted to humans and, while these viruses cause a serious illness in humans with occasional epidemics, they do not show sudden, marked changes in the antigenicity of their surface proteins. Natural infections with influenza A viruses have been reported in a large variety of animal species, including humans, pigs, horses, sea mammals and birds, occasionally producing devastating pandemics in humans.

The two surface glycoproteins of the virus, haemagglutinin (HA) and neuraminidase (NA), are the most important antigens for inducing protective immunity in the host and therefore show the greatest variation. For influenza A viruses,

16 antigenically distinct HA (H1-H16) and 9 NA (N1-N9) subtypes are recognised at present; a virus possesses one HA and one NA subtype, apparently in any combination. All subtypes, in most combinations, have been isolated from birds, but, in contrast, viruses of relatively few subtypes have been isolated from mammals; those viruses that have become **established** in mammalian species have been restricted to H1N1, H2N2 and H3N2 in humans, H1N1, H3N2 and H1N2 in pigs and H7N7 and H3N8 in horses.

Influenza A infection in humans is a serious, highly contagious disease resulting in a debilitating illness that often causes high mortality among the elderly and those suffering other predisposing illnesses. Influenza A infections in humans have been marked throughout history by serious pandemics every 10-50 years. In the 20th century, the sudden emergence of antigenically different strains in humans, termed **antigenic shift**, which resulted in pandemics occurred on four occasions, 1918 (H1N1), 1957 (H2N2), 1968 (H3N2) and 1977 (H1N1) [1]. In 1957 and 1968, the new viruses completely replaced the previous virus in the human population but, in 1977, this did not occur and currently H3N2 and H1N1 viruses both circulate.

Epidemics have occurred between the pandemics as a result of accumulated point mutations in the prevalent virus leading to gradual antigenic change, termed **antigenic drift,** which in turn results in infections in a proportion of the population that has become immunologically susceptible. The inter-pandemic influenza epidemics may have a considerable impact as a result of significant mortality, especially among the elderly and other vulnerable groups, and the severe economic cost associated with debilitating illness in a large portion of the population. Occasionally the degree of antigenic drift is sufficient for a very large proportion of the population to be susceptible and for severe epidemics to occur with worldwide spread.

By far the worst influenza pandemic for which there are accurate records was the one beginning in 1918. It has been estimated that, during the pandemic, more than 40 million people died [1]. In well developed countries such as the USA, about 0.5 % of the population died, but this figure was much higher in some communities such as Alaska and the Pacific islands.

Human/Avian Influenza Link

The RNA of influenza viruses is segmented into eight distinct genes, which code for ten proteins. Because the viral RNA is segmented, genetic reassortment can occur in mixed infections with different strains of influenza A viruses. This means that, when two viruses infect the same cell, progeny viruses may inherit sets of RNA segments made up of combinations of segments identical to those of either of the parent viruses. This gives a theoretical possible number of 2^8 (=256) different combinations that can form a complete set of RNA segments from a dual infection, although in practice only a few progeny virions possess the correct gene constellation required for viability and transmissibility.

Demonstration that the H3N2 1968 pandemic virus differed from the 1957-1968 H2N2 virus in the substitution of two genes, PB1 and the important surface glycoprotein HA gene, with genes almost certainly from an influenza virus of avian origin, led to the suggestion that antigenic shift occurred as a result of reassortment of genes in dual infections with viruses of human and avian origin [2-5]. As a result, systematic surveillance studies in the presence of influenza viruses in avian species were undertaken. These revealed enormous pools of influenza A viruses in wild birds, especially migratory waterfowl. In a series of surveillance studies involving over 20,000 birds between 1973 and 1986, virus was isolated from about 10 %, with an isolation rate of approximately 15 % from ducks and geese and 2 % from other birds [6]. More recent surveys in Europe have produced similar isolation rates. In addition, unlike mammals, where the number of subtypes that have been established appears to be limited, all 16 H and 9 N subtypes recognised currently have been recorded in birds in most possible combinations.

The isolation of so many influenza viruses of different subtypes from the bird population raised the question of why subtype changes in the human population have not occurred more frequently. However, volunteer experiments had shown that only transitory infections resulted when humans were infected with viruses of avian origin [7], and it was clear that there was some barrier to the establishment of avian influenza viruses in the human population that was related to one or more of the gene segments. Both human and avian viruses are known to infect pigs readily and it was suggested that pigs acted as "mixing vessels", in which reassortment between human and avian influenza viruses could take place with the emergence of viruses with the necessary gene(s) from the virus of human origin to allow replication and spread in the human population, but with a different haemagglutinin surface glycoprotein, so that the human population could be regarded as immunologically naive. In addition, it was shown that, while most avian influenza viruses require binding to α2-3 sialic acid receptors, compared to α2-6 for human viruses, avian viruses that had been adapted to pigs required α2-6 sialic acid receptors. The pig mixing vessel theory was also thought to explain the apparent emergence of the 1957 and 1968 pandemics in the Far East, where agricultural practices mean that high concentrations of people, pigs and waterfowl live closely together [8].

Two hypotheses have been proposed for the rhythm of occurrence of human influenza A viruses; these were termed by Shortridge [9] as an influenza circle (or cycle) and an influenza spiral. The **circulation theory** suggests there is simply a recycling of H1, H2 and H3 subtypes. If this is so, the HA subtype of the next pandemic virus would be H2. The **spiral theory** assumes that humans are capable of being infected with all HA subtypes of influenza A viruses providing the receptor demands are met and a specific constellation of the other genes is present; thus it may not be possible to predict which of the 16 H subtypes will emerge next by reassortment unless there is careful monitoring and surveillance. The theories are not mutually exclusive and, since the circulation theory does not state how the next pandemic virus will arise, it could be by reassortment.

Avian Influenza Pathogenicity

Another property of avian influenza viruses that needs considering in the context of human infections is that influenza A viruses infecting poultry can be divided into two distinct groups on the basis of their ability to cause disease. The very virulent viruses cause a disease formerly known as fowl plague and now termed highly pathogenic avian influenza (HPAI) in which mortality may be as high as 100 %. These viruses have been restricted to subtypes H5 and H7, although not all viruses of these subtypes cause HPAI. All other viruses cause a much milder disease consisting primarily of mild respiratory disease, depression and egg production problems in laying birds. Sometimes other infections or environmental conditions may cause exacerbation of influenza infections leading to much more serious disease.

The main functional glycoprotein, the haemagglutinin, for influenza viruses is produced in a precursor form, HA0, which requires post-translational cleavage by host proteases before the protein is functional and the virus particles are infectious. It has been demonstrated that the HA0 precursor proteins of avian influenza viruses of low virulence for poultry are limited to cleavage by host proteases such as trypsin and trypsin-like enzymes. They are thus restricted to replication at sites in the host where such enzymes are found, i.e. the respiratory and intestinal tracts. In contrast, virulent viruses appear to be cleavable by (a) ubiquitous protease(s), which remains to be fully identified but appears to be one or more proprotein-processing subtilisin-related endoproteases of which furin is the leading candidate [10], and this enables these viruses to replicate throughout the animal, damaging vital organs and tissues, which brings about disease and death in the infected bird.

Comparisons of the amino acid sequences at the HA0 cleavage site of avian influenza viruses of high and low pathogenicity revealed that, while viruses of low virulence have a single basic amino acid (arginine) at the site, all HPAI viruses possessed multiple basic amino acids (arginine and lysine) adjacent to the cleavage site, either as a result of apparent insertion or apparent substitution [11]. The additional basic amino acids resulted in a motif recognised and cleavable by the putative ubiquitous protease(s). Mammals, including humans, also have furin-like proteases capable of cleaving at multiple basic amino acid motifs. However, the significance of this for mammals infected with viruses with multiple basic amino acids at the HA0 cleavage site is unclear.

Human Infections with Avian Influenza Viruses (Table 1)

There were three reports of human infections with avian influenza virus in the literature before 1996. In 1959, a HPAI virus was obtained from a patient with hepatitis [12]. The second related to a laboratory worker in Australia who developed conjunctivitis after accidental exposure directly in the eye with an HPAI virus [13]. The third also related to conjunctivitis as the result of infection with an avian LPAI virus, which spread to an animal handler from an infected seal [14]. All three of these viruses were of H7N7 subtype.

In 1996, an H7N7 virus was isolated in England from the eye of a woman with conjunctivitis who kept ducks. This virus was shown to be genetically closest in all eight genes to viruses of avian origin and to have > 98 % nucleotide homology in the HA gene with a virus of H7N7 subtype isolated from turkeys in Ireland in 1995 [15].

In May 1997, a virus of H5N1 subtype was isolated from a young child who died in Hong Kong and, by December 1997, the same virus was confirmed by isolation to have infected 18 people, six of whom died [16]. There was evidence of very limited human-to-human spread of this virus [17], but clearly the efficiency of transmission must have been extremely low. The viruses isolated from the human cases appeared to be identical to those first isolated from chickens in Hong Kong in March 1997 following an outbreak of HPAI. Both human and avian isolates possess multiple basic amino acids at the HA0 cleavage site. A subsequent serological survey of poultry workers in Hong Kong after the 1997 outbreak identified 10 % seroprevalence of H5 antibodies, but without any known occurrence of clinical disease [18].

Table 1 : Human infections with avian influenza viruses.

Year	Subtype	HPAI/LPAI[1]	Country	Number infected	Symptoms	Reference
1959	H7N7	HPAI	U.S.A.	1	Hepatitis ?	[12]
1977	H7N7	HPAI	Australia	1[a]	Conjunctivitis	[13]
1981	H7N7	LPAI	U.S.A.	1[a]	Conjunctivitis	[14]
1996	H7N7	LPAI	England	1	Conjunctivitis	[15]
1997	H5N1	HPAI	Hong Kong	18	Influenza-like illness **6 deaths**	[16]
1998/9	H9N2	LPAI	Hong Kong/China	2 (+5 ?)	Influenza-like illness	[20]
2002	H7N2	LPAI	U.S.A. [Va.]	1	None	CDC website[2]
2003	H7N2	LPAI	U.S.A. [NYC]	1	Influenza-like illness	CDC website[2]
2003	H5N1	?	Hong Kong	2 (+1 ?)	Influenza-like illness **1 (+1?) death**	WHO website[3]
2003	H7N7	HPAI	The Netherlands	83 (>1000 ?)	Conjunctivitis, influenza-like illness **1 death**	[21]
2004/5	H5N1	HPAI	Thailand	17	Influenza-like illness **12 deaths**	WHO website[3]
2004/5	H5N1	HPAI	Vietnam	43[b]	Influenza-like illness **32[a] deaths**	WHO website[3]
2004	H7N3	HPAI	Canada (BC)	2	Conjunctivitis	Health Canada website[4]

1 HPAI or LPAI in chickens.
2 http ://www.cdc.gov/flu/avian/gen-info/avian-flu-humans.htm
3 http ://www.who.int/csr/disease/avian_influenza/en/
4 http ://www.hc-sc.gc.ca/english/media/releases/2004/latest_avian. htm
a As a result of laboratory accidents.
b Includes one patient infected in Cambodia.

In recent years, outbreaks in poultry as a result of viruses of H9 subtype, usually H9N2, have been widespread. During the last ten years or so, outbreaks, resulting from H9N2 subtype had been reported in Germany, Italy, Ireland, South Africa, USA, Korea, China, throughout the Middle East, Iran and Pakistan [19]; this virus continues to spread. In March 1999, two independent isolations of influenza virus subtype H9N2 were made from girls aged one and four, who recovered from flu-like illnesses in Hong Kong [20]. Subsequently, five isolations of H9N2 virus from humans on mainland China in August 1998 were reported.

In 2003, an H5N1 virus was isolated from a father and son in Hong Kong who presented with respiratory illness after returning from the Chinese mainland; the father died. A daughter had become ill and died while visiting the Chinese mainland; it is not known whether she was infected with H5N1virus.

Some genetic differences were reported between the 1997 and the 2003 H5N1 viruses (WHO website: http://www.who.int/mediacentre/releases/2003/pr17/en/).

During the 2003 HPAI H7N7 outbreaks, in The Netherlands, of 260 people involved in some aspect of the outbreak and presenting with conjunctivitis and/or influenza-like illness, 82 were confirmed as infected with H7 virus [21]. There was also evidence of three cases of human-to-human transmission within families. During this outbreak, a human fatality also occurred. The victim was a 57-year-old veterinarian who had not received prophylactic antiviral drugs and had contact with infected birds during outbreak management. He was admitted to hospital with severe headache and fever; subsequently he developed a severe respiratory condition, kidney failure and died. H7 virus was recovered from a broncho-alveolar lavage collected nine days after the onset of illness [21]. Serological surveyors of poultry farmers and others in contact with infected birds were carried out retrospectively and indicated that the true number of people infected during the outbreak in The Netherlands was in excess of 1000 [22].

Four people have been infected with avian influenza viruses in North America in recent years. Two were in the USA, both with LPAI virus of H7N2 subtype. One was involved in depopulation of a flock of poultry in Virginia USA in 2002 and showed serological evidence of infection. The other, in 2003, was in New York City and had no apparent links with poultry. The other two were associated with the HPAI H7N3 outbreaks in Canada in 2004.

From December 2003 to the present time, a series of countries in SE and E Asia (Cambodia, China, Indonesia, Japan, Lao PDR, Malaysia, Republic of Korea, Thailand, and Vietnam) reported outbreaks of HPAI as a result of H5N1 subtype and hundreds of millions of birds have been affected. In some countries, control has proved difficult and outbreaks continue to occur, possibly as a result of perpetuation of the virus in free-range commercial ducks. As indicated in Table 1, human infections with H5N1 virus have been reported in Thailand and Vietnam, but not in other affected countries, with the exception of one fatal case from Cambodia and the reports of H5 antibodies, but not clinical disease, in five people involved in the outbreaks in Japan. The reasons for infections of humans in these two countries, but not others, is not clear. Phylogenetic analysis of the viruses demonstrates that the H5N1 viruses in Vietnam and Cambodia form the same clade, which is distinguishable from viruses in other countries, but it is not clear whether the differences would be associated with the ability of the virus to infect humans. The viruses from humans in Hong Kong in 1997 do not form the same clade.

Discussion

Since 1997, 80 people have been confirmed as infected with the HPAI H5N1 virus in SE Asia and 51 (64 %) have died. Despite this high mortality, it appears that the virus has not spread systemically in the infected casualties, which was the fear because of the presence of multiple basic amino acids at the HA0 cleavage site allowing cleavage to be mediated by a furin-like protease(s) and death was primarily a result of viral pneumonia. There have, however, been two exceptions where virus was detected in organs outside the respiratory tract.

All the avian influenza viruses isolated from humans to date have shown a full set of avian genes, indicating that no reassortment had taken place. This is consistent with the very low incidence of human-to-human spread. However, the continuing worry is that, if people infected with the avian influenza viruses are infected simultaneously with a "human" influenza virus, reassortment could occur, with the emergence, as in 1957 and 1968, of a virus with internal genes from the human virus that is fully capable of spread in the human population, but with an H5, H7 or H9 HA gene, resulting in a true influenza pandemic.

In view of the consistent infections of humans with this virus in some countries, there are very real fears that, if the outbreaks of HPAI H5N1 continue in SE Asia, this will eventually occur. To date there have been no reports of surveys to determine the full extent of infections among people in contact with infected poultry, i.e. those with very mild or sub-clinical infections. The data from the surveys in The Netherlands and Hong Kong (see above) suggest that the true number of people infected in E Asia may be very large. If that is the case, it appears surprising that such reassortment has not already taken place.

It is 28 years (some would argue 37 years) since the last pandemic. The expected occurrence is approximately every 22 years with a range of 9-49 years. A new influenza pandemic in the near future seems inevitable, but will the subtype be H5, H9 or perhaps H2?

References

1 Nguyen-Van-Tam JS, Hampson AW: The epidemiology and clinical impact of pandemic influenza. Vaccine 2003; 21: 1762-1768.

2 Fang R, Min Jou W, Huylebroeck D, Devos R, Fiers W: Complete structure of A/duck/Ukraine/63 influenza haemagglutinin gene: animal virus as progenitor of human H3 Hong Kong 1968 influenza haemagglutinin. Cell 1981; 25: 315-323.

3 Gething MJ, Bye J, Skehel J, Wakefield M: Cloning and DNA sequence of double-stranded copies of haemagglutinin genes from H2 and H3 strains elucidates antigenic shift and drift in human influenza virus. Nature 1980; 287: 301-306.

4 Kawaoka Y, Krauss S, Webster RG: Avian to human transmission of the PB1 gene of influenza A virus in the 1957 and 1968 pandemics. Journal of Virology 1989; 63: 4603-4608.

5 Scholtissek C, Rohde W, von Hoyningen V, Rott R: On the origin of the human influenza virus subtypes H2N2 and H3N2. Virology 1978; 87: 13-20.

6 Alexander DJ: A review of avian influenza in different bird species. Proceedings of the ESVV Symposium on Animal Influenza Viruses, Gent 1999. Veterinary Microbiology 2000; 74: 3-13.

7 Beare AS, Webster, R.G. Replication of avian influenza viruses in humans. Archives of Virology 1991; 119: 37-42.

8 Shortridge KF, Stuart-Harris CH: An influenza epicentre? Lancet 1982; 2: 812-813.

9 Shortridge KF: Pandemic influenza: a zoonosis? Seminars in Respiratory Infections 1992; 7:11-25.

10 Stieneke-Grober A, Vey M, Angliker H, Shaw E, Thomas G, Roberts C, Klenk H-D, Garten W: Influenza virus hemagglutinin with multibasic cleavage site is activated by furin, a subtilisin endoprotease. EMBO Journal 1992; 11: 2407-2414.

11 Senne DA, Panigrahy B, Kawaoka Y, Pearson JE, Suss J, Lipkind M, Kida H, Webster RG: Survey of the hemagglutinin (HA) cleavage site sequence of H5 and H7 avian influenza viruses: Amino acid sequence at the HA cleavage site as a marker of pathogenicity potential. Avian Diseases 1996; 40: 425-437.

12 Campbell CH, Webster RG, Breese SS: Fowl plague virus from man. Journal of Infectious Diseases 1970; 122: 513-516.

13 Taylor HR, Turner AJ: A case report of fowl plague keraconjunctivitis. British Journal of Ophthalmology 1977; 61: 86-88.

14 Webster RG, Geraci JR, Petursson G, Skirnisson K: Conjunctivitis in human beings caused by influenza A virus of seals. New England Journal of Medicine 1981; 304: 911.

15 Banks J, Speidel E, Alexander DJ: Characterisation of an avian influenza A virus isolated from a human – is an intermediate host necessary for the emergence of pandemic influenza viruses? Archives of Virology 1998; 143: 781-787.

16 Shortridge KF, Gao P, Guan Y, Ito T, Kawaoka Y, Markwell D, Takada A, Webster RG: A review of interspecies transmission of influenza viruses: the Hong Kong perspective. In Proceedings of the European Society for Veterinary Virology Symposium on influenza viruses of wild and domestic animals, 16-18 May 1999, Ghent. Veterinary Microbiology 2000; 74: 141-147.

17 Buxton Bridges C, Katz JM, Seto WH, Chan PKS, Tsang D, Ho W, Mak KH, Lim W, Tam JS, Mounts AW, Bresee JS, Conn LA, Rowe T, Hu-Primmer J, Abernathy RA, Lu, X, Cox NJ, Fukuda K: Risk of influenza A (H5N1) infection among health care workers exposed to patients with influenza A (H5N1), Hong Kong. Journal of Infectious Diseases 2000; 181: 344-348.

18 Buxton Bridges C, Lim W, Hu-Primmer J, Sims L, Fukuda K, Mak KH, Rowe T, Thompson WW, Conn L, Lu XH, Cox NJ, Katz JM: Risk of influenza A (H5N1) infection among poultry workers, Hong Kong, 1997-1998. Journal of Infectious Diseases 2002; 185 (8): 1005-1010.

19 Banks J, Speidel EC, Harris PA, Alexander DJ: Phylogenetic analysis of influenza A viruses of H9 haemagglutinin subtype. Avian Pathology 2000; 29: 353-360.

20 Peiris M, Yuen KY, Leung CW, Chan KH, Ip PLS, Lai RWM, Orr WK, Shortridge KF: Human infection with influenza H9N2. The Lancet 1999; 354: 916-917.

21 Koopmans M, Fouchier R, Wilbrink B, Meijer A, Natrop G, Osterhaus ADME, van Steenbergen JE, du Ry van Beest Holle M, Conyn van Spaendonck MAE, Bosman A: Update on human infections with highly pathogenic avian influenza virus A/H7N7 during an outbreak in poultry in The Netherlands. Eurosurveillance Weekly 2003; 7:18.

22 Bosman A: Transmission of H7N7 avian influenza A virus to humans beings during the large outbreak in commercial poultry farms in The Netherlands. Lancet 2004; 363: 587-593.

Dr. D.J. Alexander, Virology Department, Veterinary Laboratories Agency Weybridge, Addlestone, Surrey KT15 3NB, United Kingdom.
E-mail: d.j.alexander@vla.defra.gsi.gov.uk

Schudel A, Lombard M (eds): OIE/FAO International Scientific Conference on Avian Influenza.
Dev Biol (Basel). Basel, Karger, 2006, vol 124, pp 85-90.

Occupational and Consumer Risks from Avian Influenza Viruses

D.E. Swayne

Southeast Poultry Research Laboratory, Agricultural Research Service, U.S. Department of Agriculture, Athens, GA, USA

Abstract: Sporadic human infections have been reported with a few select avian influenza (AI) viruses over the past 50 years. Most of the infections resulted from the H7N7 high pathogenicity AI (HPAI) virus from The Netherlands (2003) and H5N1 HPAI viruses from several Asian countries (1997-2005). Epidemiological studies have identified direct exposure to infected poultry as the primary risk factor for human infection. In The Netherlands, veterinarians, cullers and poultry farmers had an occupational risk of infection through exposure to infected commercial poultry, and presented with conjunctivitis and/or influenza-like illnesses. In Asia, most of the clinical infections involved direct exposure to poultry in the smallholder sector or live poultry markets, and not commercial poultry. However, serological data from Hong Kong during 1997 indicated H5N1 infections without clinical disease were associated with occupational exposure. No cases of human AI infection have been linked to consumption of infected or contaminated poultry products. However, HPAI virus can be present in blood, bone and meat of infected poultry, which, if consumed raw, are a potential source of virus for human infections. Cooking and pasteurisation are effective methods of killing AI viruses. Proper vaccination of poultry has been shown to prevent HPAI virus from localising in the meat.

Introduction

Over the past 50 years, avian influenza (AI) viruses have caused sporadic infections in humans as compared to the common endemic infections caused by human influenza viruses [1,2]. As of 15 April 2005, there have been 205 documented AI clinical cases in humans, of which the majority have involved two virus lineages: i.e. 89 cases with the H7N7 high pathogenicity AI (HPAI) viruses in The Netherlands (2003), and 103 cases with the H5N1 HPAI viruses in Asia (1997, 2003-2005) [3]. The other 13 cases were more sporadic and included seven cases with H9N2 low pathogenicity AI (LPAI) viruses (Hong Kong and China), two cases with H7N2 LPAI viruses (USA), two cases with H7N3 HPAI viruses (Canada), one case with H7N7 HPAI virus (USA) and one case with H7N7 LPAI virus (United Kingdom). Most concerning is the 60 fatalities, of which 59 resulted from the Asian H5N1 HPAI viruses and one from the Dutch H7N7 HPAI virus. This suggests some AI virus strains have had a greater potential to infect and cause disease in humans, and the frequency for infecting humans has been greater for HPAI than for LPAI viruses.

RISK FACTORS FOR HUMAN INFECTIONS

In general, human infections resulted from close direct contact with live or dead infected birds. Sufficient epidemiological data is available from the two larger epizootics with human infections to draw some important conclusions. First, the Dutch H7N7 HPAI epizootic resulted in clinical cases exhibiting symptoms of conjunctivitis (78 cases), flu-like illness (two cases), conjunctivitis plus flu-like illness (4 cases) and other symptoms (4 cases) [4]. There was one fatality in a poultry veterinarian, who inspected an infected chicken flock, and three cases of human-to-human contact spread were documented. Of the clinical cases, cullers and poultry veterinarians had greater infection rates (41.2 % and 26.3 %, respectively) than poultry farmers and family (14.7 %) and other persons (7.7 %). However, a seroprevalence study identified a 50 % infection rate in the at-risk population, but most lacked clinical signs [5].

During 1997, with the Asia H5N1 HPAI clinical cases in Hong Kong, the primary risk factor was exposure to live poultry in the wet market system one week before the human illness [6]. Travelling, preparing and eating poultry meat and exposure to human AI cases were not risk factors. However, in a seroprevalence survey, 10 % of poultry workers and 3 % of depopulation workers had anti – H5 antibodies, but lacked clinical disease [7]. In the early 2004 human H5N1 AI cases from Thailand and Vietnam, contact with smallholder (village) poultry was the primary exposure source, and people involved with the culling operations or workers on commercial poultry farms were not among the cases [8,9]. Specifically, of the 12 confirmed human cases in Thailand, 12 had chicken deaths within the village, nine had backyard chickens that died and eight had direct contact with dead chickens [8]. A study of early cases in Hanoi did not identify any human-to-human transmission in 87 health-care workers who had contact with five H5N1 infected patients [10], but since that time there has been some limited human-to-human transmission reported in later cases.

VARIABLES IN HUMAN AVIAN INFLUENZA INFECTIONS

Exposure to live or dead infected poultry has been the primary risk factor for development of human AI infections. However, several variables are important in determining the outcome following exposure. When exposed to the AI viruses, people can have four different results: (i) no infection; (ii) infections evident by AI-specific antibodies, but no clinical disease; (iii) mild clinical disease usually with conjunctivitis or respiratory symptoms; or (iv) severe clinical disease with death. First, the production of infection, illness and death in humans varies with the individual AI virus strain. For example, virological and serological studies of depopulation crews during the 1983-84 H5N2 HPAI outbreak in the USA, and the 1997 H5N2 and 2000 H7N1 HPAI outbreaks in Italy failed to identify human infections [11-13], while one H7N2 antibody-positive person was identified during the USA H7N2 LPAI outbreak in 2002 [14]. By comparison, depopulation crews and poultry workers in the 1997 H5N1 outbreak in Hong Kong had 3 % and 10 % seroprevalence, while the crews associated with the Dutch H7N7 HPAI outbreak had close to 50 % seroprevalence [5,7]. Second, the requirement of direct exposure to live or dead infected poultry suggests the need for a high dose of virus to achieve infection. Finally, various undefined host factors, such as young age and the presence of secondary disease conditions, may render some people more susceptible to AI virus infections [8,9,14].

Potential Mechanisms of Transmission to Humans

The potential mechanisms for exposure to AI virus that has resulted in human infections are unknown, but, based on poultry pathogenesis studies, production and marketing systems, and concepts of disease transmission, several mechanisms can be identified as those most likely involved in exposure and AI virus transmission. The respiratory secretions and faeces from infected poultry contain the HPAI H5N1 virus in high concentrations and could be the primary transmission material. The AI virus could be inhaled as dust generated from, or containing, infected particles of faeces or respiratory secretions produced in the village or small farming setting, or alternatively, through fine water droplets generated during slaughter, de-feathering, and eviscerating processes of the wet markets. Alternatively, the HPAI virus could be hand-transplanted from a surface contaminated with infected poultry faeces or respiratory secretions and transferred to oral or nasal mucus membranes or the conjunctiva. In a few cases, the exposure may have been use of oral suction to clean the clogged nasal passages of fighting cocks; this could either be inhaled or mucus membrane exposure and transmission. Finally, because HPAI viruses cause systemic infection, the consumption of raw or undercooked blood, organs or meat could be a potential mechanism, but no epidemiological evidence has been reported to support such a transmission method.

Food Safety Risks?

The question of whether AI virus can be present in poultry meat is a realistic food safety issue. In an experiment study using intranasal inoculation of specific pathogen free (SPF) broiler chickens with two different H7N2 LPAI viruses (A/chicken/Pennsylvania/21588-8/1999 and A/turkey/Virginia/158152/2002), challenge virus was isolated for the first five to seven days after inoculation from swabs or tissues of the respiratory and occasionally intestinal tracts, but not from blood, breast or thigh meat, bone marrow or bone [15]. Although surface contamination from respiratory and intestinal tissues is possible during slaughter and processing, the virus was not present within the meat. By contrast, in an experimental study using intranasal inoculation of SPF broiler chickens with H5N2 HPAI virus (A/chicken/Pennsylvania/1370/1983), challenge virus was isolated from one day post-inoculation until death of the chickens from upper and deep respiratory tracts in high titres (10^6 mean chicken embryo infectious doses [EID_{50}]/ml of media), intestinal tract in medium titres (10^4 EID_{50}/ml media), red and white blood cell fractions, breast and thigh meat, bone marrow and bone. Breast and thigh meat from these three experiments were fed to SPF broilers.

Over the 14-day observation period, the chickens fed meat from infected chickens did not become infected with the LPAI or HPAI viruses. The latter was surprising because HPAI virus was isolated from the meat fed to the chickens, but the infectious titres were low (10^3 EID_{50}/g). This suggests the quantity of virus in the meat was below the minimal infectious dose for chickens with this HPAI virus through oral exposure. In other studies, this HPAI virus was isolated from the internal contents of eggs laid by infected hens, but LPAI viruses have not been demonstrated in these eggs [16].

An additional experiment was conducted in sham (negative control) and vaccinated (inactivated H5N9 AI virus oil emulsified or live recombinant fowlpox containing an AI virus H5 gene vaccine) SPF chickens intranasally inoculated with the H5N1 HPAI virus A/chicken/S. Korea/ES/2003 (Table 1) [15]. Both vaccines prevented illness and death, and no virus was isolated from meat (Table 1). From the sham chickens, high titres ($10^{7.3}$ EID_{50}/g) of virus were recovered from the meat and feeding the meat to naïve SPF chickens transmitted the virus, resulting in a 90 % mortality rate.

Table 1: Data from SPF chickens vaccinated subcutaneously at one day of age with either a recombinant fowl poxvirus containing an H5 AI gene insert or inactivated H5N9 AI oil emulsified vaccine (A/turkey/Wisconsin/68) and challenged intranasally three weeks later with H5N1 HPAI virus (A/chicken/South Korea/ES/03).

Group	Virus isolation from meat (Log_{10} EID_{50}/gm)		Virus dose/Bird (Log_{10} EID_{50}
	Breast	**Thigh**	
Fowlpox-AIV-H5 vaccine	–	–	ND
Inactived vaccine	–	–	ND
Sham	7.3	ND	7.8

Notes: Meat samples were on day two after inoculation from euthanatised (vaccine) or dead (sham) chickens. - = no virus isolated, ND = not done [15].

Furthermore, the 2003-2004 bird and human H5N1 HPAI viruses have been demonstrated in meat obtained from both naturally and experimentally infected chickens, Japanese quail, ducks and geese [17,18] (unpublished data). This indicates HPAI viruses can be in the meat of infected poultry, and feeding meat can transmit the virus to other poultry if sufficient titres are present. However, it is unknown whether the virus titres in raw meat or other tissues/blood are sufficient to result in human infection when consumed.

A further question – would pasteurisation or cooking kill the AI viruses thus making the risk of human infection very low? In a series of experimental studies, pasteurisation of liquid egg products using standard industry combinations of temperatures and time (55.6 – 63.3C, 210 – 372 seconds) were effective at inactivating HPAI virus [16]. Furthermore, when using meat from chickens experimentally infected with the South Korean H5N1 HPAI virus, virus was recovered from samples after cooking at 70°C for one second, but no virus was recovered at five, 10, 30 and 60 seconds [19].

Conclusions

- Avian influenza is a public health threat, but the risk of human infection varies with individual virus strains. Generally, such human infections have been rare.

- The majority of clinical human cases have resulted from infections by the Dutch H7N7 (2003) and Asian H5N1 HPAI virus (1997, 2003-2005) strains, but other LP and HPAI viruses have caused sporadic human infections.
- All the fatal human cases have been associated with the Dutch H7N7 (2003) and Asian H5N1 (1997, 2003-2005) HPAI viruses.
- Direct exposure to live or dead infected poultry is the primary risk factor leading to human infections.
- Cullers, poultry workers and veterinarians have an occupational risk from the AI infections, but many of the severe human cases have not resulted from a high risk occupation – e.g. children and women.
- Asian H5N1 human AI cases from 1997-2005 have had primary exposure to infected poultry in smallholder or wet (live) poultry market sectors.
- Experimental studies have not demonstrated LPAI virus to be present in the meat, but HPAI virus has been identified in both breast and thigh meat, and the virus has been transmitted to other chickens by feeding meat from infected chickens.
- Vaccination can prevent HPAI virus from being in chicken meat.
- Cooking or pasteurisation can kill both LPAI and HPAI viruses.

Acknowledgements

The author thanks J. Beck, J. Doster and K Moresco for technical assistance.

References

1 Swayne DE, King DJ: Avian influenza and Newcastle disease. J Am Vet Med Assoc 2003; 222: 1534-1540.

2 Teates K, Brammer L, Balish A, Wallis T, Hall H, Klimov A, Fukuda K, Cox N, Katz M: Update: Influenza activity – United States and worldwide, May-October 2004. Morbidity and Mortality Weekly Report 2004; 53: 993-995.

3 Perdue ML, Swayne DE: Avian influenza virus infections in humans. Avian Dis 2005; 49: 317-327.

4 Koopmans M, Wilbrink B, Conyn M, Natrop G, van der Nat H, Vennema H, Meijer A, van Steenbergen J, Fouchier R, Osterhaus A, Bosman A: Transmission of H7N7 avian influenza A virus to human beings during a large outbreak in commercial poultry farms in the Netherlands. Lancet 2004; 363: 587-593.

5 Braakman J: Human seroprevalence in Dutch H7N7 AI outbreak. PROMED [On-line] 2004; 1015: 2808.

6 Mounts AW, Kwong H, Izurieta HS, Ho Y, Au T, Lee M, Buxton BC, Williams SW, Mak KH, Katz JM, Thompson WW, Cox NJ, Fukuda K: Case-control study of risk factors for avian influenza A (H5N1) disease, Hong Kong, 1997. J Infect Dis 1999; 180: 505-508.

7 Bridges CB, Lim W, Hu-Primmer J, Sims L, Fukuda K, Mak KH, Rowe T, Thompson WW, Conn L, Lu X, Cox NJ, Katz JM: Risk of influenza A (H5N1) infection among poultry workers, Hong Kong, 1997-1998. J Infect Dis 2002; 185: 1005-1010.

8 Chotpitayasunondh T, Lochindarat S, Srisan P, Chokepaibulkit K, Weerakul J, Maneerattanaporn M, Sawanpanyalert P: Cases of influenza A (H5N1) - Thailand, 2004 (Reprinted from MMWR, vol 53, pg 100-103, 2004). JAMA-Journal of the American Medical Association 2004; 291: 1059-1060.

9 Tran TH, Nguyen TL, Nguyen TD, Luong TS, Pham PM, Nguyen v, V, Pham TS, Vo CD, Le Thi QM, Ngo TT, Dao BK, Le Phuc P, Nguyen TT, Hoang TL, Cao VT, Le Truong G, Nguyen DT, Le Hong N, Nguyen Thi KT, Le Hoang S, Le Van T, Dolecek C, Tran TT, Jong Md, Schultsz C, Cheng P: Avian influenza A (H5N1) in 10 patients in Vietnam. New England Journal of Medicine 2004; 350: 1179-1188.

10 Liem NT, Lim W: Lack of H5N1 avian influenza transmission to hospital employees, Hanoi, 2004. Emerging infectious diseases 2005; 11: 210-215.

11 Bean WJ, Kawaoka Y, Wood JM, Pearson JE, Webster RG: Characterization of virulent and avirulent A/Chicken/Pennsylvania/83 influenza viruses: potential role of defective interfering RNAs in nature. J Virol 1985; 54: 151-160.

12 Capua I, Mutinelli F, Dalla Pozza M, Donatelli I, Puzelli S, Cancellotti FM: The 1999-2000 avian influenza (H7N1) epidemic in Italy: Veterinary and human health implications. Acta Tropica 2002; 83: 7-11.

13 Donatelli I, Campitelli L, Di Trani L, Puzelli S, Selli L, Fioretti A, Alexander DJ, Tollis M, Krauss S, Webster RG: Characterization of H5N2 influenza viruses from Italian poultry. J Gen Virol 2001; 82: 623-630.

14 CDC: Avian influenza infection in humans. http://www.cdc.gov/flu/avian/gen-info/avian-flu-humans.htm [On-line] 2005.

15 Swayne DE, Beck JR: Experimental study to determine if low pathogenicity and high pathogenicity avian influenza viruses can be present in chicken breast and thigh meat following intranasal virus inoculation. Avian Dis 2005; 49: 81-85.

16 Swayne DE, Beck JR: Heat inactivation of avian influenza and Newcastle disease viruses in egg products. Avian Pathol 2004; 33: 512-518.

17 Kishida N, Sakoda Y, Isoda N, Matsuda K, Eto M, Sunaga Y, Umemura T, Kida H: Pathogenicity of H5 influenza viruses for ducks. Arch Virol 2005; 150: 1383-1392.

18 Tumpey TM, Suarez DL, Perkins LEL, Senne DA, Lee JG, Lee YJ, Mo IP, Sung HW, Swayne DE: Characterization of a highly pathogenic H5N1 avian influenza a virus isolated from duck meat. J Virol 2002; 76: 6344-6355.

19 Swayne DE: Microassay for Measuring Thermal Inactivation of H5N1 High Pathogenicity Avian Influenza Virus in Naturally-Infected Chicken Meat. International Journal of Food Microbiology 2005, in press.

Dr. D.E. Swayne, Southeast Poultry Research Laboratory, Agricultural Research Service, U.S. Department of Agriculture, 934 College Station Road, Athens, Georgia 30605, USA.
E-mail: dswayne@seprl.usda.gov

Schudel A, Lombard M (eds): OIE/FAO International Scientific Conference on Avian Influenza.
Dev Biol (Basel). Basel, Karger, 2006, vol 124, p 91.

SESSION IV

Diagnostics

Chairperson: *D. Swayne* (APHIS, USA)
Rapporteur: *D. Senne* (APHIS, USA)

Schudel A, Lombard M (eds): OIE/FAO International Scientific Conference on Avian Influenza.
Dev Biol (Basel). Basel, Karger, 2006, vol 124, pp 93-97.

Advances in Molecular Diagnostics for Avian Influenza

I.H. Brown

Veterinary Laboratories Agency (Weybridge), Addlestone, Surrey, United Kingdom

Abstract: Recent outbreaks of avian influenza (AI) have highlighted the necessity to improve existing tests and to develop new methods, in order to detect spread or new outbreaks more quickly, which is vital for the early and successful implementation of control strategies. Conventionally, the time between clinical suspicion and laboratory confirmation of AI can be relatively long because of the logistics of sending samples to laboratories and their capacity for providing high throughput of sensitive and specific assays. Increasingly, new-generation assays based on molecular diagnostics have become available and applied successfully to disease investigation or active surveillance programmes. There has been widespread application of techniques based on the amplification of specific nucleic acid sequences by polymerase chain reaction (PCR), ligase chain reaction and nucleic acid sequence-based amplification (NASBA). The approaches generally offer high specificity and sensitivity. One of the most promising technologies is real-time PCR, which enables amplification of nucleic acids and detection of the amplified products through specific probes at the same time. A rapid diagnosis can be achieved, together with potential for high throughput resulting from process automation. Currently, microarray technology is developing rapidly and has been applied to diagnosis of influenza A virus but generally lacks the necessary sensitivity for direct application to clinical specimens. In addition, these new technologies have been increasingly applied to rapid and reliable subtyping of AI viruses. The application of molecular technologies to the " field " is now potentially an option, through the availability of portable machines for conducting such tests, with prospects for radically changing diagnostic approaches for AI in the future.

INTRODUCTION

Approaches to the diagnosis of avian influenza (AI) can be based on the detection of virus, its nucleic acid or virus-specific antibody and are described in the OIE manual of Diagnostic Tests and Vaccines for Terrestrial Animals [1]. New tools at the molecular level have revolutionised potential approaches to laboratory diagnosis with important implications for list A diseases or contagions that require a fast and accurate diagnosis to ensure timely implementation of intervention strategies. The increase in the number of influenza epidemics in poultry resulting from H5 or H7 viruses plus interspecies transmission of these viruses, including to humans, places increasing demands on the diagnostic laboratory. New initiatives globally for improved surveillance for influenza viruses in animal hosts (including as an element of pandemic preparedness) and the need to shorten the time required to provide a diagnosis of AI in the laboratory has resulted in considerable progress towards the wider use and application of molecular tools for the detection of AI viral nucleic acid.

In this paper, three technologies, real time RT-PCR, nucleic acid sequence based amplification (NASBA) and DNA microarrays will be reviewed, considering their relevance to diagnosis and surveillance for AI. The assays will be measured against fitness-for-purpose criteria that are the basis for all appropriate diagnostic assays. These criteria include: sensitivity, specificity, ease of use, rapidity and scale or throughput. In addition, new opportunities for "in-field" diagnosis will be discussed briefly.

Real Time RT-PCR (RRT-PCR)

Real time RT-PCR (RRT-PCR) extends the principle of conventional RT-PCR when the target RNA is converted into a DNA copy and amplified, with the detection of amplicon done by gel electrophoresis. RRT-PCR enables the detection of amplicon in real time using fluorogenic hydrolysis-type probes, with the additional advantage that the test can be used as a quantification tool. Samples can be analysed rapidly enabling results to be obtained in a few hours, but, because there is no post-PCR sample handling (a source of problems with conventional PCR), the opportunities for cross-contamination are much reduced, therefore improving quality assurance.

Systems developed for the detection of influenza A have largely focused on the highly conserved matrix gene [2] using **[M]**-specific primers for amplification, followed by hybridisation of a short M-specific probe to accumulate amplicon for real-time detection. The sensitivity of the test relative to virus infectivity in embryonated fowl's eggs has been estimated at 0.1 egg infectious doses 50 % (EID50) [2] equivalent to approximately ten gene copies [3].

Application to analyses of clinical specimens collected from infected turkeys reported relative sensitivity and specificity of 93.3 % and 98.4 % respectively in relation to virus isolation [4]. The assay using M detection has been validated for application to influenza subtypes H1-H15. On a flock or farm basis, the test appears to have equivalent sensitivity to virus isolation [2,4].

Application of RRT-PCR to the detection of H5 of H7 influenza viruses generally results in a reduction in sensitivity of up to 100-fold compared to the M assay [2,3], most probably because of greater heterogeneity in haemagglutinin (HA) target. Quantification is more robust and reproducible with less variation by RRT-PCR compared to infectivity titres determined in embryonated fowl's eggs [3]. Furthermore, RRT-PCR provides a powerful research tool and has been shown to be effective in discriminating among different virus strains in a mixed infection [3]. Alternative systems are under development using novel probe design that can reduce background fluorescence and increase assay sensitivity with detection limits reported down to six gene copies [5].

Overall, RRT-PCR is a highly sensitive and specific assay that has been directly applied to large-scale screening of poultry populations aiming to detect freedom from infection or early incursion of low pathogenic AI (LPAI). This is facilitated by the potential to use robotics in parts of the procedure. The assay is being used in support of confirmation of infection with highly pathogenic AI (HPAI) in Asia, so applicability and speed of result in the event of an outbreak with AI has been demonstrated. It offers a realistic improved rapid alternative to conventional PCR by increasing throughput, reducing problems of laboratory-acquired cross-contamination between samples and includes a confirmatory element using a probe, thereby minimising false positives. The unit cost of the assay compares favourably with antigen detection systems and is much cheaper than virus isolation but some specialist equipment is required. The potential for use as a multiplex assay increases application particularly for differential diagnosis. The principle disadvantages include the presence of PCR inhibitors in clinical samples, RNA degradation and variability in efficiency of RNA extraction procedures.

Nucleic Acid Sequence-Based Amplification (NASBA)

NASBA is a continuous, isothermal, enzyme-based method for the amplification of nucleic acid. During the amplification process, a complementary probe sequence with an electrochemiluminescent tag binds to an extension on one of the primers and is fully incorporated into the amplified sequence. As with RRT-PCR, samples can be analysed rapidly, with the procedure completed in approximately six hours. Reduced handling in the laboratory and the single-tube system minimise opportunities for cross-contamination.

Assay design has been applied to the detection of M, nucleoprotein (NP) HA (H5 or H7). The M-based test is specific for all tested subtypes of HA (1-15) and unreactive with a range of other avian virus pathogens [6], indicating good specificity. All assay types have been shown to have sensitivity equivalent to, or greater than, conventional PCR or virus isolation [6,7]. The approach to amplification of HA employs degenerate primers enabling detection of viruses from multiple lineages [6-8] and does not appear to produce false negative results. Generally, detection is ten- to 100-fold less sensitive than culture in embryonated eggs [6] but most data published makes comparisons with amplified virus produced in-vitro, so performance directly on clinical specimens requires thorough evaluation.

More recently, real-time NASBA has been evaluated for application to the detection of influenza A using the NP gene as target. The approach appears highly specific and potentially more sensitive than conventional NASBA with at least equivalence to RRT-PCR [9], with limits of detection approximate to 0.1 tissue culture infectious doses 50 %. Furthermore, application to detection of human influenza in clinical specimens detected 64 % more positives than conventional techniques, such as cell culture and direct immunofluorescence [9].

NASBA has been applied successfully to outbreak investigation and routine surveillance, particularly with respect to H5N1 in the Far East. The assay offers speed and has the potential for some scaling up. It provides many similar advantages to RRT-PCR but does not require thermal denaturation for DNA strand separation and is able to amplify specific single-stranded RNA target sequences in the presence of genomic DNA contaminants. Currently, unit costs are higher than for other molecular-based tests and the need for specialist equipment is likely to make the assay most suited for use in well-equipped and resourced laboratories.

DNA Microarray

A DNA microarray can, in theory, detect multiple viruses in a single hybridisation and offer the potential to provide a simultaneous screen for any of tens of thousands of nucleic acid sequences. The hybridisation of target nucleic acid to a DNA probe is visualised through fluorescence. The potential application to a virus with broad heterogeneity in many target genes, such as influenza, is possible, since large numbers of probes can be prepared to enable reliable detection of all subtypes and genotypes.

The use of this technology is still in its infancy and application to the detection of influenza A virus has been limited largely to human influenza: it has been used as a useful supplement to PCR-based methods for typing and subtyping [10]. The use of short probes is deemed critical to allow better differentiation of closely related viruses and has shown promise in confirming some genotypic properties, including identification of H1/H3 subtypes [11]. Extension of the technology to a three-dimensional (termed Flow-Thru chip) format increases binding capacity and has been applied to the detection of influenza A and B viruses including H1, H3 and H5 subtypes [12].

Whilst the technology offers promise for the future, issues of correct selection of probes is key to future success. Current systems offer much lower sensitivity than other more widely used methods and are used to analyse PCR product. Optimisation for application directly to clinical specimens remains a central challenge, together with lower costs for hardware necessary to conduct the assay.

Future Diagnostic Perspectives

Recent outbreaks of avian influenza have highlighted the necessity to improve existing tests and to develop new methods, in order to detect spread or new outbreaks more quickly: this is vital for the early and successful implementation of control strategies. Conventionally, the time between clinical suspicion and laboratory confirmation of AI can be relatively long because of the logistics of sending samples to laboratories and their capacity for providing high throughput of sensitive and specific assays. This lag between clinical suspicion and laboratory confirmation means that the virus can often spread readily and the transmission rates are such that each infected bird will infect at least one further bird. For spread to be reduced and the outbreak to be brought under control, leading to elimination, it is necessary to reduce this ratio (R0) below 1.

New molecular technologies, such as described above, offer enhanced potential for the future, because they are relatively rapid and can be scaled up to test large numbers of samples using robotic systems without compromising the quality of the result obtained. Currently, the scale of AI outbreaks can be beyond the capacity of the laboratory using conventional techniques. The use of molecular technologies can therefore permit enhanced surveillance in an infected zone, region or country without compromising necessary diagnostic examination of samples from diseased birds. This should permit earlier and more prompt detection, with implications for implementation of timely control measures in the event of an outbreak with HPAI or for detecting early incursion of LPAI in a free compartment, region or country. It is vital that proper standardisation of these 'new' technologies is conducted according to OIE guidelines [1] and it is particularly important that application to clinical specimens from the field is part of this evaluation.

The ultimate goal for rapid diagnosis is to be able to export new molecular technologies to a "field" environment. For several years, simple ELISA – or biosensor-based formats for a number of pathogens have been used, either in a basic laboratory with limited facilities or "penside" on farm. Portable machines for molecular tests are now becoming commercially available and can potentially be used to detect a range of pathogens on site, with advantages for speed and improved condition of sample as a result of no transportation. These machines are self-contained, robust and able, for example, to conduct RNA extraction and RRT-PCR. Development of machines with hand-held formats is in progress [13]. Immediate transfer of data and subsequent evaluation via the internet with web-enabled software is possible. These real possibilities have the potential radically to alter processes for diagnosis of highly contagious diseases and greatly to facilitate early detection and response, with enhanced prospects for disease control.

References

1 OIE Manual of Diagnostic Tests and Vaccines for Terrestrial Animals: Chapter 2.1.14 Highly Pathogenic Avian Influenza. Fifth Edition, 2004, OIE Paris.

2 Spackman E, Senne DA, Myers TJ, Bulaga LL, Garber LP, Perdue ML, Lohman K, Daum LT, Suarez DL: Development of a real-time reverse transcriptase PCR assay for type A influenza virus and the avian H5 and H7 hemagglutinin subtypes. J Clin Micro 2002; 40: 3256-3260.

3 Lee CW, Suarez DL: Application of real time RT-PCR for the quantitation and competitive replication study of H5 and H7 subtype avian influenza virus. J Virol Meth 2004; 119: 151-158.

4 Cattoli G, Drago A, Maniero S, Toffan A, Bertoli E, Fassina C, Terregino C, Robbi C, Vicenzoni G, Capua I: Comparison of three rapid detection systems for type A influenza virus on tracheal swabs of experimentally and naturally infected birds. Av Path 2004; 33: 432-437.

5 Di Trani L, Bedini B, Falcone E, Donatelli I, Campitelli L, Chiappini B, De Marco MA, Delogu M, Camarda A, Vaccari G, Buonavoglia C: TAQMAN-MGB probe one step quantitative real-time PCR with internal positive control for avian influenza virus RNA detection. In Proceedings of the OIE/FAO International Conference on Avian Influenza, Paris, 7-8 April 2005; 60.

6 Lau LT, Banks J, Aherne R, Brown IH, Dillon N, Collins RA, Chan KY, Wan Y, Fung W, Xing J, Yu ACH: Nucleic acid sequence-based amplification methods to detect avian influenza virus. Bioch & Biophy Res Com 2004; 313: 336-342.

7 Collins RA, Ko LS, Fung KY, Chan KY, Xing J, Lau LT, Yu ACH: Rapid and sensitive detection of avian influenza virus subtype H7 using NASBA. Bioch & Biophy Res Com 2003; 300: 507-515.

8 Collins RA, Ko LS, So KL, Ellis T, Lau LT, Yu ACH: Detection of highly pathogenic and low pathogenic avian influenza subtype H5 (Eurasian lineage) using NASBA. J Virol Meth 2002; 102: 213-225.

9 Moore C, Hibbitts S, Owen N, Corden SA, Harrison G, Fox J, Gelder C, Westmoreland D: Development and evaluation of a real-time nucleic acid sequence based amplification assay for rapid detection of influenza A. J Med Virol 2004; 74: 619-628.

10 Li J, Chen S, Evans DH: Typing and subtyping influenza virus using DNA microarrays and multiplex reverse transcriptase PCR. J Clin Micro 2001; 39: 696-704.

11 Sengupta S, Onodera K, Lai A, Melcher U: Molecular detection and identification of influenza viruses by oligonucleotide microarray hybridization. J Clin Micro 2003; 41: 4542-4550.

12 Kessler N, Ferraris O, Palmer K, Marsh W, Steel A: Use of the DNA flow-thru chip, a three-dimensional biochip, for typing and subtyping of influenza viruses. J Clin Micro 2004; 42: 2173-2185.

13 Perdue ML: Molecular diagnostics in an insecure world. Av Dis 2003; 47: 1063-1068.

Dr. I.H. Brown, Veterinary Laboratories Agency-Weybridge, Addlestone, Surrey KT15 3NB, United Kingdom.
E-mail: i.h.brown@vla.defra.gsi.gov.uk

Schudel A, Lombard M (eds): OIE/FAO International Scientific Conference on Avian Influenza.
Dev Biol (Basel). Basel, Karger, 2006, vol 124, pp 99-105.

Molecular Diagnosis of Avian Influenza during an Outbreak

G. Cattoli, I. Capua

OIE and National Reference Laboratory for Newcastle Disease and Avian Influenza
Istituto Zooprofilattico Sperimentale delle Venezie, Legnaro, Padova, Italy

Abstract: Virus isolation (VI) in specific-pathogen-free (SPF) embryonated eggs or cell cultures is traditionally considered the method of choice for the detection and identification of avian influenza (AI) viruses. However, its value is limited because it is time-consuming and not cost-effective. AI is a highly contagious disease, able to spread in a susceptible population in a short period of time. Therefore, the prompt identification of an infected flock is crucial for control and eradication purposes. During an AI outbreak, the sample processing times using the above mentioned methods are often not compatible with the demands of the poultry industry. In addition, the delay in moving birds from a premises, whilst awaiting the VI result, often results in animal welfare issues. For this reason, when dealing with an epidemic of AI, rapid and reliable laboratory tests, such as RT-PCR and real-time PCR, should be available to reveal direct evidence of infection in the flocks. Scientific reports have been published in the recent past, evaluating their use during AI monitoring and surveillance programmes and epidemics. Based on the available information, the advantages and limits concerning the application of molecular methods during AI outbreaks are discussed in this paper.

INTRODUCTION

Traditionally, laboratory protocols for the detection and identification of avian influenza (AI) viruses were based on virus isolation (VI) in SPF eggs or in cell cultures. In recent outbreaks of major proportions, the application of these methods has been limited by the fact that they are not flexible to a sudden increase in demand, not cost-effective and often require a long processing time. These characteristics hamper the management of outbreaks that occur in densely populated poultry areas (DPPA) or in cases in which there has been significant spread of infection. Experience gathered during outbreaks in Italy indicates that, under these conditions, the prompt identification of an infected flock is crucial for control and eradication purposes, and therefore alternative diagnostic strategies must be implemented.

Rapid and reliable laboratory tests are now available to demonstrate direct evidence of infection in flocks located in the areas at risk of infection. These tests include a variety of protocols for one- or two-step RT-PCR, real-time PCR and nucleic acid sequence-based amplification (NASBA) technology [1-5].

Scientific reports have been published in the recent past, evaluating the use of these tests during AI monitoring and surveillance programmes and epidemics [3,4,6,7]. Based on the available information, we discuss the advantages and limits of the application of molecular methods during AI outbreaks.

Molecular Methods During an Avian Influenza Outbreak: Why Should we Use them?

Recent outbreaks of AI occurring in Europe, the Americas and Asia, have provided field evidence of how challenging it can be to control this infection in a DPPA. In all these situations, it was observed that the movement of animals, equipment, staff and vehicles from the farm during the preclinical phase of infection represented a major risk of spreading the infection further. Therefore, the prompt identification of an infected flock is crucial for eradication purposes, since it enables the enforcement of restriction policies.

During avian influenza outbreaks, the main problems encountered by a diagnostic laboratory are:

- sudden increase in the numbers of samples to be tested;
- increased pressure for faster turn-around time (TAT);

combined with

- high-quality test performances;
- cost effectiveness.

In this respect, the possibility of diagnosing AI by using molecular methods offers important advantages over other protocols, such as VI and ELISA. The main benefits are listed and briefly discussed below.

Rapidity and flexibility

Compared to VI, molecular techniques possess TAT ranging from a few hours to one working day. In addition, when the outbreak occurs in a DPPA, a large number of samples must be processed, and sufficient SPF eggs for VI are not always available at short notice. Molecular techniques, such as one-step RT-PCR and real-time PCR are flexible and rapidly adaptable to a sudden increase in demand for testing.

Similar or faster TAT can be obtained with ELISA but, up to now, this test for AI in birds appears to be limited to tracheal or oro-pharyngeal swabs, and validated protocols for other sample types are not currently available. On the other hand, data on the performance of molecular techniques using a wide variety of samples, including tracheal, cloacal and environmental swabs and internal organs, are provided in the scientific literature, making a wider application of these protocols in the field situation possible.

Test performances

In terms of analytical and diagnostic sensitivity and specificity, the data available concerning the molecular tests for AI can be considered as optimal for their application during an outbreak, showing values of diagnostic sensitivity and specificity above 90 % [6,7]. An excellent agreement with VI was reported during an LPAI outbreak investigation [6]. Data derived from experimental studies [6] indicate that RT-PCR based methods are capable of revealing viral RNA in tracheal swabs of experimentally infected birds for ten to 15 days after challenge, similarly to VI. This period of time covers the first seven to ten days post-infection, when serology is not of diagnostic aid because of an undetectable immune response [8].

Data provided

Molecular techniques can provide a variety of data useful for outbreak investigation. Once the RNA is extracted, it is possible to gain information not only concerning the presence of influenza virus in the clinical specimen, but also about the haemagglutinin and neuraminidase gene segments, the pathotype (low pathogenic AI vs highly pathogenic AI virus) and other genomic sequencing data that can be used for molecular epidemiology. Most importantly, expensive and time-consuming *in vivo* tests for pathogenicity can be avoided, preserving laboratory animal welfare.

Logistics

Unlike VI, molecular techniques can also be applied in small laboratories, providing that the basic equipment is available. This can contribute to the extension of the diagnostic laboratory network in the affected area and to the reduction of the TAT by avoiding the submission of the samples to a distant central laboratory.

For molecular tests only, vitality and infectivity of the virus is not required. Treating the samples in order to inactivate the virus at the place of sampling (i.e. the infected flock) offers the possibility of minimising the risk of spreading the infection and of using laboratories that may not have high containment facilities or that are located in a virus-free area. In previous studies, it has been shown that most of the reagents employed in the extraction and preservation of the viral RNA inactivated many RNA viruses [9]. Nevertheless, in this regard, specific studies on AI viruses are necessary.

Cost effectiveness

The possibility of testing a large number of samples in a short period of time, employing limited laboratory personnel, makes the application of molecular methods for AI economically attractive. A cost analysis of three rapid diagnostic protocols for AI, including ELISA and RT-PCR based methods, has been reported recently indicating the cost-effectiveness of the molecular methods [6]. Market prices can vary on a country-to-country basis, however, PCR thermal cyclers, basic PCR laboratory equipment and reagents are now available in terms of cost to most developed countries. The technical development and widespread use of new technologies may well result in a reduction of the market price of these products in the near future, making them accessible to most developing countries.

Molecular methods during an avian influenza outbreak: their limits

One of the main limits to the widespread use of molecular techniques for AI diagnosis is related to the availability of skilled personnel and an adequate laboratory structure. The high sensitivity of PCR exposes these techniques to handling errors and contaminations and, therefore, laboratory technicians should be specifically trained and PCR-dedicated rooms should be accessible.

As mentioned before, for molecular assays, viable viruses are not required. As a consequence, the detection of viral RNA in the sample does not provide any information about virus infectivity.

RNA is not a stable molecule and it can be subjected to enzymatic degradation in the sample. Therefore some false negative results should be expected. In addition, sometimes it can be difficult to obtain target amplification products of good quality and in large enough amounts, for example, for sequencing purposes, directly from clinical specimens. In these cases, detailed genomic information can only be obtained once the virus has been isolated in vitro.

Developing a diagnostic strategy

Although each laboratory must determine the most suitable testing methods, it is the authors' opinion that molecular detection methods are a valuable tool for AI diagnosis in emergency situations and they should replace antigen detection tests during the monitoring and screening of large numbers of samples.

Technologies like real-time-PCR are rapid and cost-effective and valuable in testing very large numbers of samples, as in the management of an epidemic. However, real-time-PCR still requires expensive equipment and, for this reason, has the limitation of not being available in peripheral laboratories. On the other hand, the one-step RT-PCR is suitable for local laboratories primarily involved in monitoring: large numbers of samples can be processed and no expensive equipment is necessary. However, in the management of AI epidemics, some samples need to be processed urgently. In this case, the ELISA test could remain the method of choice.

In cases of suspected or confirmed outbreaks, diagnostic laboratories have to deal with surveillance programmes and controls on animal movements. Based on these considerations, a diagnostic strategy is proposed in Figures 1 and 2. These strategies were applied during the Italian LPAI H7N3 epidemic in 2002-2003. A surveillance programme in wild waterfowl and backyard flocks is currently on-going in the north-eastern part of Italy, basically following the scheme illustrated in Figure 1 [10].

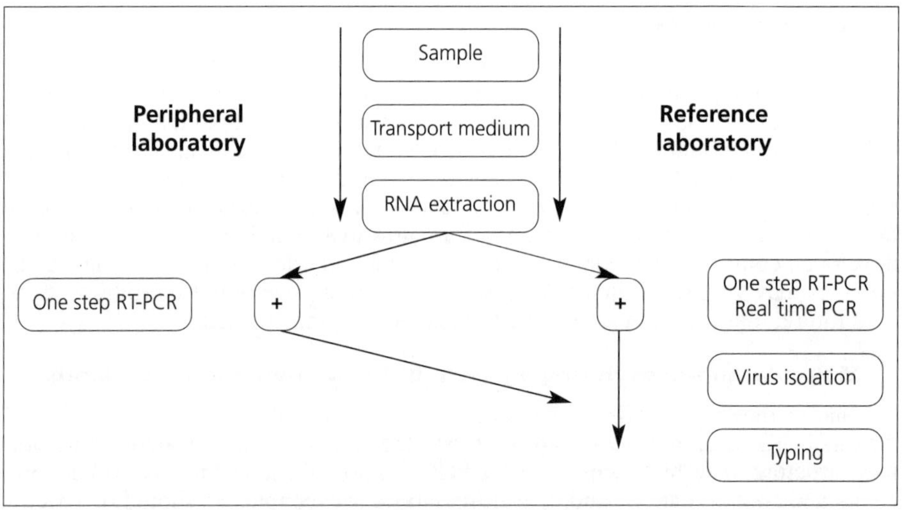

Fig. 1: Surveillance and outbreak diagnosis.

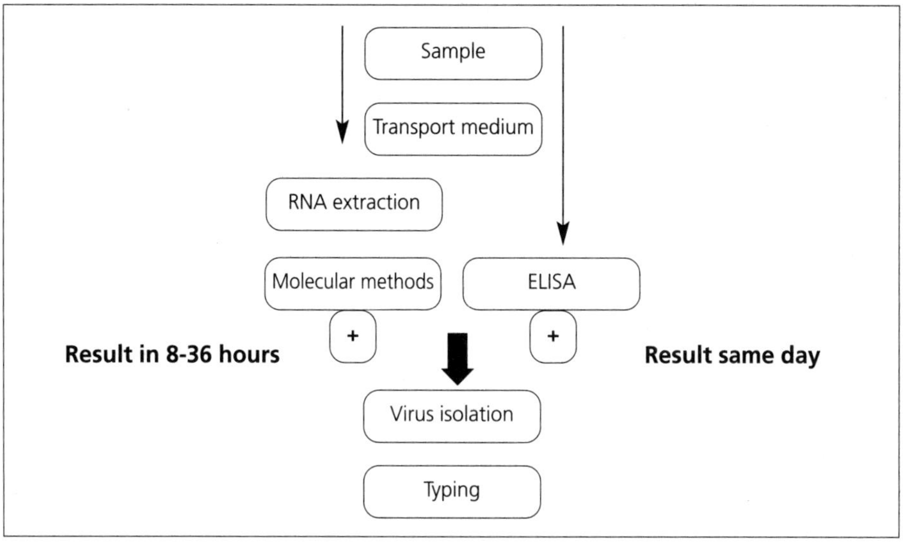

Fig. 2: Animal movements from restriction areas.

Schemes for diagnostic strategies applied during the Italian LPAI H7N3 epidemic for surveillance (Fig. 1) and animal movements (Fig. 2). RRT-PCR: real time RT-PCR.

During outbreak investigation, infection spread should be traced back in order to perform proper epidemiological studies and identify possible sources of virus. Table 1 illustrates the results of the surveillance performed by virus detection methods and serology in 209 poultry farms during the Italian LPAI H7N3 epidemic.

Table 1: Comparison between serology and virus detection methods on tracheal swab in 209 poultry flocks. By virus isolation, 37 flocks were tested positive but 36/37 were serologically negative. However, in 172 flocks virus isolation was negative but in 25/172 serology did indicate contact with the virus. Similar results were obtained by other virus detection methods.

		Serology (HI test)	
		Seropositive flocks	**Seronegative flocks**
Virus detection	**Virus isolation +**	1	36
	ELISA +	3	36
	One-step RT-PCR +	2	40
	Real-time PCR +	3	35
	Virus isolation -	25	147
	ELISA -	23	147
	One-step RT-PCR -	24	143
	Real-time PCR -	23	148

It is clear from Table 1 that neither virus detection, by any method, or serology alone can efficiently reveal the spreading of the infection within an area. Regardless of the method used, virus can be detected during the first two weeks of infection [11,12]. In contrast, serology can only reveal viral exposure starting from the second week of infection when virus detections methods are unable to. Thus, a combination of virological and serological methods should be applied for surveillance purposes.

Conclusions

In conclusion, molecular diagnosis will facilitate the management of AI outbreaks by shortening reporting time, thus being more compatible with the demands of the poultry industry and will also result in preservation of animal welfare. In addition, what appears to be of vital importance in the face of an outbreak is the development of a diagnostic strategy, which should encompass a variety of diagnostic tests and should be based on the capacities of central and peripheral laboratories in relation to the field situation.

Although molecular diagnosis has proved itself to be a valuable tool in supporting the management of major AI outbreaks, it should be complemented with other laboratory methods, including serology. Virus isolation techniques can be delayed but never abandoned, as they still remain the only diagnostic tools that enable a complete genetic and antigenic characterisation of the virus. In addition, collecting virus isolates will allow the creation of archives of fundamental importance for the selection of appropriate vaccine strains and for the study of the evolution and pathogenesis of influenza viruses.

References

1 Fouchier RAM, Bestebroer TM, Herfst S, van der Kemp L, Rimmelzwaan G F, Osterhaus ADME: Detection of influenza A viruses from different species by PCR amplification of conserved sequences in the matrix gene. J Clin Microbiol 2000; 38: 4096-4101.

2 Collins RA, Ko L, So K, Ellis T, Lau L, Yu ACH: Detection of highly pathogenic and low pathogenic avian influenza subtype H5 (Eurasian lineage) using NASBA. J Virol Methods 2002; 103: 213-225.

3 Spackman E, Senne DA, Myers TJ, Bulaga LL, Garber LP, Perdue ML, Lohman K, Daum LT, Suarez DL: Development of a real-time reverse transcriptase PCR assay for type A influenza virus and the avian H5 and H7 hemagglutinin subtypes. J Clin Microbiol 2002; 40: 3256-3260.

4 Spackman E, Senne DA, Bulaga LL, Trock S, Suarez DL: Development of multiplex real time RT-PCR as a diagnostic tool for avian influenza. Avian Dis 2003; 47: 1087-1090.

5 Lau LT, Banks J, Aherne R, Brown IH, Dillon N, Collins RA, Chan K, Fung YW, Xing J, Yu ACH: Nucleic acid sequence-based amplification methods to detect avian influenza virus. Biochem Biophys Res Comm 2004; 313: 336-342.

6 Cattoli G, Drago A, Maniero S, Toffan A, Bertoli E, Fassina S, Terregino C, Robbi C, Vicenzoni G, Capua I: Comparison of three rapid detection systems for type A influenza virus on tracheal swabs of experimentally and naturally infected birds. Avian Pathol 2004; 33: 432-437.

7 Dybkær K, Munch M, Handberg KJ, Jørgensen PH: Application and evaluation ot RT-PCR-ELISA for the nucleoprotein and RT-PCR for detection of low-pathogenic H5 and H7 subtypes of avian influenza virus. J Vet Diagn Invest 2004; 16:51-56.

8 Suarez DL, Schultz-Cherry S: Immunology of avian influenza virus: a review. Devel Compar Immunol 2000; 24: 269-283.

9 Blow JA, Dohm DJ, Negley DL, Mores CN: Virus inactivation by nucleic acid extraction reagents. J Virol Methods 2004; 119: 195-198.

10 Terregino C, Cattoli G, De Nardi R, Beato MS, Capua I, Guberti V, Scremin M: Isolation of influenza A viruses subtype H7N7 and H7N4 from waterfowl in Italy. Vet Rec 2005; 156: 292.

11 Swayne DE, Senne DA, Beard CW: Avian influenza, in Swayne DE, Glisson JR, Jackwood MW, Pearson JE, Reed WM (eds): A laboratory manual for the isolation and identification of avian pathogens, American Association of Avian Pathologists, Pennsylvania, USA, 1998 (4th edition), pp 150-155.

12 Capua I, Terregino C, Cattoli G, Toffan A: Increased resistance of vaccinated turkeys to experimental infection with an H7N3 low-pathogenicity avian influenza virus. Avian Pathol 2004; 33: 158-163.

Dr. G. Cattoli, OIE and National Reference Laboratory for Newcastle Disease and Avian Influenza, Istituto Zooprofilattico Sperimentale delle Venezie, Viale dell'Università 10, IT-35020 Legnaro, Padova, Italy.
E-mail: gcattoli@izsvenezie.it

Schudel A, Lombard M (eds): OIE/FAO International Scientific Conference on Avian Influenza.
Dev Biol (Basel). Basel, Karger, 2006, vol 124, p 107.

SESSION V

Control of Avian influenza with Focus on Vaccination

Chairperson: *I. Capua* (IZS, Italy)
Rapporteur: *I. Brown* (VLA, UK)

Schudel A, Lombard M (eds): OIE/FAO International Scientific Conference on Avian Influenza.
Dev Biol (Basel). Basel, Karger, 2006, vol 124, pp 109-115.

Control of Avian Influenza in Italy: from Stamping out to Emergency and Prophylactic Vaccination

S. Marangon, I. Capua

OIE and National Reference Laboratory for Newcastle Disease and Avian Influenza

Istituto Zooprofilattico Sperimentale delle Venezie, Legnaro, Padova, Italy

Abstract: Since 1997, north-eastern Italy has been repeatedly challenged by avian influenza (AI) infections caused by viruses of the H5 and H7 subtypes. The penetration of such infections in the industrial circuit in densely populated poultry areas (DPPAs) resulted in massive spread, and early attempts to control AI only by stamping-out and restriction policies resulted in death or culling of millions of birds. The re-emergence or the introduction of AI viruses in the same DPPA resulted in the development of an emergency vaccination programme based on the use of heterologous vaccination and a companion discriminatory test. By enabling the detection of field exposure in vaccinated animals, the application of this system, in conjunction with a monitoring programme and a well-defined territorial strategy has resulted in the eradication of H7N1 and H7N3 epidemics that occurred between 2000 and 2004. Retrospective analysis of the AI outbreaks in north-eastern Italy coupled with surveillance programmes in wild birds and in hobby flocks indicating that certain areas are at continuous high risk of infection, was the rationale for developing and implementing a bivalent H5/H7 pilot vaccination programme in a restricted area of the DPPA. Laboratory and field evidence indicate that vaccinated animals are more resistant to challenge and shed lower amounts of virus, thus acting as a tool for both prevention and control, thus limiting the impact of AI infections.

INTRODUCTION

Since 1997, Italy has been affected by seven epidemic waves of avian influenza (AI) caused by viruses of the H5 or H7 subtypes. These epidemics were caused by H5N2 HPAI (highly pathogenic AI), H7N1 (HPAI and LPAI (low pathogenicity AI)) and H7N3 (LPAI) [1].

The most severe episode was observed during 1999-2001, in which Italy was affected by four epidemic waves of AI. The first was caused by an LPAI virus of the H7N1 subtype that subsequently mutated into an HPAI virus. Following the eradication of the HPAI virus, which caused death or culling of millions of birds on infected and at-risk farms, the H7N1 LPAI virus re-emerged twice in the same densely populated poultry area (DPPA) of the Po Valley.

Following the eradication of the H7N1 virus, an LPAI H7N3 virus was introduced in the industrial poultry population of northern Italy. This strain rapidly spread among poultry flocks located in the DPPA that had been affected by the H7N1 epidemic in 1999-2001. From October 2002 to October 2003, the virus was able to infect a total of 388 poultry holdings. About one year after the elimination of the last H7N3 affected poultry flock, the virus re-emerged in the same area and the last affected farm was depopulated in December 2004.

The re-emergence or the introduction of AI viruses in the same DPPA resulted in the implementation of an emergency vaccination programme based on the DIVA (differentiating infected from vaccinated animals) strategy. By enabling the detection of field exposure in vaccinated animals, the application of this system, in conjunction with a monitoring programme and a well-defined territorial strategy has resulted in the eradication of H7N1 and H7N3 epidemics that occurred between 2000 and 2004.

Field and laboratory evidence indicate that vaccinated animals are more resistant to challenge and shed lower amounts of virus [2,3], thus vaccination can be applied both as a tool for control and for prevention, thus limiting the impact of AI infections. Taking into account the high risk of AI virus introduction and spread in the identified DPPA, since October 2004, a bivalent H5/H7 pilot vaccination programme has been implemented in a limited geographical area with the highest poultry population densities.

This paper reports the results of the vaccination strategies applied in northern Italy to deal with AI epidemics occurring in diverse conditions.

Emergency Vaccination Programmes

During 1999 to 2001, Italy was affected by four epidemic waves of AI caused by viruses of the H7N1 subtype. The first was caused by an LPAI virus of H7N1 subtype that subsequently mutated into an HPAI virus, having circulated in the industrial poultry population for approximately nine months. Following the emergence of the HPAI virus, which caused the death or culling of about 16 million birds, the eradication measures provided for in Council Directive 92/40/EEC [4] were enforced on affected and at-risk farms and areas.

Epidemiological investigations were carried out on infected farms using a standardised questionnaire to establish the possible origin of the infection and identify flocks directly or indirectly at risk. Tracing exercises carried out on affected premises allowed the identification of the possible origin of the infection in 66.3 % of the outbreaks. In particular, the origin of infection could be attributed to: movement of animals (1.0 %), indirect contacts at the time of loading for slaughter of female turkeys (8.5 %), neighbourhood spread (within 1 km radius) (26.2 %), lorries for the transport of feeds, litter and carcasses (21.3 %), and other indirect contacts (i.e. exchange of manpower, machinery, equipment) (9.4 %). Four months after the eradication of the HPAI virus, the H7N1 LPAI strain re-emerged and rapidly spread among meat turkey flocks located in the area, with the highest turkey population density located in the southern part of Verona province (Veneto region).

At this point, the application of a control policy limited to restriction and stamping-out measures was not pursuable nor applicable. The poultry industry underwent severe economic losses and would not have been able to survive; for this reason, the development of an alternative control strategy, encompassing vaccination, was required. However, the novel control strategy had to comply with certain indications specified by the EU Commission and was clearly intended as a tool to support eradication. Basically, the vaccination programme had to enable the detection of field virus circulating in the vaccinated population, was to be implemented under official control and had to be based on the use of a non-genetically modified product.

The prelude to the implementation of the vaccination programme was the establishment of a co-ordinated set of measures, including strict biosecurity and a serological monitoring programme [5]. This preparatory phase involved the recruitment of additional staff to support the public field veterinarians and liase with company veterinarians to obtain their support and develop a programme that was, within certain limits, compatible with the organisation of the poultry industry.

The vaccination strategy, now known as DIVA, was based on the use of an inactivated oil emulsion vaccine containing the same haemagglutinin (HA) subtype as the field virus, but of a different neuraminidase (NA) subtype, in this case an H7N3 strain. Clinical protection and reduction of shedding were ensured by the homologous H7 antigen, while the possibility of detecting field exposure in vaccinated animals was achieved through the development of an ad hoc serological test based on the detection of specific anti-N1 antibodies [6].

The test is based on the expression of the N1 gene in a baculovirus system and on the use of the recombinant baculovirus in H5® cells as an antigen for an indirect immunofluorescent antibody test assay (iIFA). The test was validated with 608 turkey field sera derived from: H7N1 naturally infected birds; H7 negative birds from negative flocks; H7N3 vaccinated birds. The agreement between the haemagglutinin inhibition (HI) result and the iIFA was assessed by statistical analysis, which was defined as "almost perfect agreement" between the two tests. The relative sensitivity and specificity of the iIFa compared to HI were calculated as 99.1 % and 95.7 % respectively.

The control of the field situation was to be ensured through the 'early warning' system developed in collaboration with the poultry veterinarians and through an official sero-surveillance programme aiming to detect the LPAI virus. The latter was achieved through the regular testing of unvaccinated sentinel birds in vaccinated flocks and through the application of the anti-N1 antibody detection test in vaccinated animals. To complement this approach, serological monitoring was also to be enforced in unvaccinated flocks, located both inside and outside the vaccination area. In addition, the efficacy of the vaccination schemes was evaluated in the field through regular testing of selected flocks.

From August to November 2000, the H7N1 LPAI strain infected 51 meat-type turkey farms, which housed 845,000 turkeys, and one quail farm, with a total of 429,000 quails, located in the southern part of the province of Verona. Another three quail farms, with a total of 405,000 quails, located in a contiguous province, were also affected. The latter were functionally linked to the quail farm situated in the province of Verona. All infected flocks were depopulated through stamping out or controlled marketing of slaughter birds prior to the implementation of the vaccination campaign.

Emergency Vaccination Following the Re-emergence of H7N1

The vaccination programme was to be implemented only in categories considered at high risk of exposure – meat turkeys, capons, cockerels and layers. Vaccination was implemented according to a protocol consisting of a two-shot administration in chickens and a three- to four-shot administration in turkeys on the basis of their age at slaughter. Although serological titres in chickens (layers, capons and cockerels) were satisfactory and protective (>1:16) even a year after vaccination, this was not the case in turkeys, for which high titres could be registered two weeks after vaccination, but, even following subsequent booster administrations, they decreased rather rapidly to an average titre below the minimum protective level. For this reason, a minimum of three interventions was necessary for female turkeys (slaughter age 90-100 days) and four for male birds (average slaughter age 140-150 days).

Shortly after the beginning of the vaccination programme (December 2000 to March 2001), the H7N1 LPAI virus infected three meat-type turkey farms in the vaccination area and 20 poultry holdings (19 turkey farms and one layer farm) located in a contiguous unvaccinated area. Only one vaccinated flock was affected, and the virus did not spread from this to other vaccinated farms. The last H7N1 LPAI infected poultry flock was stamped out on 26 March 2001, and the results of the serological surveillance, carried out both within and outside the vaccinated area to assess the possible presence of AI infection, demonstrated that the H7N1 AI virus strain was not circulating any longer and thus infection had been eradicated.

Although the vaccination programme was still in place, the absence of virus circulation, as demonstrated by sentinel bird monitoring combined with the application of the DIVA discriminatory test with negative results, was considered to be sufficient to lift trade restrictions on fresh meat obtained from vaccinated birds. On 30 November 2001, Commission Decision 2001/847/EC [7] authorised the marketing of fresh poultry meat originating from vaccinated birds for intra-community trade.

H7N3 LPAI Epidemic and Emergency Vaccination 2002-2003

During 2002-2003 Italy again experienced outbreaks of AI involving an H7N3 subtype influenza A virus of low pathogenicity. During October 2002, a novel H7N3 LPAI strain was introduced from the wild reservoirs in the DPPA in which the previous epidemics had occurred. The virus rapidly spread among poultry flocks, indicating that an intervention strategy encompassing vaccination could have been a valid tool to support eradication. The vaccination programme designed was based once again on the DIVA strategy and was carried out using an AI inactivated heterologous vaccine (strain A/ck/IT/1999-H7N1).

However, although the programme had been drawn up and approved by the EU Commission, the beginning of the vaccination campaign was delayed up to 31 December 2002, because of unavailability of an appropriate vaccine. From 10 October 2002 to 10 October 2003, the H7N3 LPAI virus was able to spread and infect a total of 388 poultry holdings: 332 meat-type turkey, five turkey breeder, 12 broiler breeder, 13 layer, six guinea fowl, four broiler, and three quail farms, one meat duck farm, and 12 back-yard flocks mainly located in the southern part of Veneto and Lombardy. A total of 7,660,005 birds were involved in the epidemic, and among these 4,231,452 animals were stamped out in 163 affected flocks. The remaining 3,428,553 slaughter birds were subjected to controlled marketing.

Notwithstanding the significant number of outbreaks occurring during the implementation of a vaccination campaign, of 388 outbreaks registered during the epidemic, only 88 were vaccinated flocks and all of these occurred in meat turkeys located in the a limited area of Verona province and none in layer flocks. In addition, it is interesting to point out that, despite the poultry density in the latter area, only two unvaccinated poultry farms (one broiler breeder and one meat duck farm) were affected. These farms were located in close proximity to previously vaccinated meat turkey farms that had been field exposed.

The implementation of a vaccination programme and the enforcement of strict restriction measures did not avoid the spread of LPAI virus infection among meat turkey farms located in the DPPA. Nevertheless, it was possible to prevent the massive spread of infection to poultry farms rearing birds other than turkeys and to neighbouring vaccinated areas. Only sporadic outbreaks of LPAI infection were detected in unvaccinated poultry farms, mainly located outside the vaccination area: three meat turkey, five dealer and two quail farms in Lombardy, one dealer farm in Piedmont, and two meat turkey farms and one back-yard flock in the Emilia-Romagna region. These flocks were promptly identified and stamped out. The last farm infected with H7N3 was cleared on 9 October 2003. On 13 January 2004, based on the reliability of the DIVA strategy in detecting any LPAI virus-infected flock, Commission Decision 2004/159/EC [8] authorised the marketing also of table eggs originating from vaccinated layers for intra-community trade.

From Emergency to Prophylactic Vaccination

In February 2004, the monitoring activities carried out in the areas at risk of infection enabled the detection of an LPAI virus of the H5N3 subtype in domestic ducks and geese belonging to a free-range back-yard flock located in Brescia province (Lombardy region). The flock was stamped out and no further LPAI outbreak was detected.

Given the circumstantial evidence of the risk of introduction and the difficulty in limiting virus circulation by means of restriction measures, a prophylactic vaccination programme was designed. The rationale behind the use of prophylactic vaccination is that it should be able to generate a minimal level of protective immunity in the population at risk. The immune response may be boosted if there is evidence of the introduction of a field virus.

A set of additional measures was proposed to the European Commission. It included:

- a complete reorganisation of the poultry sector in the area with the highest poultry population densities of Verona Province (long-term measure);
- a reduction of the turkey density in the same area through a temporary ban on the restocking of an established percentage of turkey farms (short-term measure).

In July 2004, the EU Commission authorised Italy to implement a prophylactic vaccination programme in the high risk areas of Veneto and Lombardy regions [9]. Italy was authorised to enforced the programme from 1 October 2004 onwards based on the availability of a bivalent (H5/H7) inactivated vaccine containing seed strains supplied by the National Reference Laboratory. Since 7 October 2004, the vaccination programme has been implemented only in categories considered at high risk of exposure – meat turkeys and layers. It was also decided to suspend the monovalent vaccination programme from 31 August 2004.

Re-occurrence of the H7N3 LPAI Virus

In September 2004, about one year after the depopulation of the last LPAI-affected flock, the AI virus of the H7N3 subtype re-emerged in the southern part of Verona province. From 15 September to 1 December 2004, the H7N3 LPAI virus infected 27 meat turkey farms and one quail farm, housing a total of 744,000 birds, located in a cluster of nine municipalities with one of the highest turkey population densities in Italy. All the affected meat turkey flocks had been vaccinated with the monovalent (H7N1) inactivated vaccine, but the majority of these flocks had been vaccinated only once or twice.

The re-occurrence of the LPAI virus in a DPPA, in which most farms are in close proximity to each other and functionally connected, required the application of strict control measures in association with the rapid implementation of a booster immunisation of the susceptible population.

The increased resistance to challenge of the vaccinated birds and the reduction of the shedding levels, combined with restrictions, biosecurity and appropriate surveillance, resulted in a significant reduction in the infectious pressure in the environment, and supported the rapid eradication of the infection. Since December 2004 there is no evidence of viral circulation in the poultry population of the high risk area.

Discussion and Conclusions

The experience gathered during the Italian 1999 to 2004 AI epidemics suggests that it is possible to use a heterologous vaccine as a DIVA vaccine for the prevention and control of AI in poultry. The sensitivity and specificity of the test validated on field sera was satisfactory in discriminating infected from vaccinated birds. The results suggest that this test can be used in the framework of a control policy for avian influenza at a population level. In fact, this system overcomes the problems linked to the use of sentinels (identification of sentinels and swapping of sentinels with healthy birds to avoid restriction measures). The implementation of the discriminatory test allows the official veterinarian to sample directly the vaccinated birds and, on the basis of the results, to establish whether or not the flocks are infected, thus allowing an accurate assessment of the field situation. The use of the discriminatory test should always be coupled with the inspection and monitoring of unvaccinated sentinels for early detection of any possible newly introduced AI virus.

It therefore appears that the combination of a DIVA control strategy with a territorial monitoring system under official control may represent an effective tool for the control of avian influenza infections in poultry, particularly in DPPAs. In addition, the application of a DIVA vaccination policy, as opposed to a conventional policy, enabled the authorities to establish that infection was no longer circulating and ultimately resulted in the possibility of marketing fresh meat and table eggs obtained from birds vaccinated against an OIE List A disease.

An accurate evaluation of the cost/benefit ratio of a vaccination programme should be carried out prior to the implementation of the campaign. This should include not only the costs of the vaccine and of vaccine administration but also the costs of monitoring, surveillance, laboratory testing and all other activities connected to vaccination.

Although the application of a DIVA vaccination strategy enables both the monitoring of the epidemiological situation in a vaccinated population and the prompt identification of infected/exposed birds and flocks, the main constraint on the use of AI vaccines is the possible impact on trade. Movement and trade restrictions to be enforced on live poultry and poultry products originating from areas where vaccination is applied should be modulated on the basis of an accurate risk assessment, and vaccination should not have unjustified repercussions on international trade. For obvious reasons, the trade implications will be clarified when the OIE and EU Commission define guidelines for the use of vaccination in the documents of their competence.

In conclusion, Italy has been challenged with several subsequent epidemics of AI and has developed and applied a vaccination programme that has resulted in eradication of infection and, given the high risk of re-introduction from the wild bird reservoir, is currently being used for the first time ever as a prevention tool.

References

1 Marangon S, Capua I, Pozza GD, Santucci U: Field experiences in the control of avian influenza outbreaks in densely populated poultry areas, in Schudel A, Lombard M (eds): Proceedings of the International Conference on the Control of Animal Infectious Diseases by Vaccination, Buenos Aires, 13-16 April 2004. Dev Biol. Basel, Karger, 2004, vol 119, pp 155-164.

2 Swayne DE, Suarez DL: Highly pathogenic avian influenza. Revue Scientifique et Technique Office International des Epizooties 2000; 20: 463-482.

3 Capua I, Terregino C, Cattoli G, Toffan A: Increased resistance of vaccinated turkeys to experimental infection with an H7N3 low-pathogenicity avian influenza virus. Avian Pathology 2004; 33: 158-163.

4 Council Directive 92/40/EEC of 19 May 1992 introducing Community measures for the control of avian influenza. Official Journal of the European Commission 1992; L167: 1-15.

5 Commission Decision 2000/721/EC of 7 November 2000 on introducing vaccination to supplement the measures to control avian influenza in Italy and on specific movement control measures. Official Journal of the European Commission 2000; L291: 33-36.

6 Capua I, Terregino C, Cattoli G, Mutinelli F, Rodriguez JF: Development of a DIVA-Differentiating infected from vaccinated animals- strategy using a vaccine containing a heterologous neuraminidase for the control of avian influenza. Avian Pathology 2003; 32: 47-55.

7 Commission Decision 2001/847/CE of 30 November 2001 amending for the third time Decision 2000/721/EC to modify the Italian avian influenza vaccination programme and current trade restrictions for fresh meat originating from vaccinated turkeys. Official Journal of the European Commission 2001; 315: 61-63.

8 Commission Decision 2004/159/EC of 16 February 2004. Official Journal of the European Commission 2004; L50: 63-64.

9 Commission Decision 2004/666/CE of 29 September 2004 on introducing vaccination to supplement the measures to control infections with low pathogenic avian influenza in Italy and on specific movement control measures and repealing Decision 2002/975/EC Official Journal of the European Commission, L303, 35-44.

Dr. I. Capua, OIE and National Reference Laboratory for Newcastle Disease and Avian Influenza, Istituto Zooprofilattico Sperimentale delle Venezie, Viale dell'Università 10, IT-35020 Legnaro, Padova, Italy.
E-mail: icapua@izsvenezie.it

Schudel A, Lombard M (eds): OIE/FAO International Scientific Conference on Avian Influenza.
Dev Biol (Basel). Basel, Karger, 2006, vol 124, pp 117-124.

Avian Influenza Vaccination in North America: Strategies and Difficulties

D.L. Suarez, C.W. Lee, D.E. Swayne

Southeast Poultry Research Laboratory, Athens, GA, USA

Abstract: Vaccination with high quality efficacious vaccines that are properly delivered can contribute to the control of avian influenza (AI) outbreaks when used as part of a comprehensive control programme that includes quarantines, animal movement controls, increased biosecurity, enhanced surveillance, and education. In North America both whole virus killed adjuvanted vaccines and fowlpox recombinant vaccines have been used to aid in the control of AI. The fowlpox recombinant vaccine is licensed in several countries including the United States (U.S.), but it has only been used in the field in Mexico and some Central American countries. The U.S., however, has considerable experience with the use of killed vaccines, primarily in turkeys. In the state of Minnesota in the 1980s and early 1990s, outbreaks of AI in range-reared turkeys were common, and vaccines were used successfully as part of a controlled marketing programme. More recently, several large layer flocks in Connecticut were vaccinated as an alternative to immediate depopulation after an H7N2 low pathogenic AI outbreak. The vaccinated flocks were intensively monitored for virus shed using sentinel birds, dead bird testing, and eventually some serological surveillance using a neuraminidase DIVA (differentiation of infected from vaccinated animal) approach. With these successes, vaccination is being considered as a valuable tool in comprehensive AI control strategies. Consideration for matching the vaccine to the field strain should also be considered to provide optimal protection including reduced shedding of virus. Antigenic drift of AI viruses after extended vaccination programmes has been observed in chickens, similar to what has been observed with human influenza viruses. Therefore, periodical evaluation of the vaccine to the field strain is necessary to maintain good protection from clinical disease and virus shedding.

INTRODUCTION

Vaccination for avian influenza has been used sparingly in the Americas for the control of avian influenza virus (AIV) outbreaks in poultry in the past. However, as the frequency of AIV outbreaks increases around the world, vaccination is being considered more commonly as an alternative control to stamping out because it is viewed as a more cost-effective strategy. In the United States (U.S.), for at least the foreseeable future, control of a highly pathogenic avian influenza outbreak will be by eradication. For control of low pathogenic AI outbreaks, vaccination is being considered on a case-by-case basis, even for H5 or H7 viruses. The U.S., although using vaccination for avian influenza relatively infrequently, does have experience with vaccination of non-H5/H7 AIVs primarily in the turkey segment of the industry [1].

Of the other countries in North America, Canada has not used vaccination as a control tool for avian influenza. Mexico, Guatemala, and El Salvador are currently using vaccination for H5N2 AIV using both killed and recombinant fowlpox virus vaccines as part of their control efforts [2]. However, for the purpose of this review, only the experiences of vaccination in the U.S. will be included. Additional discussion of the potential value of vaccination, and the different strategies that have been proposed for vaccination monitoring, will be described.

General Principles of Vaccination

The primary goal of vaccination is to prevent or reduce clinical disease from an infectious agent [3,4]. Vaccination can also be used in some cases as a control tool for the eradication of the infectious disease agent out of a region or segment of the population. Vaccination is more typically used only to manage clinical disease and not as a disease eradication tool. For example, vaccination is routinely used to manage infectious bronchitis in poultry, and influenza in swine and humans, but not as part of an eradication programme. In all three cases, the viruses are widespread in the target population, are highly infectious, and eradication would be extremely difficult to achieve. Vaccination with complete eradication has been seldom achieved with the rare exception of smallpox in humans, but it has been used successfully as a control tool to eliminate infectious disease agents from a country or even a region of the world for diseases such as foot-and-mouth disease and brucellosis of cattle. For low pathogenic avian influenza viruses, we currently use vaccination in the U.S. with both management and eradication strategies.

Vaccination also has two other potential benefits besides disease control that would be of value in a control programme. First, if vaccinated animals do become infected, they should have reduced virus shedding into the environment [5,6]. The reduction in virus shedding will decrease the likelihood of spread of infection from one herd or flock to another. The ideal vaccine would completely prevent virus infection, often called sterilizing immunity. However, sterilizing immunity is rarely if ever obtained with a commercial vaccination programme, and is extremely unlikely to be achieved with a mucosal infection like avian influenza virus. However, a good vaccine for avian influenza can reduce the amount of virus being shed, particularly from the oropharynx, by several $\log^{10}$s of virus. The minimum goal for vaccinated animals should be to reduce the amount of virus shedding by 2 $\log^{10}$s of virus at the peak of virus shedding (a 100-fold reduction in virus shedding). Peak virus shedding is often two to three days after infection. Experimental studies have in some cases shown greater than a 4 $\log^{10}$ reduction in the amount of virus shedding (a 10,000-fold reduction). This reduction in virus shedding will obviously mean less virus in the environment that can be spread to other flocks, and will also result in the more rapid elimination of virus from the environment.

The second area where vaccination can aid eradication is by increasing the minimum dose of virus that is required to infect an animal [7]. Although avian influenza is considered to be a highly infectious disease, it typically takes many viral particles (10-1000) routinely to infect a bird experimentally. This is typically defined as the minimum infectious dose 50 (MID50), or the amount of virus it takes to infect 50 % of exposed birds. At least one study has demonstrated that vaccination can increase the threshold required by infection by 10-fold or greater. This increased resistance to infection coupled with reduced shedding greatly increases the chance of breaking the infection cycle. The minimum requirement for the levels of protection needed to provide vaccination which will significantly affect the infection cycle is not clearly defined, so it is not currently possible to predict how much a vaccine has to reduce shedding or increase the resistance to infection to play a critical role in aiding an eradication programme. It cannot be emphasized enough that vaccination by itself cannot be used as an eradication programme. An eradication programme must include strict quarantines, movement controls on animals and equipment, increased biosecurity, increased active and passive surveillance, and education of the affected groups [4,5]. Without all these components in place, any eradication programme will probably fail. The use of vaccination as part of the strategy may provide a less costly alternative to an immediate stamping-out programme, but the cost will not be inconsequential.

Vaccination has typically been used for diseases that do not result in trade sanctions or restrictions. In the past vaccination has caused a presumption that infection was prevalent in the vaccinating country, and has been used as a non-tariff trade barrier for the introduction of poultry or poultry products. It is clearly the right of individual countries to ban animals or products that present a credible risk of introducing a foreign animal disease into that country. However, this ability to use disease status as a trade barrier must be done on scientific grounds. The importing country must be able to show thorough diagnostic testing that they are free of the infectious agent or that they have a continuing control programme to try and eliminate the disease from their country. There should also be evidence to suggest that movement of animals or animal products pose a real threat to introducing a disease into the country. A typical first response in considering these trade issues is for the importing country to try to assume a zero risk policy by blocking imports of all animals or animal products associated with the disease from the affected country. This approach, although effective, is often unnecessary to prevent disease introduction, and risk-based analysis can identify ways to trade both animal and animal products safely. This risk-based analysis should be science-based and should be tailored to each infectious disease agent. Mitigation strategies to the movement of poultry or poultry products may be by increased diagnostic testing, the treatment of products to ensure safety such as heating, or in some cases potentially vaccination. If vaccination is to become more accepted as a control tool, these trade barriers need to be examined to determine whether vaccinated birds can be safely traded between countries.

An additional negative aspect to vaccination is the effect that it has on serological surveillance. In the U.S., serological monitoring for avian influenza infection is routinely practised, and is an essential component of the National Poultry Improvement Plan and other monitoring programmes certifying that flocks are free of avian influenza. The killed vaccines that are available today result in measurable antibody titres to all the structural proteins, including the matrix and nucleoproteins. One or both of these two proteins are used as type-specific antigens for both commonly used antibody tests, the agar gel immunodiffusion (AGID) or commercial ELISA tests. Therefore, vaccinated birds cannot be distinguished from naturally infected birds using this approach. This loss of the ability to do surveillance has been a major inhibitor for use of vaccination in AIV control [4,8].

Vaccination in the United States of America

Vaccination has been used for low pathogenic avian influenza for both disease management and eradication in the U.S. Currently, two different types of vaccines are commercially licensed for use in the U.S., including whole virus killed oil-adjuvanted vaccines and the subunit fowlpox recombinant vaccines. Although the fowlpox recombinant vaccine for the H5 subtype is licensed in the U.S., it has never been used, and all vaccination in the U.S. has been with the killed whole virus vaccines. Even for the killed viruses, there is only a limited number of haemagglutinin subtypes that vaccine companies have available for use under a conditional licence. Alternatively, an autogenous vaccine can also be made using the outbreak strain. However, the outbreak strain must grow to high titre in embryonating chicken eggs to be cost-effective. In both situations, the vaccine companies make the vaccine based on the demand and do not have vaccine sitting on the shelf. Therefore, considerable delays will often occur before the first flocks can be vaccinated. In the U.S., as part of the conditional licence, vaccination must be authorized by either veterinary officials at the state or federal level. For low pathogenic avian influenza, except for H5 and H7 viruses, vaccination is a state control issue. For low pathogenic H5 and H7 outbreaks, vaccination must have the concurrence of both state and federal officials. Vaccination for highly pathogenic avian influenza has never been used in the U.S., but potentially could be instituted, again with the concurrence of state and federal veterinary officials.

The only routine use of avian influenza vaccination in the U.S. is to protect turkey breeder flocks from infection with swine influenza virus (SIV). Swine influenza is a common infection in swine in the U.S., and as previously mentioned, vaccination is used to manage the disease, but not to eradicate the virus. Turkeys appear more susceptible to SIV than other poultry species, and evidence of infection in turkeys is seen commonly [9]. The clinical disease is primarily a large reduction in egg production in turkey breeder flocks, and egg production typically remains depressed even after the birds are clear of the infection. Respiratory disease is not commonly seen, and flocks that are not in egg production may seroconvert without evidence of clinical disease. The use of vaccination in turkeys is widespread in areas where swine are also raised, although the amount of vaccine administered is typically only a few million doses each year.

Vaccination has also been used on many occasions as part of an eradication control programme. The most widespread use has been in turkeys in the state of Minnesota. In the 1980s until 1997, meat turkeys were commonly raised on range, where they had exposure to wild birds [10]. These range-reared turkeys were commonly infected with avian influenza in the autumn, and this timing correlated with the autumn migration of wild migratory ducks. When an outbreak of AI was detected in turkeys, the state veterinary officials would institute quarantines, movement controls, and increased surveillance in the area of the outbreak. They would also routinely use vaccination of the infected flock and other turkey flocks in the same geographical region as a control tool. The infected and vaccinated flocks were eventually sent to market under special conditions. First, the birds had to clear the active viral infection before movement. Secondly, the flocks were slaughtered at specific times to reduce the chance of virus spreading to other farms during the movement or slaughtering process [1]. Vaccination with controlled marketing was used successfully to eradicate AIVs from turkeys in Minnesota since the same subtype rarely reoccurred from year to year. With the understanding that virus was being introduced into turkeys by their exposure to wild birds, most turkey flocks in Minnesota were converted from range rearing to confinement rearing in the late 1990s. This greatly reduced the number of outbreaks of avian influenza in the state, and therefore vaccine use has also declined.

More recently vaccination was used as a control strategy in several large layer complexes in the state of Connecticut. In 2003 three large laying farms, all owned by the same company, were identified as having been infected with H7N2 avian influenza virus. The molecular epidemiology showed the viruses to be similar to what was circulating in the live bird markets in the Northeast United States. A decision was made to vaccinate these flocks to control the infection as opposed to stamping out because of the direct and indirect costs. Additionally, since Connecticut only had a relatively small poultry industry with little international export, the trade implications for vaccination was smaller than for large poultry producing states. After both state and federal agreement, the vaccination proceeded on the farms under specific agreements with the farm owner. Since not all the birds on the farm had been infected, uninfected birds and naïve pullets that were to be introduced to the farm would receive two doses of vaccine. The infected birds were also vaccinated in an effort to increase antibody levels and to provide extended protection from re-infection. As part of the vaccination agreement, certain conditions had to be met, including sending the spent layers to the rendering plant, increased biosecurity, and several levels of surveillance. First, sentinel birds were banded and placed randomly in each house. Serological surveillance was performed every two weeks on the sentinel birds. Virus isolation or real-time RT-PCR (RRT-PCR) was performed routinely on the daily mortality from each farm. Production records and daily mortality were reviewed, and abnormal changes prompted increased diagnostic testing. The initial vaccination was with a H7N2 vaccine where the seed virus was from the 1997 LPAI outbreak in Pennsylvania. This vaccine was chosen for two reasons. First, the vaccine was the same lineage of virus, and therefore was expected to be antigenically well matched to the outbreak strain. Second, 3.2 million doses were immediately available, having been produced for, but never used, during the Pennsylvania outbreak. Eventually, a heterologous neuraminidase DIVA (differentiate infected from vaccinated animals) strategy using an H7N3 vaccine was used. The H7N3 strain was from an outbreak in turkeys in Utah in 1995, had good sequence similarity for the haemagglutinin gene, and had previously been used as a vaccine seed strain. Naïve pullets were vaccinated twice before being moved into production. Although serum samples were taken for testing using the DIVA approach, the outbreak was controlled before the DIVA vaccinated birds entered production. All the surveillance done on the farm after vaccination was negative for evidence of further infection, and the vaccination programme was considered successful.

Interest in vaccination as an alternative to stamping out has increased in the U.S. because of these successful control programmes. However, because of the large amount of U.S. poultry production that goes for international export, concerns still remain about how vaccination will affect trade. Therefore interest in the use of a DIVA vaccination strategy has also increased with the goal of assuring trading partners that they are receiving a safe product. Four different strategies have been proposed for DIVA testing for avian influenza, including the use of sentinels, the use of subunit vaccines, heterologous neuraminidase strategy and the non-structural protein 1 (NS1) strategies.

The use of sentinels in vaccinated flocks have been a widely used approach to determine whether flocks have been exposed to avian influenza infections. Typically 30 or more marked or banded birds are randomly spread through a vaccinated premise and they are routinely tested for exposure to avian influenza. This is typically done by standard serological tests, but can also be done by direct virus detection methods. Sentinels are thought to provide a sensitive measure of infection of a vaccinated flock. The main disadvantage is in the management of the sentinel birds. It can be difficult to identify the sentinels in the house and keep them managed separately.

Because antibodies to the haemagglutinin and neuraminidase proteins provide the primary protection against avian influenza virus challenge, it is possible to protect birds by having only these proteins in a vaccine. Many different types of subunit vaccines, including virus vectored vaccines and vaccines using protein expressed in different culture systems, have been shown to provide protection from HPAI challenge. However, only the fowlpox vectored recombinant vaccine for the H5 subtype is available commercially. This vaccine contains the A/Turkey/Ireland/83 haemagglutinin gene, and experimentally this vaccine has been shown to be protective for many HPAI viruses [11]. Because only the HA gene is expressed in this system, the standard serological surveillance tests (AGID, ELISA) can be used to monitor whether vaccinated flocks have also been naturally infected. Although the ability to use DIVA surveillance appears to be a strength of the fowlpox-vectored system, no reports of its field application in this way have been reported.

A heterologous neuraminidase DIVA strategy is an alternative approach that has been used in several countries. This approach briefly is to vaccinate with the same haemagglutinin subtype as the field strain, but using a different neuraminidase subtype. The vaccinated birds are monitored by serology for the field viruses' neuraminidase protein and, if positive, shows exposure to the field virus. Efforts to validate this system are continuing, and its use is described elsewhere [12].

An alternative DIVA strategy that has recently been described looks at a differential immune response to the non-structural protein 1 (NS1) [13]. The NS1 protein is produced in large amounts in infected cells, but it is not packaged into the infectious viral particle. Since killed AIV vaccines are primarily whole viral particles, vaccinated birds should not have an antibody response to the NS1 protein, but naturally infected birds should develop antibodies to the NS1 protein. This DIVA approach was demonstrated previously with equine influenza viruses in horses using an ELISA format. Experimentally, the approach also works with chickens with purified killed vaccines. However, commercial avian influenza vaccines are grown in embryonating chicken eggs and are not purified, and they contain small amounts of NS1 protein from the lysed cells. Vaccinated chickens will develop some antibodies to the NS1 protein, particularly after repeated vaccinations. This small amount of NS1 antibody does make it more difficult to use the NS1 DIVA strategy, but a difference in the amount of antibody produced is evident comparing vaccinated and infected birds. By diluting the sera before testing, a clear distinction can be made between vaccinated and infected birds. For trade and surveillance purposes it is valuable not only to distinguish vaccinated from infected birds, but also to identify vaccinated and then infected birds to demonstrate to trading partners that the flock has not been exposed to infection. With the NS1 DIVA strategy, vaccinated and then infected birds do have increased levels of NS1 protein in experimentally challenged birds [13]. Continued work needs to be performed with the NS1 DIVA strategy to evaluate its performance in the field.

Vaccine Selection

For vaccination with avian influenza, little effort typically has been used to match the vaccine and the field strain. In part this is because vaccination with any H5 or H7 virus seems to provide protection from clinical disease against HPAI challenge of the same subtype, regardless of the genetic differences. This broad protection may reflect that killed vaccines typically produce high levels of serum antibody that effectively blocks the viraemia and therefore the systemic phase of infection. Vaccinated birds may still be infected and may be shedding large amounts of virus. However, when using vaccines as a control tool, both clinical protection and virus shedding are of concern. Experimental evidence demonstrates that the closer the vaccine is to the field strain, the lower the amount of virus will be shed in challenged birds. The comparison of genetic sequence of the haemagglutinin gene can provide a good estimate of the variability between the vaccine and field strain [6]. A more sensitive and time-consuming indicator is to do cross-haemagglutinin inhibition tests. This technique is commonly used for human influenza to determine probable protection and has been the primary method to determine when to change the vaccine seed strain due to antigenic drift.

Antigenic drift, which is the accumulation of point mutations in the haemagglutinin gene that results in decreased protection from vaccination, is a major problem for human, swine, and equine influenza vaccines. Antigenic drift is thought to be the result of the field virus changing, based on the antibody pressure in the host [13]. This antibody pressure may be by vaccination or natural infection, but in either case a virus will be under a selection pressure to evade the immune response, which allows the virus to replicate to higher titres in the host. The better the virus replicates, the more likely it is that the strain of virus will spread to other susceptible hosts. Until recently antigenic drift was not considered to be a problem with avian influenza. However, recent experiences with vaccination of birds in Mexico demonstrate antigenic drift to be a serious problem. Mexico has vaccinated for avian influenza since 1995 for both LPAI and HPAI. The HPAI was eliminated from their country, but LPAI remains endemic in parts of the country in spite of intensive vaccinations over the past 10 years. The virus has even spread to neighboring Guatemala and El Salvador. This outbreak provided the unique opportunity to look at long-term virus evolution in the face of vaccination. The data show that genetically, the Mexican H5N2 lineage of viruses diverged shortly after vaccination away from the vaccine strain. These divergent lineages of viruses, over time, had lower levels of cross-reactive HI antibody levels to the vaccine strain, suggesting this genetic drift was due to vaccine pressure. In the extreme examples, vaccinated birds had a 16-fold lower level of antibody protection with recent field strains of virus. Experimental studies showed that the current vaccine could still prevent clinical disease with a HPAI challenge, but it no longer provided significant protection from virus shedding. Therefore even vaccinated birds, if infected in the field, will shed large amounts of virus [14]. The data clearly show the need to update the vaccine seed strain used in Mexico.

Conclusions

Vaccination can be a valuable tool for the control of avian influenza outbreaks when done as part of a complete control programme. Recent efforts to use a DIVA vaccine strategy may be worthwhile to provide enhanced surveillance for virus infection and assure trading partners of the safety of poultry and poultry products. However, vaccines and vaccine use must be evaluated for protection, and consideration for antigenic drift must be considered for vaccines to be successful.

References

1 Halvorson DA: Strengths and weaknesses of vaccines as a control tool, in Swayne DE, Slemons RD (eds): Proceedings of the Fourth International Symposium on Avian Influenza. United States Animal Health Association, Richmond, Virginia, 1997, Vol 4, pp 223-227.

2 Villarreal-Chavez C, Rivera-Cruz E: An update on avian influenza in Mexico. Avian Diseases 2003; 47: 1002-1005.

3 Suarez DL, Schultz-Cherry S: Immunology of avian influenza virus: a review. Developmental and Comparative Immunology 2000; 24: 269-283.

4 Swayne DE: Vaccines for list A poultry diseases: emphasis on avian influenza, in Brown F, Roth J (eds): Vaccines for OIE List A and Emerging Animal Diseases. Dev Biol. Basel, Karger, 2003, vol 114, pp 201-212.

5 Swayne DE, Beck JR, Garcia M, Stone HD: Influence of virus strain and antigen mass on efficacy of H5 avian influenza inactivated vaccines. Avian Pathol 1999; 28: 245-255.

6 Swayne DE, Garcia M, Beck JR, Kinney N, Suarez DL: Protection against diverse highly pathogenic H5 avian influenza viruses in chickens immunized with a recombinant fowlpox vaccine containing an H5 avian influenza hemagglutinin gene insert. Vaccine 2000; 18: 1088-1095.

7 Capua I, Terregino C, Cattoli G, Toffan A: Increased resistance of vaccinated turkeys to experimental infection with an H7N3 low-pathogenicity avian influenza virus. Avian Pathol 2004; 33: 158-163.

8 Tumpey, T.M., Alvarez R, Swayne DE, Suarez DL: Diagnostic Approach for Differentiating Infected from Vaccinated Poultry on the Basis of Antibodies to NS1, the Nonstructural Protein of Influenza A Virus. Journal of Clinical Microbiology 2005; 43: 676-683.

9 Wright SM, Kawaoka Y, Sharp GB, Senne DA, Webster RG: Interspecies transmission and reassortment of influenza A viruses in pigs and turkeys in the United States. Am J Epidemiol 1992; 136: 488-497.

10 Halvorson DA, Kelleher CJ, Senne DA: Epizootiology of avian influenza: Effect of season on incidence in sentinel ducks and domestic turkeys in Minnesota. Applied Environ Microbiol 1985; 49: 914-919.

11 Taylor J, Weinberg R, Kawaoka Y, Webster RG, Paoletti E: Protective immunity against avian influenza induced by a fowlpox virus recombinant. Vaccine 1988; 6: 504-508.

12 Capua I, Terregino C, Cattoli G, Mutinelli F, Rodriguez JF: Development of a DIVA (Differentiating Infected from Vaccinated Animals) strategy using a vaccine containing a heterologous neuraminidase for the control of avian influenza. Avian Pathol 2003; 32: 47-55.

13 Oxford J, Eswarasaran R, Mann A, Lambkin R: Influenza – the chameleon virus, in Craig A, Scherf A (eds): Antigenic Variation. London, UK, Academic Press, 2003, pp 52-83.

14 Lee CW, Senne DA, Suarez DL: Effect of vaccine use in the evolution of Mexican lineage H5N2 avian influenza virus. J Virology 2004; 78: 8372-8381.

Dr. D.L. Suarez, Southeast Poultry Research Laboratory, 934 College Station Rd, Athens, GA 30605, U.S.A.
E-mail: dsuarez@seprl.usda.gov

Schudel A, Lombard M (eds): OIE/FAO International Scientific Conference on Avian Influenza.
Dev Biol (Basel). Basel, Karger, 2006, vol 124, pp 125-126.

Control and Eradication Strategies of Avian Influenza in Mexico

C.L. Villarreal

Dispositivo Nacional de Emergencia de Sanidad Animal (DINESA), Mexico-United States Commission for the Prevention of Foot and Mouth Disease and other Exotic Animal Diseases (CPA). Animal Health General Directorate, Senasica, Sagarpa, Mexico.

Key words: Strategies, Mexico, avian influenza.

Abstract: In December 1994, a highly pathogenic (HP) avian influenza (AI) outbreak occurred in Mexico, caused by the subtype H5N2, affecting two main regions of egg and poultry-meat production. At that time, governmental actions included immediate stamping out of the affected flocks, disinfection of affected premises, quarantine measures in the region, strict movement controls on poultry and their products and vaccination. With these policies, the disease was eradicated in a relatively short time. The last case of HPAI was detected in June 1995 and the country was declared as free of HPAI virus in January 1996 to the World Animal Health Organisation (OIE). Since then, Mexico has maintained a control programme against low pathogenic (LP) AI virus that is based on a zoning classification, movement controls and other strategies.

INTRODUCTION

Within Mexican livestock production, the poultry sector is the most developed; its production in 2004 was 2.3 million metric tons of poultry meat and 1.9 million metric tons of egg, which represented 40.2 % of the livestock internal net product of the country. The national poultry inventory covers 3,800 commercial farms, among which the mainly poultry-meat producers are the states of Jalisco, Guanajuato and the Region Lagunera and the mainly egg producers are Jalisco, Puebla and Sonora, although the other states also produce eggs but in less quantity. The annual consumption per cápita is 19.22 kg of egg and 22.94 kg of chicken meat.

AVIAN INFLUENZA IN MEXICO

A Low Pathogenic Avian Influenza (LPAI) subtype H5N2 outbreak was first recognised on commercial farms in central Mexico in May 1994. Subsequently, an HPAI outbreak occurred in December 1994, caused by the same subtype, in the states of Puebla and Querétaro, which are important regions of egg and poultry-meat production [1].

At that time, government actions included immediate stamping out of the affected flocks, disinfection of affected premises, quarantine measures in the region, strict movement control of poultry and their products, and vaccination. With these policies, the disease was eradicated in a relatively short time. The last case of HPAI was detected in June 1995 and the country was declared to OIE to be free of HPAI virus (HPAIV) in January 1996.

Current Situation of Avian Influenza

Since then, Mexico has continued with an LPAI virus (LPAIV) control programme based on a zoning classification of free and under-eradication states or regions. This programme consists of systematic monitoring and, in the endemic zone, there was established: an "AI-free flock/farm certificate"; surveillance and laboratory diagnosis by haemagglutination inhibition, agar gel immunodiffusion, viral isolation and its filogenesis, virus subtypification and pathogenecity determination; movement control of poultry and their products; vaccination under official authorisation, which only applies to the menace resulting from LPAIV presence and to protect flocks in the case of a virus mutation to HPAIV [2].

Vaccination Strategies

The current vaccines are made from the HPAIV found in 1995 from an inactivated virus emulsion subtype H5N2; in 1998, a recombinant vaccine (fowl poxvirus as carrier) was developed and authorised [3]. To use the vaccine, poultry producers have to request an official authorisation for its use it on their farms, and it is a requirement to have sentinel birds for the surveillance of AI.

Conclusions

The subtype H5N2 is the only AI virus that has been detected in Mexico. The best tool against high pathogenic AI virus in Mexico was vaccination.

Vaccine does not prevent infection of low pathogenic AI virus but prevents its mutation to high pathogenic and diminishes viral elimination in infected birds.

References

1 Flores-Hernández AO, Villarreal-Chavez CL, Flores-Crespo R, Garcia-Garcia J, Lopez-Hinojosa R, Medina-Alvarez P, Solis-Sanchez S, Rivera-Cruz E: La Influenza aviar en Mexico (Memoria). SAGAR, 1997.

2 Secretaría de Agricultura, Ganadería y Desarrollo Rural: Norma Oficial Mexicana, NOM-044-ZOO-1995, Campaña Nacional contra la influenza aviar. Diario Oficial de la Federacion, 1996.

3 Secretaría de Agricultura, Ganadería y Desarrollo Rural: Norma Oficial Mexicana, NOM-055-ZOO-1995, Requisitos mínimos para la elaboración de vacunas emulsionadas inactivadas contra la influenza aviar subtipo H5N2. Diario Oficial de la Federacion, 1998.

Dr. C.L. Villarreal, Dispositivo Nacional de Emergencia de Sanidad Animal (DINESA), Mexico-United States Commission for the Prevention of Foot and Mouth Disease and other Exotic Animal Diseases (CPA). Animal Health General Directorate, Senasica, Sagarpa, Mexico.
E-mail: coor.tec@senasica.sagarpa.gob.mx

Schudel A, Lombard M (eds): OIE/FAO International Scientific Conference on Avian Influenza.
Dev Biol (Basel). Basel, Karger, 2006, vol 124, pp 127-132.

Development of a Recombinant Fowlpox Virus Vector-Based Vaccine of H5N1 Subtype Avian Influenza

C. Qiao, K. Yu, Y. Jiang, C. Li, G. Tian, X. Wang, H. Chen

Animal Influenza Laboratory of the Ministry of Agriculture and National Key Laboratory of Veterinary Biotechnology, Harbin Veterinary Research Institute, Chinese Academy of Agricultural Sciences, Harbin, P. R. China

Key words: Avian influenza, recombinant fowlpox virus, vaccine.

Abstract: The genetic stability of the recombinant fowlpox virus (named rFPV-HA-NA) was confirmed by serial passage on chicken embryo fibroblast (CEF) cells. The immune efficacy, safety, the minimum immunising dose, the time of immunity induced and the immune duration of the vector-based vaccine was evaluated in specific-pathogen-free (SPF) chickens. The recombinant virus vaccine containing 100 plaque form units (PFU) could induce complete protection against challenge with H5N1 highly pathogenic avian influenza virus (HPAIV). The immune efficacy, protecting chickens from clinical signs and death after challenge, was obtained one week after the immunisation with this vaccine. Protective immunity could last for 40 weeks post-immunisation. So the recombinant fowlpox vaccine is a safe and highly effective gene engineering vaccine candidate, and will be used to prevent H5 subtype avian influenza in the future.

INTRODUCTION

H5N1 subtype highly pathogenic avian influenza virus (HPAIV) first caused 18 human infection and six deaths in 1997 in Hongkong [1]. Continuing outbreaks of highly pathogenic avian influenza (HPAI) in a number of Asian countries, caused by H5N1 subtype virus, represent a serious risk for animal and public health worldwide. Thus, the development of a highly effective influenza virus vaccine for chickens would be of benefit to both veterinary and human health.

An inactivated vaccine derived from A/turkey/England/N-28/73 (H5N2) was used to prevent H5N1 avian influenza in 2004 in China. Now a novel inactivated vaccine composed of H5N1 AIV, a genetically modified reassortant H5N1 low pathogenic avian influenza virus generated by reverse genetic system has been developed (data unpublished). Furthermore, a recombinant fowlpox virus co-expressing H5 HA and N1 NA genes has been constructed. The protective immunity, evaluated in specific-pathogen-free (SPF) chickens, demonstrated that immunisation with rFPV-HA-NA could induce complete protection against challenge with H5N1 [2]. In the present study, the immune efficacy, safety, the minimum immunising dose, the time of immunity induced and the immune duration of the vector-based vaccine was evaluated in SPF chickens. It will provide the theoretical and experimental gist for the field application of the recombinant vaccine.

Materials and Methods

Chickens

SPF chickens used in this study were obtained from the Experimental Animal Center of HVRI, and housed in negative-pressure filtered-air isolation cabinets in a biosafety level 3 (BSL-3) agriculture facility.

Challenge virus

A/Goose/Guangdong/1/96 (H5N1) [GD1/96] is a highly pathogenic isolate of AIV. This virus was propagated in the allantoic cavities of nine- to ten-day old SPF embryonated chicken eggs, titrated in six week old SPF chickens using standard methods. All the challenge experiments were conducted under BSL-3 containment conditions.

Vaccines

A recombinant fowlpox virus (rFPV-HA-NA) vaccine containing a cDNA copy of the HA and NA gene of A/Goose/Guangdong/3/96 (H5N1) [GD3/96] was used. The parent fowlpox virus, S-FPV-017, a less attenuated FPV strain was used in the sham vaccination group.

Genetic stability of the recombinant fowlpox virus rFPV-HA-NA

The recombinant fowlpox virus was serially passaged to passage 25 on SPF chicken embryo fibroblast monolayer. Three passages of recombinant fowlpox viruses, 5, 15 and 25 were selected to examined the genetic stability. The HA gene and NA gene were amplified by polymerase chain reaction (PCR) and sequenced. Meanwhile, the immunogenicity of the recombinant virus was evaluated by immunising SPF chickens.

Experimental design

Experiment 1: Immune efficacy assay

A total of thirty-four-week old SPF chickens were randomly assigned three groups, one group was immunised with rFPV-HA-NA vaccine by wing web puncture with a double needle used for commercial vaccination of poultry with FPV. Approximately 50μL inoculum containing 2×10^3 PFU of rFPV was given to each chicken. The other two groups, vaccinated with S-FPV-017 and unvaccinated, were used as controls. All the chickens were bled weekly after immunisation. Challenge was conducted three weeks after vaccination, with 0.2mL of allantoic fluid containing $100LD_{50}$ of GD1/96 isolate by intranasal route. The chickens were monitored daily for two weeks for death and infection. Four days after challenge, cloacal swabs were collected for virus re-isolation.

Experiment 2: Safety evaluation

Ten one-day old SPF chickens were vaccinated with ten-time the dose of recombinant vaccine by wing-web puncture, five chickens unvaccinated were used as control. All the chickens were observed for two weeks for absence of clinical signs of disease or local lesions.

Experiment 3: Determination of the minimum immunising dose

The minimum immunising dose was determined in four-week old SPF chickens. Sixty chickens were allocated into six distinct groups. Five of the groups were individually vaccinated with 1×10^4PFU, 1×10^3PFU, 1×10^2PFU, 10PFU, 1PFU, respectively, of recombinant fowlpox virus contained in a volume of 0.05ml of vaccine. The sixth group was kept as control for challenge. All the chickens were challenged three weeks post-vaccination (p.v.) by intranasal administration with $100LD_{50}$ of GD1/96 isolate. The specific HI antibody induced by the vaccine was checked thee weeks after immunisation.

Experiment 4: Determination of the time of immunity induced

Eighty four-week old SPF chickens were randomly allocated into eight groups. Eight chickens of each group were vaccinated with 0.05ml vaccine containing 2×10^3PFU of rFPV-HA-NA. Another two were kept as control for challenge. Haemagglutinin inhibition (HI) antibody detection and challenge experiments were carried out at the same time, respectively, 3, 7, 10, 14, 18, 21, 28 and 35 days after immunisation.

Experiment 5: Detection of the immune duration

Eighty four-week old SPF chickens were randomly assigned ten groups. Eight chickens in each group were immunised with an immune dose of vaccine containing 2×10^3PFU of rFPV-HA-NA, another two were kept as challenge control. Individual serum was collected at 2, 4, 8, 10, 15, 20, 25, 30, 35 and 40 weeks after vaccination for HI antibody surveillance. Challenge experiments were carried out, respectively, 10, 20, 30 and 40 weeks after immunisation.

Serological tests

All the serum samples collected weekly after immunisation and challenge were stored frozen so that all tests were conducted simultaneously. The HI test was performed as described previously; in it, four HA units of GD1/96 virus was used as antigen, the HI titres were determined as reciprocals of the highest serum dilution in which inhibition of haemagglutination was observed.

Virus isolation

Cloacal swabs were taken from the surviving chickens four days after challenge with HPAIV and shaken in phosphate-buffered saline (PBS), then treated with antibiotics. Samples for virus isolation were inoculated into nine- to 11-day old embryonated SPF chicken eggs via the allantoic cavity (AC) route.

Results

Genetic stability of the recombinant fowlpox virus rFPV-HA-NA

After 25 passages, the HA and NA gene derived from 5, 15 and 25 passage recombinant virus, were sequenced, respectively. The immunogenicity of these three passages of recombinant virus were tested by inoculating SPF chickens. The results demonstrated that the sequences of these two genes remained the same, and the recombinant virus retained its immunogenicity with the passage of the virus.

Immune efficacy of the recombinant vaccine

Serum samples were collected weekly after immunisation for detection of HI antibody response. HI antibody was observed one week post-immunisation (p.i.), and rose up to 7.0log2 two weeks p.i. of chickens vaccinated with rFPV-HA-NA vaccine. In comparison, no detectable HI antibodies were present in chickens vaccinated with S-FPV-017 and unvaccinated control. Meanwhile, morbidity, mortality and reduction of viral shedding were also detected following experimental infection. Vaccinated chickens were protected from virus-shedding, clinical disease signs and death after being challenged with H5N1, while the control chickens died within two weeks.

Safety evaluation

Among the ten chickens immunised with the recombinant vaccine, no chicken was dead, and no clinical signs were observed after vaccination. So this recombinant vaccine was safe, even though one-day old SPF chickens were vaccinated with ten-times the immunising dose.

Determination of the minimum immunising dose

First, the recombinant virus vaccine was titrated on CEF cells by numbering PFU. The different dilution of recombinant virus was inoculated into SPF chickens. HI antibody was induced in each group of chickens immunised with different doses of rFPV-HA-NA vaccine. Lethal challenge with H5N1 was conducted three weeks after immunisation. The chickens immunised with 100PFU rFPV-HA-NA vaccine were 100 % protected from virus-shedding, clinical signs and death (shown in Table 1). So the minimum administration dose of the recombinant virus vaccine was 1×10^2PFU.

Table 1: Immune efficacy induced by different doses of rFPV-HA-NA vaccine.

Groups (inoculation dose, PFU)	HI Ab (log2)	No. positive/no. tested	No. sick/total	No. dead/total
10000	7.14	0/10	0/10	0/10
1000	6.33	0/10	0/10	0/10
100	4.60	0/10	0/10	0/10
10	3.32	1/10	0/10	0/10
1	3.57	2/10	2/10	1/10
Control	*	10/10	10/10	10/10

* HI antibody could not be detected.

Determination of the time of immunity appearence

HI antibodies detection and challenge trials were carried out at the same time. The HI antibodies were detected one week after vaccination titred as high as 3.58log2. Complete protection was achieved, and no chicken was sick and died, while all the control chickens died (Table 2).

Table 2: Immunity induced by the vaccine at different times after vaccination.

Time of Ab detection and challenge (days)	HI Ab (log2)	No. challenged	No. sick	No. dead	No. virus-shedding
3	0	10	10	8	10
7	3.58	10	0	0	0
10	6.09	10	0	0	0
14	6.56	10	0	0	0
18	6.80	10	0	0	0
21	6.68	10	0	0	0
28	6.92	10	0	0	0
35	6.87	10	0	0	0

Determination of the duration of immunity

Antibody titres were tested periodically after vaccination. The HI antibody titre was 6~7log2 from two to ten weeks after immunisation. The level of HI antibody titre decreased 4.5log2 25 weeks post-vaccination. The antibody titre was 3~4log2 25~40 weeks after immunisation. Challenge experiments were conducted ten, 20, 30 and 40 weeks after immunisation. All the chickens survived the lethal challenge with GD1/96.

Discussion

Although the inactivated whole virus AI vaccines have shown efficacy against the outbreak of HPAI, they induced immune responses to the group-specific influenza A nucleoprotein (NP) antigen that negates detection of natural infection [3]. Several studies were conducted on the basis of development of a novel vaccine strategy. HA and NA are the major surface glycoproteins of influenza A virus primarily involved in induction of specific humoral immunity. Functionally distinct roles have been attributed to the humoral response elicited by these two viral proteins. A variety of vaccines derived from HA and NA genes of AIV, including recombinant virus vaccine, subunit haemagglutinin protein and DNA vaccines [4-7] have been shown experimentally to be effective for immunisation against influenza. The immunogenicity of a recombinant fowlpox virus expressing HA and NA genes of avian influenza virus has been discussed in a previous paper [2]. This paper has focused on evaluating the safety and immune efficacy of this recombinant fowlpox virus vaccine.

Humoral immunity plays the key role in the immunology of avian influenza. HI antibodies could neutralise the infection of the virus, and NI antibody could restrict the replication of the infective viruses [8-9]. The level of HI antibody induced by the whole virus inactivated vaccine is correlated to the observed protection, and a level that can be considered a cut-off for susceptibility is 4log2. For the recombinant virus vaccine, the criterion may not be applicable. From our results, the HI antibodies titred as low as 3log2, the complete protection could also be achieved after vaccination with this vaccine. Even though no HI antibody could be detected, the chicken immunised with the vaccine would survive the lethal challenge with H5N1. This result was consistent with the document that recombinant vaccinia virus expressed HA gene of AIV could induce complete protection against the lethal challenge, accompanied by HI antibody titre of 1~2log2 [5]. These results confirmed that the cellular immunity of AI is also very important for the protection of chicken from the challenge. When the antibody is insufficient to induce protection, the cellular immunity could decrease the morbidity and mortality of the immunised chickens to a certain extent, though it could not protect chicken from infection by the challenge virus.

When compared to the inactivated vaccines, the recombinant fowlpox virus vaccine has three advantages. First, it does not interfere with surveillance studies monitoring natural infection in which antibodies to NP are used as marker. Secondly, the domestic poultry are, when necessary, vaccinated against fowlpox; the use of a fowlpox vector has another important advantage that it can be used to produce multivalent vaccines providing protection against both AI and fowlpox. Finally, the recombinant vaccine avoids the adjuvant, a component of an inactivated vaccine, which makes it much safer than the latter for public health.

The recombinant fowlpox virus vaccine can provide excellent protection against the lethal challenge with H5N1. If the chicken was preimmunised with a fowlpox vaccine or infected with fowlpox virus, how about the immune efficacy of the recombinant fowlpox virus vaccine? SPF chickens were infected with fowlpox virus named S-FPV-017, then they were immunised with recombinant fowlpox vaccine at various time intervals. The results showed that, whether the immunisation with recombinant vaccine and infection with S-FPV-017 was at the same time or at an interval of more than four weeks there was no effect of infection by fowlpox virus on the immune efficacy of the recombinant fowlpox virus vaccine (data unpublished). This is inconsistent with the previous report that the use of FPV-based vector vaccine is only effective in chickens without prior vaccination against FPV and prior exposure to field strains of FPV would also be expected to limited protection induced by this vaccine [10].

In conclusion, our results demonstrate the development of a safe and effective vaccine to prevent the outbreak of H5 subtype AI.

References

1 Subbarao K, Klimov A, Katz J, Regnery H, Lim W, Hall H, Perdue M, Swayne D, Bender C, Huang J, Hemphill M, Rowe T, Shaw M, Xu X, Fukuda K, Cox N: Characterization of an avian influenza A (H5N1) virus isolate from a child with a fatal respiratory illness. Science 1998; 297: 393-396.

2 Qiao CL, Yu KZ, Jiang YP, Jia YQ, Tian GB, Liu M, Deng GH, Wang XR, Meng QW, Tang XY: Protection of chickens against highly lethal H5N1 and H7N1 avian influenza viruses with a recombinant fowlpox virus co-expressing H5 haemagglutinin and N1 neuraminidase genes. Avian Pathology 2003; 32: 25-31.

3 Beard CW, Schnitzlein WM, Tripathy DN: Protection of chickens against highly pathogenic avian influenza virus (H5N2) by recombinant fowlpox viruses. Avian Disease 1991; 35: 356-359.

4 Kodihalli S, Sivanandan V, Nagaraja KV, Shaw D, Halvorson DA: A type-specific avian influenza virus subunit vaccine for turkeys: induction of protective immunity to challenge infection. Vaccine 1994; 12: 1467-1472.

5 Chamber T, Kawaoka Y, Webster RG.: Protection of chickens from lethal influenza infection by vaccinia expressed hemagglutinin. Virology 1988; 167: 414-421.

6 Kodihalli S, Goto H, Kobasa DL: DNA vaccine encoding hemagglutinin provides protective immunity against H5N1 influenza virus infection in mice. Journal of Virology 1999; 73: 2094-2098.

7 Chen Z, Kadowaki S, Hagiwara Y, Yoshikawa T, Matsuo K, Kurata T, Tamura S: Cross-protection against a lethal influenza virus infection by DNA vaccine to neuraminidase. Vaccine 2000; 18: 3214-3222.

8 Deroo T, Jou WM, Fiers W: Recombinant neuraminidase vaccine protects against lethal influenza. Vaccine 1996; 14 (6): 561-569.

9 Wood JM, Kawaoka LA, Newberry E: Standardization of inactivated H5N2 influenza vaccine and efficacy against lethal A/Chicken/pennsylvania/1370/83 infection. Avian Disease 1985; 29 (3): 867-872.

10 Swayne DE, Beck JR, Kinney N: Failure of a recombinant fowlpox virus vaccine containing an avian influenza hemagglutinin gene to provide consistent protection against influenza in chickens preimmunized with a fowl pox vaccine. Avian Disease 2000; 44: 132-137.

Dr. Hualan Chen, National Avian Influenza Reference Laboratory, Animal Influenza Laboratory of the Ministry of Agriculture, Harbin Veterinary Research Institute, CAAS, 427 Maduan Street, Harbin 150001, P.R. China.
E-mail: hlchen@hvri.ac.cn

Schudel A, Lombard M (eds): OIE/FAO International Scientific Conference on Avian Influenza.
Dev Biol (Basel). Basel, Karger, 2006, vol 124, pp 133-143.

Use of Avian Influenza Vaccination in Hong Kong

T.M. Ellis[1], *L.D. Sims*[1], *H.K.H. Wong*[1], *C.W. Wong*[1], *K.C. Dyrting*[1], *K.W. Chow*[1], *C. Leung*[2], *J.S.M. Peiris*[2]

[1] Agriculture Fisheries and Conservation Department, Kowloon, Hong Kong SAR
[2] Department of Microbiology, The University of Hong Kong, Hong Kong SAR.

Abstract: Outbreaks of H5N1 highly pathogenic avian influenza (HPAI) that occurred in Hong Kong up until February/March 2002 were controlled by stamping out. With endemic presence of the virus in the region and large daily importation of poultry to Hong Kong, the Administration considered that further risk management measures, in addition to improved biosecurity and enhanced surveillance, were necessary to prevent outbreaks. Vaccination using a killed H5N2 vaccine was evaluated over a 12-month period in the district with the last HPAI cases in the early 2002 outbreak. The vaccination trial showed that farmer-administered killed H5N2 vaccine produced suitable flock antibody responses; vaccinated birds were protected against H5N1 HPAI virus challenge and excreted significantly less H5N1 virus; and vaccination was able to control virus excretion in flocks during field outbreaks.

Universal vaccination of local chicken farms was introduced in June 2003 and by the end of 2003 all chickens entering the live poultry markets in Hong Kong were vaccinated by killed H5N2 vaccine. In addition to vaccination, an enhanced biosecurity programme on farms and in live poultry markets and a comprehensive surveillance programme in poultry, wild birds, recreation park birds and pet birds were in place. Vaccination use and performance is closely monitored. This programme was successful in protecting local farms and live poultry markets from H5N1 outbreaks during the regional H5N1 outbreaks in 2004.

INTRODUCTION

A major outbreak of H5N1 highly pathogenic avian influenza (HPAI) occurred in 1997 in Hong Kong during which the virus directly infected humans, causing 18 influenza cases with death in six people and resulted in the total depopulation of the poultry population (1.3 million birds) [1]. As a result of the socio-economic and public health impacts of this outbreak the Administration of Hong Kong SAR and the re-established poultry industry progressively enhanced risk control measures to prevent further outbreaks of avian influenza. From 1998 the farming of ducks and geese stopped and imported live waterfowl entered Hong Kong via sea-routes to a separate wholesale market and were centrally slaughtered so no live waterfowl entered the retail live poultry markets.

However further outbreaks occurred in chickens and other gallinaceous poultry in 2001, 2002 and 2003 [2,3]. The 2001 the retail poultry market H5N1 HPAI outbreak resulted in the culling of 440,000 birds in poultry markets, closure of the markets and culling of 800,000 unaffected older market age chickens on farms. The H5N1 HPAI outbreaks on 22 farms in February-March 2002 resulted in the culling of 900,000 chickens. In December 2002 exceptional outbreaks of H5N1 HPAI occurred in waterfowl (geese, ducks and swans) and other wild water birds (Little Egrets *Egretta garzetta*, and captive Greater Flamingo *Phoenicopterus ruber*) at two recreation parks in Hong Kong as well as two dead wild Grey Heron (*Ardea cinerea*) and a Black – headed Gull (*Larus ridibundus*) [3]. At the time of the second waterfowl outbreak there were also outbreaks in some retail poultry markets and in late December 2002-January 2003 there were outbreaks on five chicken farms (three districts).

After the 2001 outbreak the poultry farm and market biosecurity measures and monitoring systems in place since 1998 were further enhanced. Detailed epidemiological study of the February-April 2002 H5N1 HPAI outbreak by an Investigation Team recommended further measures to improve farm and market biosecurity. All these measures have now been included in individual farm biosecurity plans for all local poultry farms and these form part of the poultry farm licence conditions.

Chicken farms in Hong Kong are generally family run farms growing the slow-growing Shek-kee or yellow chicken that reaches market age at 90-100 days. Most are grower farms receiving one-day old chickens imported from Mainland China but recently some farms are now also breeding and hatching in Hong Kong for their own supply and supplying one-day old chickens to other farms. From about three-four weeks the chickens are reared in A-frame cages and batches of the same age are segregated from other batches. At present there are 148 licensed farms with a licence capacity for between 3.0 and 3.7 million birds depending on market age and current bird numbers at 2.9 million birds. All birds are sold through a central live poultry wholesale market and then move to retail live poultry markets located in wet markets throughout Hong Kong where birds are purchased live and killed and dressed within the market stall. Before 2004 the local industry supplied approximately 25 % of the demand for chickens with the remainder imported mostly from Mainland China, but since then local farms have been supplying approximately 50 % of the demand.

After the additional outbreaks of H5N1 HPAI in 2001 and early 2002 and due to the large daily movement of poultry into Hong Kong from southern China and the endemic presence of H5N1 virus in the region, the Administration considered H5 avian influenza vaccine may be an additional risk management measure that could be considered along with enhanced biosecurity and surveillance activities.

Vaccines have been used in other countries to assist in the control of avian influenza. Countries using vaccines against influenza viruses include Italy [4], USA [5], Mexico and Pakistan [6]. Mostly vaccination has been directed against low pathogenic strains of avian influenza virus but Mexico and Pakistan have successfully used vaccine against highly pathogenic H5 or H7 avian influenza viruses. Experimental studies have shown that commercially available H5 avian influenza vaccines could protect poultry from 1997 Hong Kong strains of H5N1 HPAI virus [7].

The year-long field evaluation trial of a commercial killed H5N2 vaccine on chicken farms in Hong Kong is reported. The effect of vaccination in the face of an outbreak was also examined in three chicken farms which were not included in the original vaccination evaluation trials. The current avian influenza control programme including vaccination, biosecurity on farms and in live bird markets and the surveillance programme for early detection and the monitoring of the programme, are discussed.

Materials and Methods

The vaccine used in Hong Kong

The vaccine used in these evaluations was Nobilis® Influenza H5, an inactivated avian influenza Type A H5N2 virus (A/Chicken/Mexico/232/94/CPA) water-in-oil emulsion vaccine (Intervet International, Boxmeer, The Netherlands) given as a 0.5 ml dose subcutaneously into the neck in young chickens and intramuscularly into the breast muscle of older chickens. The vaccination was farmer-administered but advice on technique was given by the Agriculture, Fisheries and Conservation Department (AFCD) staff.

The initial evaluation trial was conducted on chicken farms in the district involved in the last four cases of H5N1 HPAI in the February-April 2002 outbreak (Phase 1). After H5N1 HPAI outbreaks in waterfowl parks and wild birds in December 2002, the vaccination programme was extended to farms considered at higher risk from wild bird transmission (Phase 2). Subsequently, with H5N1 HPAI outbreaks on five unvaccinated chicken farms, vaccination was used during the outbreak on three farms and its effect was evaluated (Phase 3).

Phase 1 vaccination programme

Phase 1 vaccine evaluation was conducted on 22 chicken farms in the Pak Sha district of the New Territories in Hong Kong and located within 2 kms of the last four chicken farms infected with H5N1 virus in the February-April 2002 outbreak. Vaccinations commenced in April 2002 and the programme continued on these farms until March 2003. In the first round all chickens between eight and 55 days of age were vaccinated and revaccinated four weeks later. Subsequently, all new batches of chickens were vaccinated at eight-10 days of age and again four weeks later. Each batch had a group of 30 individually identified chickens left unvaccinated (sentinels).

Blood was collected from the 30 unvaccinated sentinel chickens and 30 individually identified vaccinated chickens four weeks after the first and second dose of vaccine and again within five days of sale. Serum was tested by standard haemagglutination inhibition test for antibody to H5 avian influenza using avian influenza A/chicken/Hong Kong/97 (H5N1) virus antigen. Sentinel or vaccinated chickens that died were subjected to necropsy examination and tested for the presence of avian influenza virus by standard procedures [8]. Before sale a sample of 60 chickens per batch had cloacal swabs collected and tested for presence of H5 virus by NASBA [9] or real-time RT-PCR [10].

Empirically set criteria for successful use of vaccine in this farmer-administered vaccination programme were based on the World Health Organisation reported success rate for human influenza vaccines in vaccinated adult populations [11]. The criteria for successful vaccination was ≥ 70 % of chickens per batch had a HI titre ≥ 16 and the geometric mean titre (GMT) by HI test of the batch was ≥ 20 after two doses of vaccine. Statistical analysis was conducted on post-vaccination antibody responses on the vaccinated flocks from these farms using analysis of covariance with repeated measures.

Experimental challenge procedures

An experimental challenge with a current H5N1 virus was conducted in a biosafety level 3 laboratory using 71 day-old vaccinated and sentinel chickens from a single batch of chickens from one vaccinated farm. The virus used was a H5N1 (Z genotype) virus isolated from a dead chicken from a retail poultry market in April 2002. The virus was inoculated via the eye, nose and beak into 10 vaccinated chickens and 10 sentinel chickens so that each chicken was challenged via eyes nares and orally with approximately 15,000 ($10^{4.2}$) egg infectious doses (EID) of virus per chicken.

After challenge all chickens were examined daily for signs of disease and swabs were collected daily from cloaca and throat of all surviving chickens for the duration of the trial (10 days). Virus infectivity in the swabs was titrated in nine-11 day old SPF chicken embryos via the allantoic route. Surviving chickens were tested for antibody at 10 days post-challenge.

In parallel with challenge studies conducted in Hong Kong, a similar challenge was conducted by Professor Robert Webster at the WHO Animal Influenza Reference Laboratory, Memphis using the same vaccine administered at the same ages to Leghorn chickens and challenged with 10 or 100 Chicken Lethal Dose$_{50}$ (CLD_{50}) 21 days post-vaccination with H5N1 (Z genotype) virus isolated from the index farm from the February-March 2002 outbreak [12].

Phase 2 vaccination programme

In late December 2002 a decision was taken to extend the H5N2 vaccination programme to areas around the initial 22 farms and to farms deemed to have a high potential risk of exposure to wild birds (Phase 2 vaccination programme). This was done in response waterfowl wild bird and retail poultry market outbreaks.

Vaccination commenced on 53 farms from 23 December 2002. As with the Phase 1 (Pak Sha) vaccination trial, initially all chickens up to 55 days of age were vaccinated twice at a monthly interval and then subsequent batches of chickens were vaccinated at eight and 36 days of age. Antibody response was measured a month after the second vaccination to determine the proportion of batches with ≥ 70 % of chickens with HI antibody titre ≥ 16 and the overall percentage of chickens with HI antibody titre ≥ 16.

Phase 3 – vaccination of chicken flocks during an outbreak

In late December 2002 to the end of January 2003, outbreaks of HPAI caused by H5N1 virus occurred on five previously unvaccinated chicken farms. Immediate quarantine and movement control was initiated and two farms were completely depopulated. On three farms affected sheds were depopulated and strict biosecurity procedures, vaccination and close daily monitoring of other sheds and surrounding farms started. In two farms (TKP1 and TKP2) infection spread to adjacent sheds before vaccination had time to induce an immune response. This enabled monitoring of the effect of the vaccine in the face of field challenge with virulent H5N1 virus as reported previously [13].

Universal vaccination and monitoring programme in Hong Kong

After completion of the vaccine evaluation programme and detailed assessment and consideration, the Administration approved universal vaccination of chickens entering the live poultry markets as an additional risk management procedure to enhanced biosecurity on farms and in markets and a comprehensive early detection surveillance programme for the control of avian influenza in Hong Kong. Universal vaccination with killed H5N2 vaccine in Hong Kong farms commenced in June 2003 with birds receiving two doses (eight-10 days and 38-40 days of age); breeder birds also received booster injections at 12 and 18 weeks and then six-monthly boosters. The monitoring of vaccine usage on local chicken farms involved close monitoring of bird numbers in batches by AFCD field staff by farm inspection and farm data bases with licensed farm capacity, data on number of day-old chickens entering farms and number of birds sold to market. The vaccine supply is restricted to local chicken farmers and is controlled by an industry organization (New Territories Chicken Breeders Association – NTCBA) and based on the number of day-old chickens entering the farm. The vaccine sales records are provided to AFCD for entry to the farm database and on the inspection visits the farmers return the empty vaccine vials to AFCD staff as evidence of use.

The inspection and testing process on local farms includes the use of 60 individually tagged unvaccinated sentinel chickens in every batch of chickens on farm and these are dispersed randomly throughout the shed. Any sick/dead sentinels must be reported and investigated, including virology testing. Fourteen vaccinated and 14 sentinel chickens are blood sampled at day 64 (one month after the second vaccine dose) and tested for antibody to H5 avian influenza by HI test to monitor vaccine response in vaccinates and to check for absence of H5 low pathogenic avian influenza virus and to check that the farmer has not vaccinated the sentinels. A database of vaccine antibody responses for batches of chickens from every farm is maintained by AFCD and summary data are monitored to check that the vaccine efficacy is being maintained. If a batch of chickens shows a poor antibody response a third dose of vaccine must be given and arrangements are made with NTCBA to supply additional vaccine to the farmer.

Within five days of sale the number of sentinels is counted by AFCD staff and 14 sentinels are again bled and tested for H5 antibody. If there is an unexplained loss of sentinels or any evidence of H5 antibody responses in sentinels, virological investigation is conducted on cloacal swabs from 60 birds from the batch by RRT-PCR. All testing must be passed before a sale approval is provided by AFCD for that batch of chickens.

To address concerns that vaccination may mask the presence of infection with H5 viruses a surveillance programme was introduced, whereby each month 100 swabs of fresh faecal droppings are randomly collected from the cages from 13 farms and these undergo virus culture in nine-11 day-old SPF chicken embryos.

Experience with H5N2 vaccination of waterfowl in a recreation park in Hong Kong

The waterfowl collection in Kowloon Park was a valuable zoological collection of mature waterfowl species from around the world and when the H5N1 outbreak was detected on 20 December 2002, strict quarantine was instigated, with the separation of sick birds to an isolation area for nursing. To attempt to salvage some of the collection, emergency vaccination of 163 healthy birds was undertaken on 20-21 December using a standard 0.5 ml dose of the above killed H5N2 vaccinen. Cloacal and throat swabs were collected from these birds at the time of vaccination. A second vaccination was given to 80 surviving birds on 10 January 2003 and swabs were again collected for virus culture. Subsequently a sub-sample of ducks at Kowloon Park and from another zoological waterfowl collection at Hong Kong Zoological and Botanical Gardens (HKZBG) that were similarly vaccinated had blood collected for H5 antibody testing by HI test.

Results

Antibody responses and virus monitoring on Phase 1 farms

In total, 248 batches of chickens involving 1.35 million birds were vaccinated and fully tested by 31 March 2003. No clinical outbreaks of disease associated with H5N1 virus were detected on any of these vaccinated farms. Nor was any H5N1 virus detected in tests conducted on the chickens from these farms before sale or on dead sentinel chickens. Ninety-eight percent of batches had detectable antibody after the first dose of vaccination and 80 % of the 248 batches of chickens developed satisfactory antibody levels after two doses of vaccination. The monthly breakdown of results for field vaccinations are shown in Table 1.

Analysis of the data showed associations between the vaccination of older chickens, farm of origin and batch variation with poor responses to vaccination and this

Table 1: Results of Phase 1 vaccination in Pak Sha based on the month when chickens received the first dose of vaccine.

Month given first dose	Number of successful batches	Total batches vaccinated	Proportion successful batches (%)	Mean no. antibody positive[a]	Mean antibody titre[b]
April 2002	21	42	50 %	70 %	31.0
May 2002	14	21	67 %	76 %	37.7
June 2002	17	27	65.4 %	70 %	39.3
July 2002	17[c]	23	73.9 %	82 %	49.3
August 2002	16	17	94.2 %	86 %	50.6
Sept. 2002	23	25	92 %	87.7 %	75.2
Oct. 2002	25	28	89.3 %	84.8 %	69.6
Nov. 2002	25	29	86.2 %	84.4 %	66.4
Dec. 2002	16	20	80.0 %	77.5 %	43.4
Jan. 2003	13	16	81.3 %	85.2 %	53.8
Total	**188**	**248**	**75.8 %**	**80.5 %[d]**	**50.9[d]**

[a] % of birds with HI titre $\geq$ 16 at one month after second vaccination.

[b] Mean geometric mean titre of batches at one month after second vaccination.

[c] Five of these batches were very marginally below the success target.

[d] Weighted mean allowing for numbers of batches per month.

may have been related to the presence of immunosuppressive diseases in 20-50 day-old chickens that were detected in investigations of dead birds from vaccinated batches of chickens in these farms during the evaluations as reported previously [14].

Experimental challenge

The H5 HI titres in the vaccinated chickens at challenge ranged from 32 to 256. No sentinel chickens had antibody to H5 influenza virus. After challenge, none of the vaccinated chickens became ill, whereas all the unvaccinated sentinel chickens died within three days. This indicated a highly significant level of protection (Chi-square = 20, p = 0.00000). Vaccinated chickens excreted markedly reduced titres of virus via cloaca or throat. Throat swabs from unvaccinated chickens contained an average of 18,000 EID of virus. No vaccinated chickens had detectable virus in throat or cloaca on day two or any other day except for day four post-infection when two vaccinated chickens had low levels of virus in the throat ($10^{1.0}$ EID) (Table 2).

Table 2: Summary of results of experimental H5N1 challenge in Hong Kong.

Group	Proportion infected (mean days to first signs)	Proportion dead (mean death time)	HI antibody positive 10 days post-challenge	Cloacal virus (titre on day two)[a]	Throat virus (titre on day two)[a]
Not vaccinated	10/10 (2)	10/10 (2.3)	None survived	7/10 ($10^{2.03}$)	10/10 ($10^{4.25}$)
Vaccinated (GMT = 119)	0/10	0/10	10/10 (GMT = 239)	0/10	0/10[b]

[a] Virus titre = Log_{10} embryo infectious doses (EID) per swab via chicken embryo allantoic route.

[b] Virus was detected in two vaccinated birds at low level ($10^{1.0}$ EID) on day four only.

Similar results were obtained from Professor Webster's Laboratory in Memphis with respect to protection from disease and reduction in the level of virus excretion in vaccinated chickens after one or two doses of this vaccine and challenged with a similar H5N1 HPAI (Z genotype virus) [12].

Phase 2 – vaccination programme

A total of 60 batches of chickens were vaccinated during the evaluation period. Thirty-two batches (53.3 %) had ≥ 70 % of chickens with HI antibody titre ≥ 16 and overall 69.2 % of the chickens had HI antibody titre ≥ 16.

No clinical outbreaks of disease associated with H5N1 virus infection were detected on any of the Phase 2 vaccinated farms, no H5N1 virus was detected in tests conducted on any dead or sick chickens submitted from these farms as part of the sentinel and surveillance programme and none of the sentinel chickens gave positive H5 antibody results. Some 1.55 million vaccine doses were given to chickens on these farms with no adverse effects apparent from use of this killed vaccine.

The vaccination response in Phase 2 was not significantly different from that for the first round of Phase 1, which also involved vaccination of birds ranging from eight to 55 days of age. In Phase 2 nearly half (28/60) the batches received their first dose of vaccine when older than 21 days of age and only 19 batches received their first vaccination at eight-10 days of age. Problems of vaccination technique with older chickens and immuno-suppressive diseases are likely to have had a similar effect on the first round of vaccination on these farms as they did with the Phase 1 farms.

Phase 3 – vaccination of chicken flocks during an outbreak

As reported previously [13], on farm TK1 infection spread fairly quickly to nine out of 10 sheds which had all been depopulated by day nine post-vaccination. H5N1 infection was detected with low levels of mortality in the more remote shed two on day nine post-vaccination (p/v) and low rates of H5N1 mortality continued to be detected until day 18 p/v. However, subsequently no sick or dead birds were diagnosed as H5 avian influenza in shed two and no subclinical infection with H5N1 virus was detected by virus culture of 1080 randomly collected cloacal and throat swabs from this shed by AFCD or staff from the Department of Microbiology from the University of Hong Kong. Sequential H5 HI antibody measurement in vaccinated chickens in shed two showed that by day 15 p/v 53.3 % of chickens were HI test positive (Titre ≥ 16) and by day 22 p/v 81.7 % of chickens were positive with a GMT of 33.9. By this time there had been no mortalities due to H5 avian influenza or H5 virus isolations for four days.

Similarly on farm TK2, dead bird monitoring showed that a small number of chickens in three sheds died of H5N1 HPAI when the birds were 13-17 days p/v and there was only limited disease in these sheds over a two-day period. Subsequently virus culture testing of cloacal swabs collected from 700 randomly sampled chickens was negative for H5N1 viruses. Sequential H5 HI antibody measurement in vaccinated chickens in one shed at day 10 p/v showed 42.9 % of chickens were HI test positive (Titre ≥ 16), in another shed at day 13 p/v showed 28.6 % of chickens were positive, and in both sheds by days 30 to 33 p/v all chickens were HI test positive.

Monitoring of H5N2 vaccination in Hong Kong

No further outbreaks of H5N1 avian influenza or evidence of H5N1 infection has occurred in Hong Kong chicken farms since universal killed H5N2 vaccination was added to other control measures and there have been no further isolations of H5 viruses in the comprehensive live poultry market surveillance despite the widespread H5N1 outbreaks in the region in 2004 and 2005 so far. During this period H5N1 HPAI viruses have been isolated in Hong Kong from migratory wild birds including individual Peregrine Falcon in January 2004, individual Grey Herons in November and December 2004, and a Chinese pond Heron in January 2005.

The serological monitoring of vaccine antibody responses in local chicken farms for 2004 has continued to indicate similar antibody responses to those present during the vaccine evaluation phase, as indicated in Table 3.

Experience with H5N2 vaccination of waterfowl during H5N1 outbreak

The daily mortality graph for the waterfowl at Kowloon Park during the H5N1 outbreak (Fig. 1) indicates that new cases of disease stopped by days 11-12 p/v. Species previously shown to be susceptible to lethal H5N1 infection were still present in the remaining waterfowl population at this time. However, antibody responses to the vaccine in a ducks from a non-exposed waterfowl collection (HKZBG) were considerably poorer than ducks from Kowloon Park that had been exposed to H5N1 virus and vaccinated (Table 4). At the time of the first vaccination 27/163 apparently healthy waterfowl were H5N1 virus-positive but by the time of the second vaccination 21 days later, all 80 vaccinated waterfowl were H5N1 virus-negative.

Table 3: Monthly summary of post-vaccination H5 antibody responses in H5N2 vaccinated chicken farms in Hong Kong in 2004.

Month	Batches that reached target serology %[a]	Batches that reached target GMT ≥ 20	Mean of GMT
January	182/257 (70.8 %)	170/257 (66.1 %)	44.45
February	159/224 (71 %)	164/224 (73.2 %)	51.43
March	206/251 (82 %)	204/251 (81.3 %)	61.54
April	81/109 (74.3 %)	80/109 (73.4 %)	63.69
May	36/55 (65.5 %)	38/55 (69.1 %)	40.54
June	60/80 (75 %)	63/80 (78.8 %)	55.00
July	77/83 (92.8 %)	80/83 (96.4 %)	82.88
August	109/122 (89.3 %)	109/122 (89.3 %)	82.51
September	263/309 (85.1 %)	276/309 (89.3 %)	76.72
October	232/242 (95.9 %)	235/242 (97.1 %)	94.53
November	210/239 (87.9 %)	222/239 (92.9 %)	84.78
December	220/270 (81.5 %)	228/270 (84.4 %)	77.21

[a] Target serology % is ≥ 70 % of batch with H5 haemagglutination inhibition (HI) test titre ≥ 16.

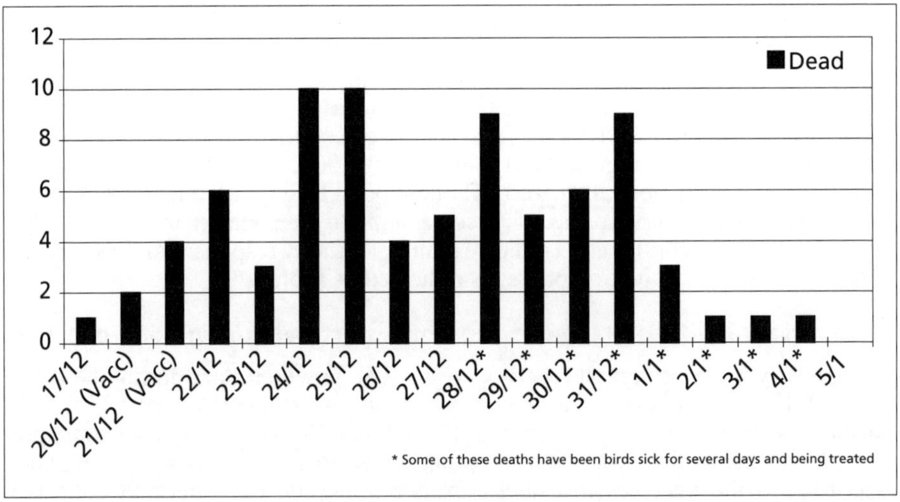

Fig. 1: Waterfowl deaths at Kowloon Park during H5N1 outbreak.

Table 4: H5 antibody responses by HI tests after killed H5N2 vaccine in ducks in Hong Kong.

Time post-vaccination[a]	Exposed to H5N1 virus and vaccinated (Kowloon Park)	Time post-vaccination	Not exposed but vaccinated (HKZBG)
42 days	21/24 antibody + ve[b]	37 days	3/10 antibody + ve
131 days	10/13 antibody + ve	127 days	2/6 antibody + ve

a Time after first dose of vaccination course of two doses of vaccine given at 21 days interval.

b Antibody positive indicates HI titre ≥ 16.

Discussion

The vaccine evaluation study vaccine showed that the commercially available killed H5N2 avian influenza could protect vaccinated chickens against highly pathogenic avian influenza caused by the H5N1 (Z genotype) viruses involved in the 2002 outbreak in Hong Kong and produce a very significant reduction (> 1000-fold) in the excretion of infectious H5N1 virus in vaccinated compared with unvaccinated chickens. As a farmer-administered vaccination programme, good flock H5 antibody responses resulted for most batches of chickens when immunosuppressive infectious diseases were under control and when used in the face of field challenge, the vaccine was able to protect chickens and interrupt virus transmission by 13-18 days p/v.

Concerns that needed to be addressed before the decision to add universal vaccination to the risk management programme in Hong Kong included: (i) whether the H5N2 vaccine would continue to be efficacious against newly evolving strains of H5 avian influenza virus in the region; (ii) whether continued virus shedding in vaccinated chickens would go undetected; (iii) whether emerging virus strains would go undetected in vaccinated chickens; and (iv) whether vaccination may undermine the efforts to improve biosecurity on farms and in live poultry markets. Experimental studies have shown that antibodies generated to a H5 subtype-specific vaccine can cross-protect against field strains varying up to 13 % in the haemagglutinin-deduced amino acid sequence [6] so it could be expected that the H5N2 vaccine would continue to have efficacy against evolving H5 virus strains in the region. Recent challenge studies with this killed H5N2 vaccine against a 2003/2004 H5N1 (Z genotype) HPAI virus from Vietnam by Dr. D. Swayne at the South East Poultry Research Laboratory, USDA, showed protection from disease and > 10,000-fold reduction of virus shedding in vaccinated birds given a heavy experimental challenge. Monitoring for continuing vaccine efficacy and the other concerns were addressed by ensuring that a comprehensive system of virus surveillance was in place for early detection and characterization of H5 viruses circulating in vaccinated flocks and by linking individual farm biosecurity and live poultry market biosecurity plans to farm or market licences, then enforcing compliance.

After consideration of the vaccine evaluation results and the above concerns the Administration approved universal vaccination of chickens on local farms and negotiated vaccination of land-based poultry on farms from Mainland China that supply the Hong Kong market. Universal H5N2 vaccination commenced on local farms in June 2003 and by the end of the year in Mainland farms. A comprehensive virus monitoring and surveillance programme was put in place to detect the presence of H5N1 and other avian influenza viruses in poultry farms, wholesale and retail live poultry markets, wild birds (particularly water birds), captive birds, especially waterfowl in recreational parks, pet birds, imported aviary birds and imported chilled or frozen poultry products. Any H5 viruses isolated will be genetically and antigenically characterized.

Biosecurity procedures on poultry farms are incorporated into an individual farm biosecurity plan which forms part of the farm licence and penalties or even cancellation of the farm licence can be imposed for failure to adhere to biosecurity requirements. Currently there are 58 biosecuity conditions applied to chicken farms in Hong Kong, including bird-proofing of all sheds, foot baths at shed doors, vehicle washing points on entry gates, and strict control on the use of washed and disinfected transport cages. Adherence is monitored by AFCD staff during inspection visits for vaccine monitoring or pre-sale inspection visits. Similarly, live poultry market stalls have biosecurity and hygiene conditions imposed, including the implementation of two rest days per month where all markets stalls and the wholesale market on those days are completely emptied of birds, cleaned and thoroughly disinfected. Failure to comply can result in the loss of stall licences and adherence is monitored by the Health Inspectors from the Food and Environmental Hygiene Department.

With concerns about control strategies for H5N1 infection in farmed ducks in South-East Asia, the results of vaccination of ducks in the Kowloon Park outbreak with the killed H5N2 vaccine are interesting. By 11-12 days p/v mortality had stopped and by 21 days p/v no further virus shedding occurred. In ducks that were exposed to virus then vaccinated at Kowloon Park, 87 % were H5 antibody-positive three weeks after a second and 77 % were positive three months later, whereas for HKZBG ducks not exposed to virus but vaccinated with the same vaccine, only 30 % were antibody positive. This vaccine is not currently licensed for use in ducks but recent information provided from the manufacturer (Intervet) indicated that increasing the vaccine dose to 1.0 ml resulted in acceptable HI antibody responses in eight out of nine ducks vaccinated at three weeks of age (Dr. V. Leong, personal communication).

Conclusions

The programme for control and risk management of H5N1 avian influenza in Hong Kong will continue to be based on enhanced biosecurity on poultry farms and in live poultry markets, a comprehensive surveillance and monitoring programme for early detection of virus incursions and the universal use of the killed H5N2 vaccination. This programme is expected to remain in place until comprehensive regional surveillance indicates this virus has been effectively controlled. The efficacy of the vaccine will be continually monitored and if the level of protection and control against potential newly emerging H5 virus strains falls, more appropriate vaccine strains will be considered.

Acknowledgements

We wish to acknowledge the excellent technical support provided by the staff of the Avian Virology, Serology and Molecular Biology Laboratories at Tai Lung Veterinary Laboratory and Livestock Farm Division of AFCD and the Leisure and Cultural Services Department staff at Kowloon Park and HKZBG for their support during investigations of the waterfowl outbreak. We also acknowledge the advice and support from Directorate staff, Dr. K. K. Liu and Mr. Lai Ching-Wai and from Import/Export Division staff led by Dr. Richard Rubira from AFCD.

References

1 Shortridge KF, Gao P, Guan Y, Ito T, Kawaoka Y, Markwell D, Takada A, Webster RG: A review of interspecies transmission of influenza viruses: the Hong Kong perspective. Veterinary Microbiology 2000; 74: 141-147.

2 Sims LD, Ellis TM, Liu KK, Dyrting K, Wong H, Peiris M, Guan Y, Shortridge KF: Avian influenza in Hong Kong 1997-2002. Avian Diseases 2003; 47: 832-838.

3 Ellis TM, Bousfield RB, Bissett LA, Dyrting KC, Luk GSM, Tsim ST, Sturm-Ramirez K, Webster RG, Guan Y, Peiris JSM: Investigation of outbreaks of highly pathogenic H5N1 avian influenza in waterfowl and wild birds in Hong Kong in late 2002. Avian Pathology 2004; 33: 492-505.

4 Capua I, Terregino C, Cattoli G, Mutinelli F, Rodriguez JF: Development of a DIVA (Differentiating Infected from Vaccinated Animals) strategy using a vaccine containing a heterologous neuraminidase for the control of avian influenza. Avian Pathology 2002; 32: 47-55.

5 Halvorson DA: The control of H5 or H7 mildly pathogenic avian influenza: a role for inactivated vaccine. Avian Pathology 2002; 31: 5-12.

6 Swayne DE, Suarez DL: Highly pathogenic avian influenza. Revue of Science and Technology of the Office International des Epizooties 2000; 19: 463-482.

7 Swayne DE, Beck JR, Perdue ML, Beard CW: Efficacy of vaccines in chickens against highly pathogenic Hong Kong H5N1 avian influenza. Avian Diseases 2001; 45: 355-365.

8 Alexander DJ: Highly Pathogenic Avian Influenza, in OIE Manual of Standards for Diagnostic Tests and Vaccines. Fourth Edition. Paris: Office International des Epizooties. 2000, pp 212-220.

9 Collins RA, Ko LS, So KL, Ellis T, Lau LT, Cheung HY: Detection of highly pathogenic and low pathogenic avian influenza subtype H5 (Eurasian lineage) using NASBA. J Virol Methods 2002; 103: 213-225.

10 Spackman E, Senne DA, Myers TJ, Bulaga LL, Garber LP, Perdue ML, Lohman K, Daum LT, Suarez DL: Development of a real-time reverse transcriptase PCR assay for type A influenza virus and the avian H5 and H7 hemagglutinin subtypes. J Clin Micro 2002; 40: 3256-3260.

11 Anon.: Studies with inactivated influenza virus vaccines, in Weekly Epidemiological Record. World Health Org, Geneva, 2003, vol 9, p 60.

12 Liu M, Wood JM, Ellis T, Krauss S, Seiler P, Johnson C, Hoffmann E, Humberd J, Perez D, Hulse D, Zhang Y, Webster RG, Perez DR: Preparation of a standardized, efficacious, agricultural H5N3 vaccine by reverse genetics. Virology 2003; 314: 580-590.

13 Ellis TM, Leung YHC, Chow KWM, Bissett LA, Wong W, Guan Y, Peiris JSM: Vaccination of chickens against H5N1 avian influenza in the face of an outbreak interrupts virus transmission. Avian Pathology 2004; 33: 405-412.

14 Ellis TM, Sims LD, Wong HKH, Bissett LA, Dyrting KC, Chow KW, Wong CW: Evaluation of vaccination to support control of H5N1 avian influenza in Hong Kong, in Koch G, Schrijver R (eds): Wageningen UR Frontis Series: Avian influenza, prevention and control. Dordrecht, Kluwer Academic Publishers, 2004, pp 75-84.

Dr. K. Dyrting, Agriculture Fisheries and Conservation Department, 303 Cheung Sha Wan Road Kowloon, Hong Kong SAR.
E-mail: k_c_dyrting@afcd.gov.hk

Schudel A, Lombard M (eds): OIE/FAO International Scientific Conference on Avian Influenza.
Dev Biol (Basel). Basel, Karger, 2006, vol 124, pp 145-150.

Use of Strategic Vaccination for the Control of Avian Influenza in Pakistan

K. Naeem, N. Siddique

Central Avian Influenza Monitoring Laboratory, National Reference Laboratory for Poultry Diseases, Animal Sciences Institute, National Agricultural Research Centre, Islamabad, Pakistan

Key words: Avian influenza, vaccination, disease control.

Abstract: The first outbreak of highly pathogenic avian influenza (HPAI) virus caused by subtype H7N3 appeared in Pakistan in 1995. A homologous aqueous-based vaccine prepared from the field isolate employed as ring vaccination around the epicentre of the outbreak helped in controlling the disease. Later, in 1998, an outbreak of avian influenza virus (AIV) subtype H9N2, particularly affecting the broilers and broiler-breeders, was dealt with using the same vaccination approach. However, this time, the virus could not be successfully contained in the affected areas. Later on, low pathogenic avian influenza (LPAI) virus subtype H7N3 re-emerged in the broiler-breeder flocks in different poultry estates of the northern area of the country during 2000. This prompted the introduction of a vaccine strategy, whereby both aqueous and oil emulsion vaccines were routinely employed in and around the affected areas. This helped in the control of disease in this region. However, no AI monitoring and control strategy could be launched on a sustainable basis in these areas. In November 2003, new outbreaks of HPAI subtype H7N3 occurred specifically in commercial layers in the southern part of the country, which were never vaccinated against AI in the past. In many cases, subtype H9N2 was also recovered from the diseased flocks, with or without the presence of subtype H7N3. The disease caused heavy losses in the south. An emergency plan to control this outbreak was developed with the help of FAO in this regard. Under this plan, a nationwide AIV monitoring and vaccination strategy was developed. This paper discusses the role of vaccine type and vaccination schedule in the control of HPAI in this country.

INTRODUCTION

In most of the trading countries, eradication by stamping out has been the preferred method for dealing with OIE list A diseases, such as highly pathogenic avian influenza (HPAI). This has resulted in the depopulation of millions of chickens at various places during the past few years alone. The past experience has shown that choosing a control strategy based on culling chickens that are infected or suspected of being infected may not be sufficient to avoid the spread of infection. This is particularly applicable in the areas that have a high density of chickens. There is an increased risk of disease-spread in these areas and the financial consequences of any occurring outbreak are severe [1]. Based on the economic situation of a country, for many poultry diseases, including those on list A, judicious use of vaccines has been part of prevention, control and/or eradication programmes.

The earlier approved definition of avian influenza was confined to the disease caused by HPAI virus of subtype H5 or H7, however, the revised definition includes all avian influenza viruses of the H5 and H7 subtype, regardless of their virulence and pathogenicity [2]. This further encourages the use of vaccines for the prevention or control of avian influenza in poultry.

Pakistan has been affected by two major outbreaks of HPAI, in 1995 and in 2003-04 caused by H7N3 subtype. During 1998, an outbreak of low pathogenic avian influenza (LPAI) virus subtype H9N2 appeared in the southern part of the country [3]. A short-lived outbreak of LPAI subtype H7N3 also occurred in 2000 in the north. The outbreaks of 1995, 1998 and 2000 remained confined to distinct poultry estates affecting broiler-breeders, broilers, and broiler-breeders, respectively [3]. However, the HPAI outbreak of 2003-04 primarily affected the commercial layers. Subsequently, during 2004, the LPAI caused by H7N3 also appeared in broiler-breeders in the northern areas of the country. Unfortunately, the outbreaks of 2004 coincided with the H5N1 outbreak in Far East countries. The name bird flu was used by the local press to reflect any outbreak of avian influenza anywhere in the world, irrespective of its involvement in human infection. This resulted in creating fear in the public in Pakistan about using chicken meat and chicken products. As a result, several establishments, such as broiler production units, hatcheries, feed mills, and allied businesses were forced to stop functioning, causing heavy economic losses. Furthermore, economic losses resulted from the export ban imposed on the infected region and heavy mortality and loss of production at the farms. The characteristics, consequences and control policies applied in these outbreaks are reported below.

Outbreaks of 1995 and 2000

The outbreak of 1995 was caused by HPAI virus subtype H7N3 and in 2000 by an LPAI virus subtype H7N3 in the northern areas of the country, primarily affecting broiler-breeders. On both occasions, the disease remained endemic and was controlled by introducing stringent bio-security measures along with the use of ring vaccination around the affected areas. In this regard, an aqueous-based vaccine, using field isolates of HPAI subtype H7N3, was developed and used in the field in 1995, whereas, during the 2000 outbreak, ring vaccination with aqueous-based vaccine followed by an oil-based preparation was employed in broiler-breeders in the affected area. This helped in the control of avian influenza in the affected areas.

Epidemic of 1998

The epidemic of LPAI subtype H9N2 appeared in the southern part of the country in summer 1998, primarily affecting broilers. The disease caused severe respiratory signs and heavy mortality in broilers of all ages [4]. A homologous aqueous-based vaccine was employed for its control in broilers. The disease later appeared in broiler-breeders reared in the northern areas, severely affecting their egg production. An oil-based vaccine was introduced in the affected areas, which helped to control the further spread of disease.

Epidemic of 2003-04

During 2003, Pakistan was affected by a devastating epidemic of HPAI, caused by H7N3 that originated from the mutation of an LPAI virus of the same subtype. The low path AI virus was first isolated in the south in April 2003 in the coastal town of Karachi, where 70 % of the country's commercial layers are raised. The flocks that were initially affected by LPAI of subtype H7N3 showed a 70 % decline in production and 20 % mortality. The LPAI virus was repeatedly isolated from ten other flocks in the vicinity; however, since this virus did not qualify under the international standards of controllable avian influenza, any voluntary restriction of bird movement, controlled marketing or quarantine policies could not be implemented.

In November 2004, the HPAI subtype H7N3 emerged in the Karachi area, with a sudden increase in mortality at some farms. The virus was confirmed as HPAI with an IVPI index of 2.8. At some places, low path avian influenza virus subtype H9N2 was also isolated from the same flocks. The H7N3 subtype was found to affect commercial layers specifically, since no outbreak was recorded from broiler flocks raised in the close vicinity. During the next four weeks, the disease had spread throughout the commercial layer estates within a radius of 80 kilometres. This resulted in very heavy mortality among the affected flocks ranging from 70-80 %. A disease-control strategy was developed at this stage, which included:

(i) Voluntary depopulation, cleaning and adoption of bio-security measures.

(ii) Introduction of vaccination policy.

(iii) Setting up a national AIV surveillance programme.

(i) Voluntary depopulation, cleaning and adoption of bio-security measures

Because there is no compensation policy, it was not practical to demand that the affected farmers destroy their flocks. However, with the help of the Pakistan Poultry Association (PPA), a number of farmers with multi-age flocks at the same farms were pursued to slaughter the affected flocks, clean and disinfect the premises and leave them empty for the next 60 days. Before restocking the premises, basic bio-security measures were also introduced at most of the farms.

(ii) Introduction of vaccination policy

A vaccination policy against avian influenza was developed at this stage in co-ordination with the poultry industry, vaccine manufacturers and officials of the Ministry of Food, Agriculture and Livestock (MINFAL). Under this plan, both short-term and long-term vaccination strategies were worked out (Table 1). Initially, all the commercial-layer flocks in the affected poultry estates were vaccinated with an aqueous-based AIV H7 + H9 combined vaccine, aided by aluminium hydroxide [5]. These flocks were subsequently given oil-based vaccines three weeks later. The flocks were monitored for sero-conversion against H7 and H9 subtypes, revealing higher antibody levels (Table 2). However, it is apparent that high antibody titres in some cases could be a result of the unnoticed field challenge of the prevailing serotypes of AIV. After two months of high mortality in this area, the intensity of the disease started to decline.

Table 1: Vaccination strategy against avian influenza outbreak of 2003-04 in Pakistan.

A) During the outbreak of HPAI (Nov 03-Feb 04)	1. Vaccination in layers using AIV aqueous H7 + H9 vaccine and AIV oil-based H7 + H9 vaccine in disease-affected areas of Karachi poultry Estates
	2. Mass vaccination in broiler-breeders in northern areas, with three oil-based shots of combined AIV H7 + H9 vaccine
B) After the outbreak of HPAI (March 04 onward)	1. In Karachi, mass vaccination in layers with AIV oil-based H7 + H9 vaccine
	2. In northern parts, regular mass vaccination with AIV oil-based H7 + H9 vaccine among broiler-breeders

HPAI = highly pathogenic avian influenza.

AIV H7 + H9 = avian influenza subtypes H7N3 and H9N2.

Table 2: Sero-conversion against avian influenza virus subtype H7 + H9 combined vaccine employed within the disease-outbreak zone.

Vaccine type	**No. of flocks tested***	**HI-antibody titre range (GMT log2) at weeks post-vaccination**			
		Virus subtype	**0**	**3**	**6**
AIV H7 + H9 (A) (Shot # 1)	20	AIV-H7	0-4.4	3.3-7.1	–
		AIV-H9	0-7.5	2.5-10.2	–
AIV H7 + H9 (O) (Shot # 2)	20	AIV-H7	3.3-7.1	4.1-7.5	4.2-8.1
		AIV-H9	2.5-10.2	3.5-11.0	3.1-11.0

Shot #2 was given three weeks after the first shot.

* Sample size = 24 sera/flock.

AIV H7 + H9 = avian influenza virus subtype H7 and H9.

A = aqueous-based O = oil-based GMT = geometric mean titre.

From November to March 2004, more than 80 % of the commercial layers were vaccinated against AIV H7 + H9 in the Karachi area alone. In the mean time, a mass vaccination was launched by the PPA in the major breeding-stock rearing areas in the northern parts of the country, where a three-shot, oil-based vaccination was used in the breeding stocks. The required protective antibody levels were successfully achieved in the vaccinated flocks against AIV subtype H7 and H9 (Table 3).

(iii) Setting up avian influenza monitoring

As a part of avian influenza control strategy, a disease-monitoring set-up was established with the financial and technical assistance of FAO. For this purpose, a number of Influenza Monitoring Labs set up throughout the country were linked together under a Central Monitoring Lab to carry out sampling from healthy or sus-

Table 3: Sero-conversion against avian influenza virus subtype H7 + H9 combined vaccine employed outside the disease-affected zone.

Vaccine type and time	No. of flocks tested*	HI-antibody titre range (GMT log2) at weeks post-vaccination			
		Virus subtype	0	3	6
AIV H7 + H9 (O) Shot # 1 (at 0 week)	20	AIV-H7	0.0	0-2.8	–
		AIV-H9	0.0	0-2.5	–
AIV H7 + H9 (O) Shot # 2 (3 weeks post 1st shot)	20	AIV-H7	0-2.8	1.4-5.3	3.2-7.4
		AIV-H9	0-2.5	1.7-4.9	2.4-7.1
AIV H7 + H9 (O) Shot # 3 (9 weeks post 2nd shot)	20	AIV-H7	3.3-7.4	4.0-8.8	3.8-8.9
		AIV-H9	2.2-7.4	3.1-8.1	3.2-8.3

In new flocks Shot # 1 was employed at between three and five weeks of age.

* Sample size = 24 sera/flock.

GMT = geometric mean titre.

AIV H7 + H9 = avian influenza virus subtype H7 and H9.

O = oil-based.

pected flocks in the area for serologic and virologic evaluation. Once an infected flock was identified, an epidemiological investigation was carried out on the affected farms by means of a standardised questionnaire to establish the possible origin of infection. To assess the performance of the vaccine and identify undiagnosed LPAI infection, the flocks located both in the affected areas and outside were tested serologically and virologically. In vaccinated flocks reared outside the affected areas, at least ten sentinel birds per flock were serologically tested every six weeks for seroconversion and virus shedding against H7 and H9 subtypes of AIV.

Based on the information generated from AI monitoring, in April 2004, shedding of LPAI subtype H7N3 was discovered among the breeding stocks in the north, however, no overt signs of disease have occurred so far in this area. The surveillance data collected from other poultry-rearing areas of the country have not revealed the presence of any avian influenza virus in their poultry.

Discussion

The information presented here indicates that the emergency vaccination in the face of an outbreak, coupled with increased bio-security and intensive surveillance can be helpful in controlling the spread of avian influenza. The use of aqueous-based vaccine alone during the outbreak of HPAI in 1995 and LPAI in 2000 provided a protective immune response in the field to check further spread of the virus. The same strategy was used while combating HPAI virus subtype H7N3 in 2003 in

Karachi. It appears from the data presented here that aqueous-based AI vaccine produces faster though short-lived immunity against HPAI under field conditions. There appears to be no stress induced by this vaccination when given in the face of an outbreak.

The comparison between rate of spread observed during the outbreak of LPAI virus H9N2 in 1998 and that of LPAI H7N3 in 2003, with the limited spread of HPAI virus H7N3 in 2004 from Karachi to other parts of the country, indicates that bio-security, surveillance and vaccination are effective tools for the control of LPAI. Use of homologous vaccine specially prepared from the LPAI field isolates has been shown to be quite efficacious under field conditions. This is probably because of the production of higher antigen mass by the field strain selected for vaccine production locally [5]. However, it may not be able to distinguish between the field exposure and a vaccination titre, as proposed elsewhere [1].

In conclusion, our experience of using homologous vaccines from local field isolates since 1995 against HPAI virus subtype H7N3 has revealed that a co-ordinated set of control measures along with vaccination can be successful in controlling the circulation of HPAI viruses. This may also be helpful in averting any new mutation within the circulating subtype on account of introducing a new vaccine strain with different N-type or pathotype.

Acknowledgements

This work was partly funded by a grant from FAO (FAO/TCP/PAK/3002) and financial assistance from the Chinese Government for the control of avian influenza to Pakistan.

References

1 Capua I, Marangon S: Avian influenza in Italy (1999-2000): a review. Avian Pathology 2000; 29: 289-294.

2 Capua I, Marangon S: The use of vaccination as an option for the control of avian influenza. Avian Pathology 2003; 32 (4): 335-343.

3 Bano S, Naeem K, Malik SA: Evaluation of pathogenic potential of avian influenza virus serotype H9N2 in chickens. Avian Diseases 2003; 47: 817-822.

4 Naeem K, Ullah A, Manvell RJ, Alexander DJ: Avian influenza A subtype H9N2 in poultry in Pakistan. Veterinary Record 1999; 145: 560.

5 Naeem K, Baqi S: Development of effective vaccine and vaccination strategy to combat avian influenza in poultry, in proceedings of XXII World's Poultry Congress. Istanbul Convention and Exhibition Centre, Istanbul, Turkey, 2004, pp 777.

6 Swayne DE, Beck JR, Garcia JR, Stone HD: Influence of virus strain and antigen mass on the efficacy of H5 avian influenza inactivated vaccines. Avian Pathology 1999; 28: 245-255.

Dr. K. Naeem, Central Avian Influenza Monitoring Lab., National Reference Laboratory for Poultry Diseases, Animal Sciences Institute, National Agricultural Research Centre, Park Road, Islamabad-45500, Pakistan. E-mail: nrlpd@isb.comsats.net.pk

Schudel A, Lombard M (eds): OIE/FAO International Scientific Conference on Avian Influenza.
Dev Biol (Basel). Basel, Karger, 2006, vol 124, pp 151-155.

Making Avian Influenza Vaccines Available, an Industry Point of View (IFAH)

P. van Aarle

Intervet International, Boxmeer, The Netherlands

Abstract: Vaccination against avian influenza (AI) has proved to be an efficient tool in the reduction of virus excretion and in increasing the threshold for infection. Vaccination in outbreaks, as part of a complete programme, has proved to be an essential component of control and eradication programmes.

Avian influenza is a serious threat to public health. In contingency plans for outbreaks of highly pathogenic AI (HPAI), the option of emergency vaccination, using inactivated or recombinant vaccines, should be considered. The availability of suitable vaccines has to be ensured in 'peace time' in a contract for a vaccine or antigen bank.

Unlike the human influenza vaccines, poultry AI vaccines have proved to provide protection against a wide range of strains within the same H-subtype. However, in case new H5 or H7 strains emerge in poultry, there is no regulatory guideline to support a swift reaction by the vaccine industry.

Production of HPAI virus should take place in facilities with a Biosafety Level 3 (BSL3) to safeguard containment of virus and to prevent infection of manufacturing staff. Vaccine strains for inactivated vaccines should preferably be low pathogenicity AI (LPAI).

In a new outbreak, it is essential to determine early which vaccine strain will provide protection against the field virus. Sequencing does not predict the protective capacity of vaccines. Challenge studies, providing essential information, take too much time and can be carried out only in BSL3 facilities. Serological matching of vaccine and field strains would provide a faster system. It is recommended that a matching system be developed and validated.

IFAH

IFAH is the International Federation for Animal Health representing manufacturers of veterinary medicines, vaccines and other animal health products in both developed and developing countries across five continents.

Introduction

The primary goal of the battle against avian influenza (AI) is to eradicate the disease. In countries where the disease is endemic, eradication might not be feasible in the short term and control of the disease might have to be the first step towards eradication. Stamping out [1], vaccination [2] or a combination of these have proved to be essential tools in an eradication strategy. Once eradication has been achieved, it is of prime importance to prevent re-introduction.

Vaccines and their Efficacy

Several vaccines are available in the market: inactivated vaccines; recombinant fowl pox H5 vector; combination vaccines of two AI strains [3]; and combination vaccines against AI and Newcastle disease. Vaccines, as part of an overall strategy against AI, have proved to be efficient in the control and eradication of AI.

Inactivated vaccines protect against clinical disease and mortality and, more importantly, reduce the ability of the AI virus to replicate in chickens, resulting in decreased excretion of virus after challenge [4]. Vaccination, in addition to quarantine, depopulation and biosecurity measures, was applied in the face of an outbreak in Hong Kong [5]. In two farms, the infection spread to vaccinated sheds with low rates of H5N1 mortality; the chickens were between nine and 18 days post-vaccination. After 18 days post-vaccination, no more H5N1 mortality occurred and intensive monitoring showed no evidence of asymptomatic virus shedding. It is concluded that this is an important aspect when dealing with a virus, which poses a significant risk to human health.

Inactivated vaccines can be used at all ages. Protection starts to develop at two weeks after vaccination and reaches a maximum from three weeks after vaccination. For a long duration of immunity, revaccination is recommended.

Recombinant fowlpox vaccine, containing an H5 influenza haemagglutinin gene insert, protected chickens against clinical signs and death following challenge with nine different field viruses [6]. The vaccine reduced detectable infection rates and shedding titres. There was a significant positive correlation in haemagglutinin sequence similarity between challenge viruses and vaccine, and the ability to reduce titres of challenge virus isolated from the oropharynx, but no similar correlation for reducing cloacal virus titres. The recombinant fowlpox vaccine is injected at day 1 and is typically indicated for vaccination of replacement birds.

Monitoring of Infection in Vaccinated Flocks

As long as AI virus circulates, the chance exists of a strain emerging that is infectious and pathogenic for people, carrying with it the risk of a new global influenza pandemic. Virus detection, in combination with measures to control virus circulation, is therefore essential. Although there is significantly less excretion of virus from vaccinated birds, circulation can still occur and it is important to monitor this.

Sentinel birds

A number of birds in the flock are left unvaccinated. The sentinel birds will show morbidity/mortality immediately when highly pathogenic AI (HPAI) is circulating in the vaccinated flocks. Sentinel birds will show antibodies if low pathogenicity AI (LPAI) virus is in circulation in a vaccinated flock.

DIVA approach

Differentiating infected from vaccinated animals (DIVA) is possible through the use of a vaccine that contains a neuraminidase (NA) that is different from that of the field strain [7]. Antibodies against the neuraminidase of the field virus indicate infection. This approach generally is combined with the use of sentinel birds.

Non-structural protein (NS) test

Conventional inactivated vaccines induce antibody titres against non-structural proteins that are considerably lower than the antibody titres after infection [8]. Field sera from poultry, vaccinated with commercial AI vaccines, were positive for antibodies in the Agar Gel Precipitin (AGP) test but negative on the NS1 Elisa. Sera from infected poultry were positive for both AGP and NS1 antibodies.

Serological methods for recombinant fowlpox vaccine

The vaccine only expresses the haemagglutinin of the AI virus and does not interfere with antibody tests against other antigens of the AI virus. As a result, a wide range of diagnostic methods can be used: classical AGP or nucleoprotein- or matrix-based ELISA, NA- and NS-based tests.

Evolution of AI Strains and Necessity for Vaccine Updates

Avian influenza virus does not seem to undergo frequent antigenic drift. In a challenge study with inactivated vaccines, vaccinated birds were challenged with North American viruses isolated over a period of 27 years from separate geographical areas. In this study, there was no positive correlation between the genotype (haemagglutinin) of the vaccine and challenge strain and the ability of the vaccine to reduce the quantity of virus shedding from the cloaca and oropharynx [9].

The recombinant fowlpox vaccine also provided good protection against a wide range of challenge viruses [6]. There was a significant positive correlation in haemagglutinin sequence similarity between challenge viruses and vaccine, and the ability to reduce titres of challenge virus isolated from the oropharynx but no similar correlation for reducing cloacal virus titres.

The evolution of the Mexican field virus seems to show signs of antigenic drift [10]. Serologic analysis using the haemagglutination inhibition test and virus neutralisation tests showed major antigenic differences among isolates belonging to different sub-lineages. These results were confirmed in vaccine protection studies, which demonstrated that the vaccine used was not able to prevent virus shedding when chickens were challenged with antigenically different isolates.

Clearly the antigenic evolution of human influenza viruses is more rapid than that of the avian influenza viruses. Potential reasons might be: differences in the human and avian population; differences in the vaccine antigen and adjuvants between human and avian vaccines.

In spite of the low tendency for antigenic evolution of avian influenza virus, it is essential for vaccine efficacy to monitor the antigenic match between vaccine- and field-virus. At this moment, challenge studies are the model to test for antigenic variation, and the most important criterion is the ability of the vaccine to reduce virus shedding. Challenge has to be carried out in BSL3 facilities and requires time for the planning, preparation and virus isolation.

It is recommended that further research is done towards development of a model of serological matching that correlates with virus shedding after challenge. Such a system is used for Foot and Mouth Disease and is a fast and convenient method for matching field- and vaccine-virus.

Containment of AI Virus Production

The OIE Manual of Diagnostic Tests and Vaccines for Terrestrial Animals (Appendix I.1.6.1.) describes the regulations for "International Transfer and Laboratory Containment of Animal Pathogens". HPAI is a list A disease with potentially serious public health implications. Fully virulent HPAI virus should therefore only be handled in a BSL3 laboratory and vaccine production from HPAI strains must be in high containment facilities.

Because of the possible negative consequences, both for the poultry industry and public health, production of commercial inactivated vaccines should be based on LPAI production strains, which require normal containment standards for vaccine production.

Emergency Preparedness

There is no proper regulatory framework for licensing emergency vaccines. For example, in Europe, emergency vaccines can be used under article 8 of the EU Directive for licensing [11]. In the event of a serious disease epidemic, a country may decide to use a non-licensed product. However, there is no regulation or guidance on the conditions for such a decision.

In countries free of a serious disease, there is generally a non-vaccination policy. In countries with a non-vaccination policy, which would only consider limited use of vaccines in case of an outbreak, there is no justification for a commercial company to invest in full-scale development and licensing of a vaccine. Emergency vaccination is included in most contingency plans and the availability of a licensed vaccine would greatly facilitate the political decision to use vaccination.

It is recommended that special and simplified legislation be developed for vaccines that are only used in case of emergency. Alternatively, governments should support the industry financially to fully license emergency vaccines.

There is no regulatory framework in the veterinary field for a speedy update of influenza vaccine strains. For every vaccine strain and for every update of the vaccine strain, a new registration is required. It is recommended that legislation is developed that allows, as is the case for human influenza vaccines, a speedy update of vaccine strains, should the need arise.

If vaccination is seen as an option in contingency plans, the availability of vaccines needs to be addressed. It is recommended that the availability of vaccines is arranged in a contract between the government and the industry in "peace time".

References

1 Stegeman A, Bouma A, Elbers AR, de Jong MC, Nodelijk G, de Klerk F, Koch G, van Boven M: Avian influenza A virus (H7N7) epidemic in The Netherlands in 2003: Course of the epidemic and effectiveness of control measures. J Infect Dis 2004; 190: 2088-2095.

2 Capua I, Marangon S: The use of vaccination as an option for the Control of Avian Influenza. 71st General Session of the International Committee of the World Organisation for Animal Health, Paris, 18-23 May 2003. http://www.oie.int/downld/71SG_2003/A_71% 20SG_12_CS3E.pdf.

3 EU Commission Decision of 29 September 2004 on introducing vaccination to supplement the measures to control infections with low pathogenic avian influenza in Italy and on specific movement control measures and repealing Decision 2002/975/EC. EU Commission Decision 2004/666/EC.

4 Swayne DE, Beck JR, Perdue ML, Beard CW: Efficacy of vaccines in chickens against highly pathogenic Hong Kong H5N1 Avian Influenza. Avian Dis 2001; 45: 355-365.

5 Ellis TM, Leung CYHC, Chow MKW, Bissett LA, Wong W, Guan Y, Peiris MJS: Vaccination of chickens against H5N1 avian influenza in the face of an outbreak interrupts virus transmission. Avian Path 2004; 33 (4): 405-412.

6 Swayne DE, Garcia M, Beck JR, Kinney N, Suarez DL: Protection against diverse highly pathogenic H5 avian influenza viruses in chickens immunized with a recombinant fowlpox vaccine containing an H5 avian influenza hemagglutinin gene insert. Vaccine 2000; 18: 1088-1095.

7 Capua I, Terregino C, Cattoli G, Mutinelli F, Rodriguez JF: Development of a DIVA (Differentiating Infected from Vaccinated Animals) strategy using a vaccine containing a heterologous neuraminidase for the control of avian influenza. Avian Path 2002; 32: 47-55.

8 Tumpey TM, Alvarez R, Swayne DE, Suarez DL: Diagnostic approach for differentiating infected from vaccinated poultry on the basis of antibodies to NS1, the non-structural protein of influenza A virus. J of Clin Microbiol 43 (2): 676-683.

9 Swayne DE, Beck JR, Garcia M, Stone HD: Influence of virus strain and antigenic mass on efficacy of H5 influenza inactivated vaccines. Avian Path 1999; 28: 245-255.

10 Lee CW, Senne D, Suarez DL: Effect of vaccine use in the evolution of Mexican lineage H5N2 avian influenza virus. J Virol 2004; 78 (15): 8372-8381.

11 Directive 2001/82/EC of the European Parliament and of the Council of 6 November 2001 on the Community code relating to veterinary medicinal products. EU Commission Directive 2001/82/EC.

Dr. P. van Aarle, Intervet International b.v., P.O. Box 31, NL-5830 AA Boxmeer, The Netherlands.
E-mail: paul.vanaarle@intervet.com

Schudel A, Lombard M (eds): OIE/FAO International Scientific Conference on Avian Influenza.
Dev Biol (Basel). Basel, Karger, 2006, vol 124, p 157.

SESSION VI

Improvement of Management Tools

Chairperson: *P. Vannier* (AFSSA, France)
Rapporteur: *D. Suarez* (SEPRL, USA)

Schudel A, Lombard M (eds): OIE/FAO International Scientific Conference on Avian Influenza.
Dev Biol (Basel). Basel, Karger, 2006, vol 124, pp 159-162.

OIE Laboratory Standards for Avian Influenza

S. Edwards

Veterinary Laboratories Agency, New Haw, Addlestone, Surrey KT15 3NB, United Kingdom

Abstract: The principles are outlined by which the Office International des Epizooties (OIE) recognises diagnostic laboratory test procedures, based on the validation data and the fitness for purpose of any given test. The latest proposals for a definition of notifiable avian influenza are described, together with the place of vaccination, as part of the effort to control influenza in domestic poultry.

INTRODUCTION

The members of the Biological Standards Commission of the Office International des Epizooties (OIE) are elected for a term of three years by the International Committee of the OIE. They are required to have experience in veterinary laboratory diagnostics and/or vaccine standardisation. The Commission provides technical advice to the OIE on laboratory diagnostics and vaccines for diseases of mammals, birds and bees; in doing so, it is able to draw on the accumulated knowledge and experience of experts world-wide through the OIE network of reference laboratories and collaborating centres.

A major output from the Commission is the OIE Manual [1], which provides a series of general introductory chapters on aspects of laboratory standards, followed by disease-specific chapters on diseases listed by the OIE and a number of others of veterinary or public health importance. The Manual is fully revised every four years, while intermediate updates to individual chapters are made annually to the on-line edition. This paper describes the approach adopted in the Manual both in general principle and in regard specifically to the chapter on avian influenza.

VALIDATION PRINCIPLES

The OIE "Principles of validation of diagnostic assays for infectious diseases" are set out in one of the introductory chapters to the Manual. These principles are based on the work of Jacobson [2] and attempt to provide a practical approach to validation for diagnostic laboratories, while maintaining a sound statistical basis. A key point is that validation is not a one-off event but a continuous process, refining the test parameters as additional data are accumulated. Another fundamental principle is that validation is related to the purpose for which the test is to be used, and the same assay may be tuned to different levels of diagnostic sensitivity and specificity according to the application. This is termed "fitness for purpose".

Most attention has been paid to the validation of serological assays, although even here it is recognised that many established tests are accepted as valid on the basis of historical usage, experience and consensus. Thus many such tests which are described in the Manual are not supported by formal validation dossiers. New tests, or new variants of established tests, are not accepted for inclusion in the Manual unless such a dossier is provided. The OIE will also seek expert opinion on the dossier and, as with all its standards, circulate new Manual texts to Member Countries for comment before seeking approval by the International Committee.

Test Recognition by the OIE

Particular attention has been focused on the specification for "Prescribed tests", which are recommended by the OIE for use in screening animals before they are accepted for international trade or movement. In this respect, the laboratory standards for prescribed tests as described in the Manual complement the requirements of the OIE Terrestrial Animal Health Code [3]. A second category of "Alternative test" is provided for methods that do not fully meet the requirements of a prescribed test but may be useful in international trade and can be applied following bilateral agreement between countries.

In the case of avian influenza, the Code does not require testing before international movements and therefore there are no prescribed tests. This does not imply that the tests described in the Manual are not useful or relevant, simply that they are not required for the specific application of international trade testing. Prescribed tests will be proposed in accordance with changes in the requirements of the Code.

Beginning in 2005, the OIE is establishing a new register of diagnostic tests that have been validated as "fit for purpose". To gain entry to the register, a test validation dossier must be submitted to the OIE with an explanation of the purposes for which the test is designed and validated. A template is available for submissions. The dossier will be evaluated by a panel of experts appointed by the OIE. This extends the relevance of the Manual and provides guidance to readers on how and when to apply diagnostic tests in specific situations, for example, to support clinical diagnosis, to conduct population surveys, or to differentiate vaccinated animals from those potentially infected with the wild-type disease agent.

Avian Influenza – Definition of Pathogenicity

The 2004 edition of the Manual [1] refers principally to "Highly pathogenic avian influenza" (HPAI), which up till now has been the only form of the disease included on the OIE list (formerly List A). HPAI strains of the virus have been defined either by their pathogenicity for four to eight week old chickens, assessed by either of two methods as described in the Manual or, in the case of H5 and H7 viruses of low pathogenicity, the demonstration of multiple basic amino acids in the sequence at the cleavage site of the haemagglutinin protein.

To date, almost all HPAI strains have been of H5 or H7 types, and it is considered that highly pathogenic strains arise in the field by mutation from low pathogenicity strains. For this reason "potentially pathogenic" strains of H5 and H7 possessing the characteristic amino acid sequence have been included by the OIE since 1992 within the definition of HPAI. Depending on whether or not the OIE International Committee adopts the new version of the Code chapter on avian influenza in May 2005, either the current definition of HPAI in the Manual will continue, or a new version will be proposed that complements the new Code*.

In the new version of the Manual, the same laboratory methods will be used to assess pathogenicity as at present, but all isolates of H5 and H7 will become notifiable, regardless of their pathogenicity, and the nomenclature will be changed as follows:

- Highly pathogenic notifiable avian influenza (HPNAI) – isolates that meet the criteria for pathogenicity by intravenous inoculation of four to eight week old chickens, or H5 and H7 isolates that possess multiple basic amino acids at the haemagglutinin cleavage site.
- Low pathogenicity notifiable avian influenza (LPNAI) – isolates of H5 and H7 that are neither pathogenic in chickens nor possess multiple basic amino acids at the cleavage site.
- Low pathogenicity avian influenza (LPAI) – low virulence isolates (non-notifiable) of subtypes other than H5 and H7.

Avian Influenza – Use of Vaccines

The current version of the Manual describes the production and product control procedures for conventional inactivated vaccines, based primarily on experiences in the U.S.A. An expanded section of the chapter is proposed for adoption in 2005, which provides more detail on how such conventional vaccines have been used in different countries, using LPNAI and LPAI strains to prepare the vaccines for use in either chickens or turkeys. A fundamental consideration which should be constantly emphasised is that vaccination alone is not the solution to the control of avian influenza, where eradication (from domestic poultry) is the preferred approach. Where vaccine is used without supporting surveillance and control measures, the likelihood is that wild-type virus will continue to circulate and become endemic in poultry populations [4].

A new text is also provided on the differentiation of infected from vaccinated animals (the "DIVA" strategy). This combines the use of a vaccine with homologous haemagglutinin subtype to the circulating field virus, and serological surveillance for natural infection using tests for antibodies to other proteins – either neuraminidase where a heterologous N subtype is used for the vaccine as adopted in Italy [5], or non-structural proteins that are absent from the vaccine. The latter approach has so far been evaluated only at laboratory level [6], but it may be a future option for field use. Strategic use of vaccination combined with DIVA diagnostics can enable control and eradication without the need for mass culling used in traditional control systems.

* The new version was adopted by the OIE in May 2005.

Finally, an introduction is provided on recombinant vaccines to avian influenza. So far these have been constructed in heterologous live vector viruses (either fowlpox or infectious laryngotracheitis) into which the appropriate influenza haemagglutinin has been inserted. They are inherently suitable for combination with a DIVA strategy as the vaccine contains only one influenza protein. While such vaccines have many advantages in terms of ease of manufacture and administration, their limitation is the widespread pre-existing immunity to the vector viruses in poultry populations, so they are recommended only for use in day-old chicks. Even here, the possible interference by maternal immunity has not been fully evaluated, although there is some evidence that it does not prevent vector virus replication. Also, in the case of infectious laryngotracheitis, this virus does not replicate in turkeys, so those vaccines are not suitable for this species. Recombinant fowlpox vector-based vaccines have been extensively used in the field in Mexico and Central America [7]. For the future, it is anticipated that novel vaccines may be produced, for example, using protein expression systems in baculovirus, or DNA-based vaccines.

Conclusions

The OIE Manual provides internationally approved standards for diagnostic laboratories and vaccine manufacturers. The Biological Standards Commission of the OIE liaises closely with experts in reference laboratories and puts forward proposals to update the standards as appropriate. In the case of avian influenza, the current proposal is to modify the requirements for notification to the OIE, and to update the information on vaccines.

References

1 Anon: Manual of Diagnostic Tests and Vaccines for Terrestrial Animals (mammals, birds and bees). Paris, OIE, 2004, 5th edition, pp 1178.

2 Jacobson RH: Validation of serological assays for diagnosis of infectious diseases. Rev sci tech Off int Epiz 1998; 17: 469-486.

3 Anon: Terrestrial Animal Health Code. Paris, OIE, 2004, 13th edition, pp 554.

4 Lee CW, Senne DA, Suarez DL: Effect of vaccine use in the evolution of Mexican lineage H5N2 avian influenza virus. J Virol 2004; 78: 8372 – 8381.

5 Capua I, Alexander DJ: Avian influenza: recent developments. Avian Pathol 2004; 33: 393-404.

6 Tumpey TM, Alvarez R, Swayne DE, Suarez DL: Diagnostic approach for differentiating infected from vaccinated poultry on the basis of antibodies to NS1, the nonstructural protein of influenza A virus. J Clin Microbiol 2005; 43: 676-683.

7 Villareal-Chavez C, Rivera Cruz E: An update on avian influenza in Mexico, in: Proceedings of the 5th International Symposium on Avian Influenza. Georgia Center for Continuing Education, University of Georgia, Athens, Georgia, USA, 14 – 17 April 2002. Avian Dis 2003; 47: 1002-1005.

Prof. S. Edwards, Veterinary Laboratories Agency, New Haw, Addlestone, Surrey KT15 3NB, United Kingdom.
E-mail: s.edwards@vla.defra.gsi.gov.uk

Schudel A, Lombard M (eds): OIE/FAO International Scientific Conference on Avian Influenza.
Dev Biol (Basel). Basel, Karger, 2006, vol 124, pp 163-169.

Surveillance and Compartmentalisation as a Tool to Control Avian Influenza

C. Zepeda

USDA-APHIS-VS Centers for Epidemiology and Animal Health/Animal Population Health Institute, Colorado State University. Fort Collins, CO, USA

Abstract: Surveillance for avian influenza can have several objectives. Generally, these are to detect the presence of infection or to declare disease freedom. Claims for disease freedom can refer to an entire country, a zone within a country, or a compartment. Disease freedom cannot be demonstrated absolutely; however, through a multi-pronged approach employing different surveillance strategies, sufficient confidence in the absence of infection can be achieved. The recently developed OIE guidelines for surveillance for avian influenza offer different approaches to meet these goals. The guidelines are not intended to be prescriptive but rather offer options that countries may apply depending on their epidemiological situation. Compartmentalisation is a new concept that allows the recognition of populations of different health status based on management as opposed to geographic factors (regionalisation). A proposed approach for the application of this novel concept is presented.

INTRODUCTION

Surveillance is the basis for detecting the occurrence of disease promptly and instituting actions for control and eradication. Avian influenza has been an important disease affecting poultry production world-wide and limiting trade of poultry and poultry products. The emergence of the H5N1 subtype of avian influenza virus (AIV) as a significant public health concern in many countries in South East Asia has highlighted the importance of developing reliable and efficient disease surveillance systems world-wide. Avian influenza has triggered trade restrictions by many countries. The proposed OIE Code chapter on avian influenza that is likely to be approved during the next OIE General Session in May 2005 clearly establishes the differences between highly pathogenic notifiable avian influenza (HPNAI) and low pathogenic notifiable influenza (LPNAI). The proposed chapter recommends different measures for safe trade in poultry and poultry products from countries, zones, or compartments. The OIE recently developed guidelines for surveillance for avian influenza in support of the Code chapter. This paper presents the new proposed guidelines for surveillance for avian influenza and outlines a proposal for the application of the concept of compartmentalisation.

OIE Guidelines for Surveillance for Avian Influenza

The OIE Scientific Commission developed General Guidelines for Animal Health Surveillance that will be included in the OIE Code [1]. On the basis of these general guidelines, specific guidelines for avian influenza have been proposed [2]. In general, the philosophy of the guidelines for surveillance is to avoid excessively prescriptive recommendations and instead to provide a set of approaches and strategies that each OIE member country can tailor to suit their particular conditions.

At the level of a country, zone or compartment, surveillance may have two objectives:

- To determine the presence or absence of notifiable AIV (NAIV) infection.
- To determine the prevalence of NAIV.

When determining disease freedom, there is an explicit recognition that no country can declare itself free from AIV in wild birds. Therefore, the guidelines for surveillance for avian influenza are based on the OIE definition for poultry: "all birds reared or kept in captivity for the production of meat or eggs for consumption, for the production of other commercial products, for restocking supplies of game, or for breeding these categories of birds" [3].

Different countries may have very different production systems or poultry raised under different types of production systems. For example, in most developing countries, intensive poultry farming co-exists with backyard production. By the same token, many developed countries have gradually shifted from intensive systems of production and have increased significantly the number of birds raised under free-range extensive systems. These changes have resulted in poultry subpopulations with different levels of exposure to AIV. In addition, some production systems may include more than one susceptible species. Clearly, there is a need for a flexible approach to surveillance that is adaptable to each country's characteristics.

It is scientifically impossible to demonstrate disease freedom in absolute terms. However, sufficient confidence in disease freedom can be achieved through a combination of approaches and strategies.

Two approaches for surveillance have been widely used: random and targeted. For either of these approaches, clinical, serologic or virologic methods can be applied.

Random surveillance relies on statistically based surveys, usually applying serologic testing. In the case of AI, seropositive findings must be followed by virologic methods for confirmation. Targeted surveillance generally is aimed at high risk groups, i.e. those in which we expect a higher frequency of disease occurrence. In these subpopulations, serologic and virologic methods should be used concurrently.

Clinical surveillance is based on the detection of clinical signs of AI at the flock level. Clinical surveillance is important for HPNAI, but is less effective for LPNAI because of the frequent absence of clinical signs. Positive clinical findings must be followed by serologic and virologic surveillance. Similarly, positive serologic results should be further investigated by clinical surveillance.

Virologic surveillance is used to monitor populations at risk, for instance, by testing "normal" daily mortality to ensure early detection of infection in the face of vaccination or in establishments epidemiologically linked to an outbreak. Virologic methods are used also to confirm clinically suspect cases and to follow up positive serologic results.

Serologic surveillance is most useful in non-vaccinated flocks. In vaccinated flocks, a strategy that allows the differentiation of infected and vaccinated animals (DIVA) [4] and/or sentinel birds should be used. Any finding of seropositive flocks clustered geographically or in time should always be thoroughly investigated using virologic, serologic and clinical methods.

In vaccinated flocks, the choice of strategy is dependent on the type of vaccine used. Two types of AIV vaccine exist:

- Inactivated whole AIV.
- Haemagglutinin expression-based vaccines.

Birds vaccinated with inactivated whole virus will develop antibodies that are indistinguishable from those resulting from infection. A DIVA strategy using a vaccine virus that shares the haemagglutinin of the field virus but has a different neuraminidase will allow differentiation of vaccinated and infected birds. Irrespective of the type of vaccine used, sentinel birds that are unvaccinated and permanently identifiable are an excellent means of detecting antibodies resulting from infection.

Figures 1-4 describe the diagnostic processes to confirm NAIV using serologic methods in vaccinated and unvaccinated populations, as well as virologic methods including virus isolation, nucleic acid detection and antigen detection.

Compartmentalisation

Compartmentalisation is a relatively new concept for disease management. As in the case of regionalisation, compartmentalisation seeks to recognise animal populations of different health status. Regionalisation uses geographic criteria, frequently an administrative border or natural barriers; compartmentalisation relies on management practices to distinguish these populations. In both cases, the idea is to establish a biosecurity border separating infected from non-infected populations.

Recently, at the request of the OIE Scientific Commission, an approach for the application of this concept was developed by USDA-APHIS based on the process currently used for regionalisation [5]. Nine factors were identified.

1) Definition of the compartment

The compartment must be defined clearly based on functional relationships of all its components and the degree of separation with other compartments of higher risk. Some examples of potential compartments include:

- Commercially produced poultry.
- Backyard poultry.
- Poultry produced for the live-bird market system.
- Wild birds.
- Slaughter plant and all related establishments supplying birds.

2) Documentation of factors critical to the compartment definition

To support the definition of a compartment as a separate entity, evidence describing the biosecurity measures that are applied, surveillance methods and results, and management practices must be submitted.

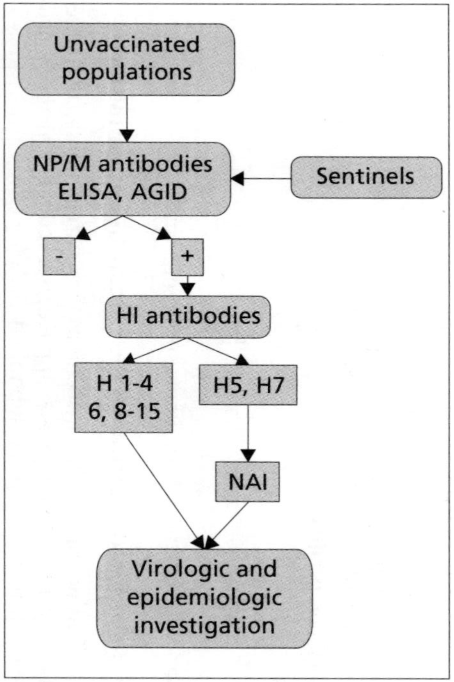

Fig. 1: Diagnostic process for serologic testing in vaccinated populations
(NP – nucleo-protein, M – matrix, ELISA-enzyme linked immunosorbent assay, AGID- agar gel immunodiffusion test, HI haemagglutination inhibition).

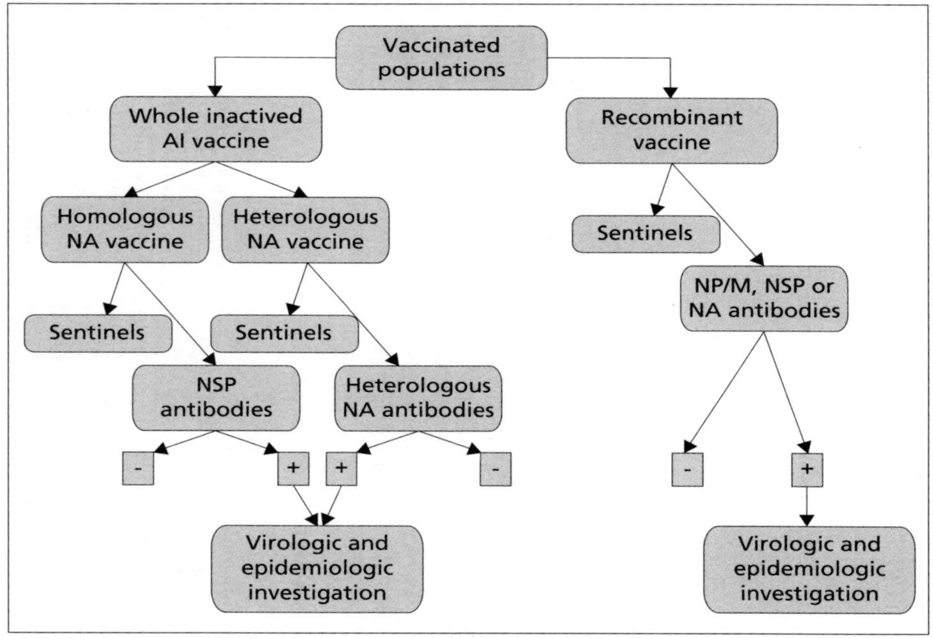

Fig. 2: Diagnostic process for serologic testing in vaccinated populations.

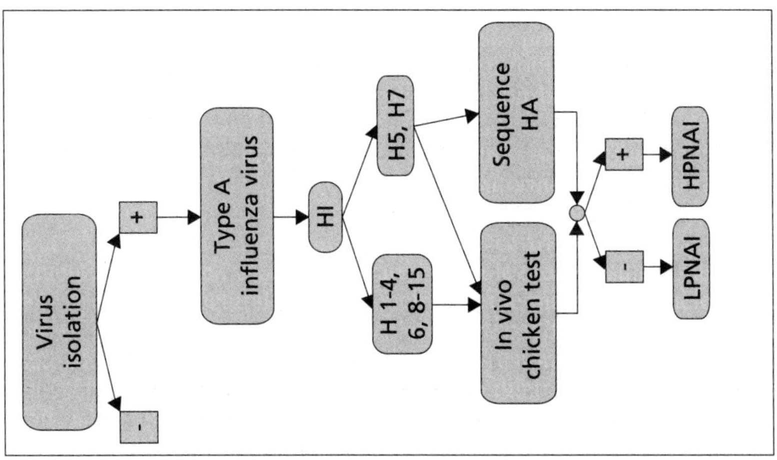

Fig. 3: Diagnostic process for virologic testing using virus isolation.

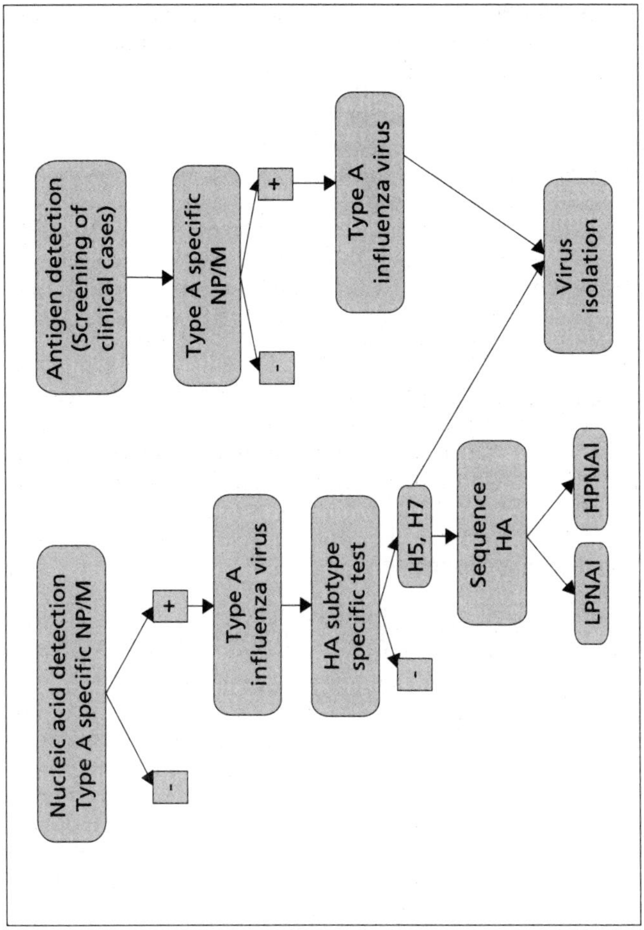

Fig. 4: Diagnostic process for virologic testing using nucleic acid detection or antigen detection.

3) Oversight of the compartment

The key difference between regionalisation and compartmentalisation is the responsibility for maintenance of the biosecurity border. In regionalisation, the oversight of the application of all measures is dependent on the official veterinary service, whereas, in compartmentalisation, the measures are applied by the private sector. Therefore, there is a need for supervision from the official veterinary services to ensure that the biosecurity measures, surveillance, and any other measure deemed necessary to maintain the separation of the compartment are applied effectively.

To document this factor, a thorough description of the authority, organisation, and infrastructure of the veterinary services organisation and industry management that have oversight of the compartment is required.

4) Disease status of the compartment

The burden of proof is on the disease-free compartment. Documentation on the date of last occurrence, control methods applied, and evidence supporting the absence of infection should be submitted for review.

5) Vaccination status of the compartment

If vaccination is applied, the vaccination programme should be described, including the type of vaccine used, frequency of application, and species vaccinated.

6) Epidemiologic separation of the compartment

These factors relate to pathways of disease transmission, mitigations to prevent exposure, disease-specific factors, and environmental factors that affect exposure and propagation of the disease agent. All potential pathways for disease introduction should be assessed and corresponding biosecurity measures should be included in a comprehensive biosecurity plan. Other factors, such as the physical, geographic, or location factors that affect the status of biosecurity in the compartment, demographics, and marketing practices, should be taken into consideration.

7) Surveillance for the agent

Surveillance in the disease-free compartment should be continuous. This will help minimise the time between introduction and detection in the event of introduction of the virus of concern. Details on the number and type of samples collected as well as the methods of collection and the supervising authority should be analysed. Surveillance should follow the OIE guidelines for surveillance for avian influenza.

8) Diagnostic capabilities

All samples should be tested using internationally recognised tests as described in the OIE Manual of Standards for Diagnostic Tests and Vaccines [6]. Information on the number of laboratories, both official and accredited, in the requesting country should be presented. In the case of accredited laboratories, i.e., privately managed laboratories allowed to perform official tests under supervision of the veterinary services, details on the accreditation procedures should be submitted.

9) Emergency response, control, and notification capability

One of the most important factors that will reduce the risk of spreading a disease is early detection. For this to occur, effective disease-reporting mechanisms need to be in place, incorporating producers, private veterinarians, and official veterinarians. Outbreak investigation and emergency response procedures should be documented clearly.

Conclusions

The proposed guidelines for surveillance allow flexibility in the choice of approaches to achieve the desired level of confidence in disease-freedom claims. The persistent challenge of AIV introduction posed by wild bird populations requires that continuous surveillance is applied to domestic poultry populations. These guidelines provide support to the new proposed chapter on AI in the OIE Code.

The OIE Code recently introduced the concept of compartmentalisation. The concept, although relatively new in its definition, has been applied for quite some time by official veterinary services world-wide. The idea of compartmentalisation is helpful particularly for diseases that have a wild animal component, such as avian influenza. Application and monitoring of biosecurity measures are the key to successful implementation.

References

1 OIE. General Guidelines for Animal Health Surveillance. OIE Scientific Commission, 2004.

2 OIE. Guidelines for the surveillance of avian influenza. OIE Scientific Commission, 2004.

3 OIE. Terrestrial Animal Health Code. OIE, 2004.

4 Capua I, Terregino C, Cattoli G, Mutinelli F, Rodriguez JF: Development of a DIVA (Differentiating Infected from Vaccinated Animals) strategy using a vaccine containing a heterologous neuraminidase for the control of avian influenza. Avian Pathology 2002; 32: 47-55.

5 Scott A, Garber L, Zepeda C, Smith J, Swayne D, Rhorer A: Compartmentalization concept paper. Paper submitted to the OIE Scientific Commission, 2004.

6 OIE. Manual of Standards for Diagnostic Tests and Vaccines. OIE, 2004.

Dr. C. Zepeda, USDA-APHIS-VS Centers for Epidemiology and Animal Health/Animal Population Health Institute, Colorado State University. 2150 Centre Av., Bldg. B, Fort Collins, CO 80526, USA.
E-mail: cristobal.zepeda@aphis.usda.gov

Schudel A, Lombard M (eds): OIE/FAO International Scientific Conference on Avian Influenza.
Dev Biol (Basel). Basel, Karger, 2006, vol 124, pp 171-176.

Social, Economic and Policy Issues in the Long-Term Control of HPAI

A. McLeod, E. Guerne-Bleich

Animal Production and Health Division (AGA), FAO, Rome, Italy

Abstract: Prevention and control of HPAI in Asia is a long term problem with important economic and policy consequences. The macro level impact of a single national outbreak is greatest for an exporting country, ranging in 2003-5 from $65 million to over $400 million. No estimates are available for the impact of market disruption if endemic disease changes the pattern of regional and international trade. In countries with minimal exports, the total financial impact may be much smaller, but there can be serious losses to vulnerable sectors of society at several stages of the market chain. The economies of the region are growing and some countries could finance recurrent costs of AI control, but substantial investment in veterinary services is required. National and regional financing structures need to be reviewed. AI control strategies should include a broad financial support system that addresses education, credit, compensation and social relief programmes. Some strategies may result in restructuring of the industry, or affect the wider development of rural areas and local food security.

Introduction

At the Second FAO/OIE regional meeting on Avian Influenza Control in Asia, held in Bangkok in February 2005, a number of recommendations were made on economic and policy issues, which included the following:

- Analyses should be made of the potential social and economic impacts of AI control measures…
- The structure of animal health financing should be reviewed…
- Planning for AI control should include a broad financial support system…

This paper reviews each of the above topics in turn.

Methodology

The paper draws on three sources of information. The first is a review of the literature, mainly for estimates of macro-economic impact. The second is a study that was funded by FAO during 2004 and carried out in five affected countries (Cambodia, Indonesia, Lao PDR, Thailand and Vietnam). A total of 1806 farmers and 234 stakeholders have been interviewed so far, using questionnaires and semi-structured interviews. The analysis for four countries is complete, the work in Thailand is still continuing. One summary report has been produced [1] and a paper has been submitted for publication [2]. Finally, during 2004, an FAO consultative process funded five national workshops in affected countries to discuss responses to AI, a further regional workshop to discuss issues of common concern, and a workshop drawing particpants from six countries to discuss social, economic and policy issues [3].

Results

The majority of studies to date have considered the impacts of outbreaks over a relatively short period. There does not appear to have been any assessment of the long term effects of "endemic" avian influenza, with smaller but repeated outbreaks over a number of years. There has also been limited work on the social and economic impacts of strategies to control HPAI. The figures presented here consider the loss of agricultural production but not the loss of human life or the impact on households of losing an economically productive family member.

Macro level effects

For an exporting country, a single large outbreak of HPAI may result in a reduction of up to 1.5 % of GDP growth. In Thailand, agricultural growth may have halved during the 2003-4 outbreak, according to estimates made by the Thai Development Research Foundation. In Vietnam, predictions were made of the costs of the 2003-4 outbreaks that were initially estimated at 0.3 %-1.8 % of GDP, depending on the spread of disease and the time taken to control the outbreak [4]. Based on GDP estimates for 2004, this would have been the equivalent of US$76m-450m. The final estimate of losses was approximately $118 million. Two outbreaks in the USA were estimated to have cost US$65 and US$140 million. The cost of the 1997 outbreak in Hong Kong, it is suggested, may have been hundreds of millions of US$ including knock-on effects, but the very strict control measures applied may have prevented large scale human infection. Countries not infected in a regional outbreak can experience temporary gains, for example in 2004 The Philippines temporarily increased exports of day-old chicks and dressed chicken.

Micro level effects

The countries affected by AI in 2003-4 have in common large rural populations, many with low incomes (Table 1) and wide ownership of poultry, over 60 % of the rural population, making an estimated total of at least 136 million poultry owners in the five countries shown. In these countries, ducks are10-15 % of the poultry population and are found in three systems: commercial; migrating and seasonally herded in rice paddies and wet areas; and small backyard flocks mixed with chickens.

One case study in a Vietnamese village [5] paints a typical picture of losses at the household level. The death of birds, loss of 2.3 months of production and loss of home consumption were estimated to have cost US$ 69-108 for households involved in the outbreak – a large sum when compared to an income per person of $2 per day or less.

Indirect impacts were experienced by poultry farmers even in villages that did not experience HPAI outbreaks, as a result of reduced prices for poultry and eggs during outbreak periods. Figure 1 shows the changes in chicken and duck broiler prices during the HPAI outbreak in Cambodia. Chicken prices fell sharply, while duck prices were hardly affected. Early in 2004, the role of ducks in carrying and

Table 1: Population and household income in five countries affected by HPAI.

Country	Population 2004 (million)	% hholds < US$ 2/person/day	% rural	% labour in agriculture
Cambodia	13.4	(36.1)	81.5	75
Indonesia	238.5	55.4	52.3	45
Lao PDR	6.1	73.2	69.9	80
Thailand	64.9	32.5	75.3	49
Viet Nam	82.7	63.7	71.7	63

Sources: CIA website, 2004; FAOSTAT, 2004; UNDP website, 2004.

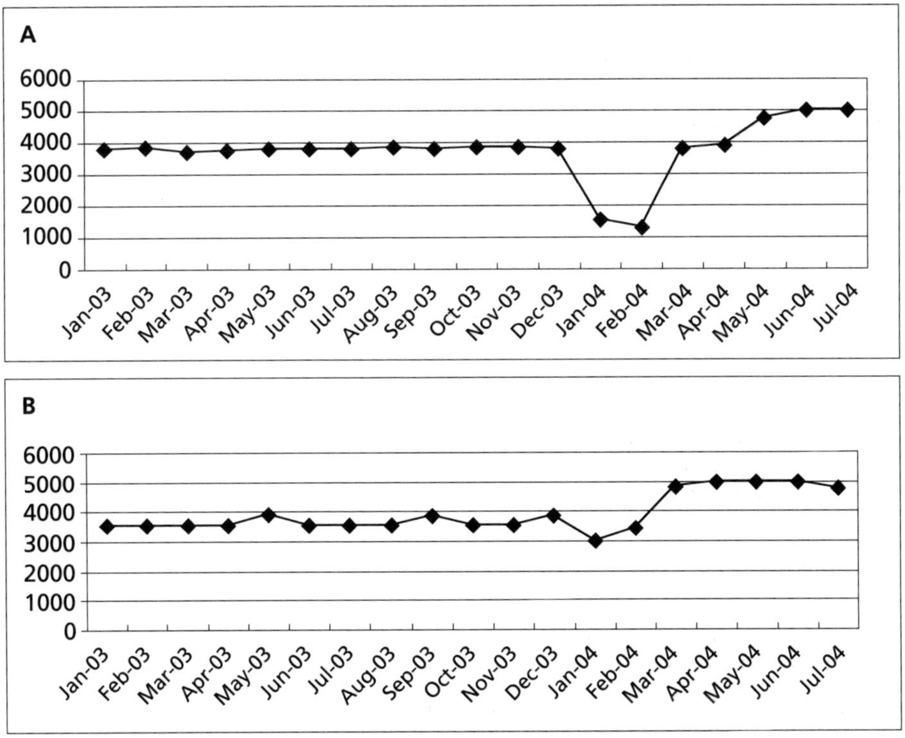

Fig. 1: Chicken and duck prices in Cambodia during and after an HPAI outbreak.
a) Chicken broilers, price per kg in riels; b) Duck broilers, price per kg in riels.
Source: Vétérinaires Sans Frontières [6].

spreading HPAI was not widely known. Egg prices showed a similar pattern to chickens. Data from the Indonesian Poultry Information Centre database [7] showed a fall in the price of chicken broilers over about two months after the HPAI outbreak was known, and a slow recovery over approximately another two months.

The impact of an HPAI outbreak varies along the poultry market chain and with the type of chain. Table 2 summarises quantitative and qualitative information from the FAO funded studies in 2004 and general literature on poultry production to suggest the likely impacts at different points.

Table 2: Potential impacts of an HPAI impact along a poultry market chain.

	Losers	Neutral	Winners
Input supply	Feed industry Day Old Chick suppliers		Animal health providers Vaccine producers
Production	Producers with high investment in fixed capital and loans Producers not compensated for poultry loss	Producers not directly affected (depending on price swings)	Producers of meat that substitutes for chicken
Marketing	Sole traders of poultry in affected areas	General traders of livestock	Traders of other livestock
Processing	Poultry abattoirs (especially for export) Workers in poultry export & processing	General abattoirs	Other livestock abattoirs. Workers in other livestock processing
Consumers	Urban poor Rural poor in areas affected by HPAI	Rural poor in areas not affected by HPAI Consumers who can afford other protein	
General	Families of people who have died. Tourism industry		

Sources: Rushton et al [2].

The scale of impact can be expected to vary with the type of chain. Five types, or variants of them, can commonly be found in South and East Asia, namely:

- industrial, vertically integrated (not found in all countries);
- large commercial farms supplying a chain that leads to a slaughterhouse;
- small commercial producers supplying a chain that leads to a "wet markets" or slaughter point – these include herded flocks of ducks found in wet, rice growing areas of Thailand, Vietnam and China;
- backyard scavenging poultry supplying local consumers within the same village.

At the time of writing this paper no comprehensive study had been done to assess differential impacts in each type of chains.

Restructuring

Some approaches to reducing HPAI risk that are now being considered, such as increased confinement of birds, concentration of production and processing into larger units, compartmentalization, and even recording to improve traceability, may require or result in restructuring of the industry. Smallholder production systems may reduce in importance or eventually be excluded altogether, if farmers are unable or unwilling to meet new requirements for risk reduction. They will need to make the choice to increase biosecurity and survive, or stop poultry production.

Wider impacts

Poultry production in rural areas is linked to pig and rice production. Changes in the poultry sub-sector can be expected to affect the wider development of rural areas and local food security. However, little was known at the time of writing about the impact of HPAI through the rural economy.

Discussion

More work is needed to estimate differential impacts arising from HPAI outbreaks, their prevention and control along the different types of poultry market chain. Ideally this would be based on multi-disciplinary analysis, conceptualised in Figure 2. More work is also needed on the impacts of HPAI and its control on the wider rural economy. If concern about human-to-human infection grows, wider economy effects may increase, for example a fall in income from tourism.

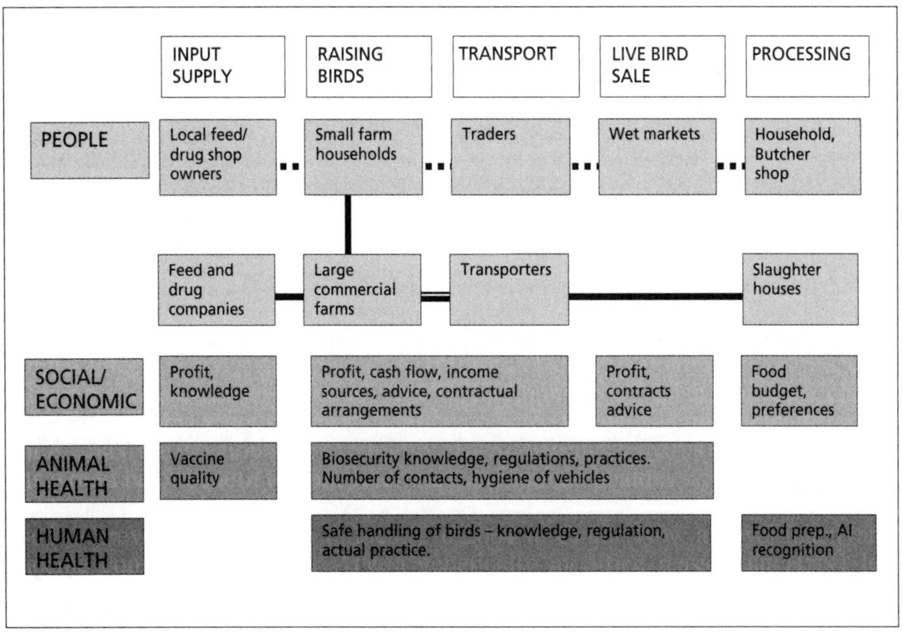

Fig. 2: Poultry market chain model showing issues that might be investigated by different disciplines.

National poultry subsectors are connected. Thailand, Indonesia and The Philippines all trade regionally. In the Mekong Delta there is informal as well as formal movement of birds between countries. This means that, as well as strengthening regional disease control initiatives, it is important to conduct regional economic studies and for economists within the region to co-ordinate the work they do on HPAI control.

Economic estimates of the impact of HPAI and its control will need to consider funding sources and the sustainable financing of control measures that may need to be carried out over a number of years. On a positive note, the economies of the region are growing. Some countries have a taxable GDP large enough to finance recurrent costs of AI control, although most would need assistance with investment. However, national financing structures for animal health control tend to be weak and face the additional challenge of decentralisation. Regional financing structures for regional control activities could offer economies of scope and scale. Reviews of funding mechanisms will need to take into account the role of stakeholders in financing different elements of AI control, possible options for revenue generation, and transparent fund management.

With the assumption that some farmers may need to upgrade their systems while others will leave poultry farming, economic analysis of HPAI control strategies will need to consider financial support in broad terms. Most programmes are likely to include compensation as an element of outbreak stamping out, although not all countries support this concept or can afford to implement it. An alternative may be credit accessible to all poultry farmers, including smallholders. Subsidized credit is highly problematic to implement, but micro-credit through farmer groups may be appropriate. For the really poor who are unable to continue poultry farming, social relief programmes may be necessary.

REFERENCES

1 Dolberg F: Emergency Regional Support for Post-Avian Influenza Rehabilitation, TCP/RAS/3010 (E). Summary of project results and outcomes, February 2005. FAO AGAP, 2005.

2 Rushton J, Viscarra R, Guerne-Bleich E, McLeod A: Impact of avian influenza outbreaks in the poultry sectors of five South East Asian countries (Cambodia, Indonesia, Lao PDR, Thailand, Viet Nam) outbreak costs, responses and potential long term control. World Poultry Science Journal 2005; 61(3): 491-514.

3 FAO: Workshop on social and economic impacts of avian influenza control, 8-9 December 2004, Siam City Hotel, Bangkok, Thailand. FAO AGAL, 2004.

4 World Bank: The impact of the avian influenza epidemic on the Vietnamese economy: an estimate by the World Bank in Vietnam, http://www.worldbank.org.vn/news/press40_01.htm, 2004.

5 Delquigny T, Edan M, Nguyen DH, Pham TK, Gautier P: Evolution and Impact of Avian Influenza Epidemic and Description of the Avian Production in Vietnam. World Bank, 2004.

6 Vétérinaires Sans Frontières: Review of the poultry production and assessment of the socio-economic impact of the highly pathogenic avian influenza epidemic in Cambodia. Final Report for FAO's TCP/RAS/3010 "Emergency Regional Support for Post Avian Influenza Rehabilitation". FAO, Rome, Italy, 2004.

7 Hartono D: Economic impact of AI on price and supply of poultry product. Paper presented at National Workshop on Post Avian Influenza Recovery (October 4-5, 2004). PINSAR Unggas Nasional (Indonesian Poultry Information Center). Direkorat Jenderal Bina Produksi Peternakan and Food and Agriculture Organization, 2004.

Dr. A. McLeod, Animal Production and Health Division (AGA), FAO, Viale delle Terme di Caracalla, IT-00100 Rome, Italy.
E-mail: anni.mcleod@fao.org

Schudel A, Lombard M (eds): OIE/FAO International Scientific Conference on Avian Influenza.
Dev Biol (Basel). Basel, Karger, 2006, vol 124, p 177.

General Conclusions and Recommendations

Chairperson: *B. Vallat* (OIE)
Rapporteur: *J. Domenech* (FAO)
Panel: *I. Capua* (IZS, Italy), *S. Edwards* (VLA, UK), *K. Sakamoto* (NIAH, Japan), *A. Thiermann* (OIE)

Schudel A, Lombard M (eds): OIE/FAO International Scientific Conference on Avian Influenza.
Dev Biol (Basel). Basel, Karger, 2006, vol 124, pp 179-186.

Recommendations

OIE/FAO International Scientific Conference on Avian Influenza
OIE Paris, France, 7-8 April 2005

CONSIDERING THAT

1. Preventing the spread of pathogens through international trade in animals and animal products is one of the primary missions of the World Organisation for Animal Health (OIE). This is accomplished by establishing and updating international standards and guidelines that prevent spread of pathogens while avoiding unjustified sanitary barriers.
2. The OIE works in close association with FAO in helping countries implement such standards and guidelines.
3. The FAO has as its foremost mission to alleviate poverty through the promotion of sustainable agricultural production, food security and safe and wholesome food products in the market places, and response to crises caused by animal diseases including zoonoses. This is particularly relevant to the FAO priority programme EMPRES (Emergency Prevention System for the Prevention of Plant and Animal Pests and Diseases), and specifically to the Emergency Centre for Transboundary Animal Diseases (ECTAD).
4. The OIE standards for terrestrial animals are contained in the *Terrestrial Animal Health Code* (the *Terrestrial Code*) and the *Manual of Diagnostic Tests and Vaccines for Terrestrial Animals* (the *Terrestrial Manual*).
5. The collection, analysis and dissemination of veterinary scientific information is also one of the main missions of the OIE. Comprehensive analysis of agro-ecological factors, production parameters, and demographics, including animal census, as done at FAO, provides additional understanding in disease occurrences and offers opportunities to develop strategic intervention measures.
6. The standards developed by the OIE are recognised as international standards for animal health and zoonoses by the Agreement on the Application of Sanitary and Phytosanitary Measures (SPS Agreement) of the World Trade Organization (WTO); the OIE also serving as a partner with the FAO/WHO Codex Alimentarius on animal production food safety. Implementation of these standards by

Member Countries also has benefits for public health (including food safety) and improvement of animal production.

7. Infectious animal diseases and zoonoses such as highly pathogenic avian influenza (HPAI) represent a major constraint to efficient poultry production and regional and international exchanges, and present a threat to the livelihood of farmers, especially in developing countries, to public health, and to national economies.
8. During the past few years, the world has witnessed the emergence of a severe avian influenza epidemic that has had a major impact on animal health and the potential for serious human health outcomes. This has severely affected the economies of developed as well as developing countries
9. FAO emergency implementation of some 19 projects at national, regional, and supra-regional level for HPAI prevention, control, and eradication is recognised and has improved the current outlook, with the publication of Guiding Principles for Surveillance and Recommendations taking into account OIE standards, supported by WHO and the donor community.
10. Recent research has confirmed that certain aquatic birds (particularly domestic ducks) can act as reservoirs of infection for HPAI H5N1 with or without clinical signs and are capable of excreting viruses into the environment.
11. Many of the countries infected or threatened by AI are under-resourced and lack the capacity of Veterinary Services for an effective early detection and response to the epidemic in poultry.
12. New scientific and technological knowledge for the prevention and control of AI will contribute to the development of safer and more efficacious measures for the final control and eradication of the disease.
13. For ethical, ecological and economic reasons, it is no longer considered acceptable to control and eradicate diseases mainly by applying mass killing of animals.
14. Safe and effective vaccines, if used appropriately, can help to improve animal health, public health, animal welfare, and agricultural sustainability and to protect the environment, maintain biodiversity, and protect consumers of animal products.
15. The OIE has incorporated wherever possible into its standards and guidelines the most up-todate scientific knowledge on the use of appropriate diagnostic tests, disease prevention and control methods including vaccination, and has reviewed, commented, and endorsed the FAO Recommendations for the Control of HPAI in Asia.
16. Recent scientific advances in the diagnostic field, in particular the possibility of differentiating vaccinated animals from infected animals, have been recently incorporated into the *Terrestrial Manual*. Their implications have already been reflected in the review of the *Terrestrial Code* for disease control using appropriate vaccination and for recovery of disease-free status after occurrence of a disease.
17. The Conference has provided an opportunity for the exchange of the latest scientific information at the global level that will also assist in the evaluation and improvement of the current OIE standards and FAO guidelines for better control

of avian influenza and safety of regional and international trade of poultry and poultry products, implementation of strategies, and requirements for effective disease management.

18. To this effect, the OIE/FAO have acted in collaboration with WHO, with which a long and valuable tradition for confronting zoonotic diseases exists.
19. There is a need to harmonise communication on risk assessment and risk management.
20. FAO has underlined the links and risks between farming systems, market chains, socioeconomic status, and epidemiology of HPAI in Asia, indicating that multidisciplinary approaches are required to tackle the epidemic in poultry adequately and prevent infection spread to humans.
21. It is necessary to protect human health by controlling the disease as a matter of priority at source, i.e. on farms and markets. It is essential to provide national and international support for the improvement of the efficiency of Veterinary Services for that purpose.
22. Long-term prevention and control of AI need to be compatible with social, economic and technical considerations,
23. Effective AI prevention and control require actions from local, national, regional, and international levels,
24. The recently renewed agreement between OIE and FAO has led to synergistic approaches to fight transboundary animal diseases, particularly through the joint initiative GF-TADs,
25. Research into better tools (diagnostics, vaccines, anti-virals, adjuvants, disinfectants, for instance) and virus dynamics (excretion, pathogenesis, virulence genes) that will assist in developing control strategies and prevention measures as well as better epidemiological studies in the country where the disease prevails, is needed.
26. The role of wild birds in the spread of HPAI H5N1 viruses remains unresolved. Circumstantial evidence suggests limited local infection of resident wild birds, but transfer of H5N1 HPAI viruses outside the outbreak zones by migratory birds has not been substantiated.

Conference attendees of the OIE/FAO International Scientific Conference on Avian Influenza recommend the following

Session I: Ecology and Epidemiology

1. Preventing the spread of AI viruses to unaffected areas/countries.
2. Country/regional specific studies should be conducted to establish the ecology and epidemiology of the AI virus in reservoir and spill-over species of poultry for the purpose of developing control programmes to stop virus cycling and re-infection.
3. Surveillance and epidemiological studies in migratory and resident wild birds should be conducted to assess the role of wild birds in the maintenance and dissemination of HPAI viruses.

4. Developing sustainable risk-based surveillance programmes for poultry for early identification of AI virus transfer from reservoir species to agricultural systems in order to know if and which AI viruses are present in poultry and to develop rapid mitigation and elimination strategies, if required.
5. Encourage national laboratories to join multi-national and international laboratory networks to share AI virus isolates, data and expertise in order to understand AI virus ecology and develop effective control strategies.
6. Support pathogenesis studies in other farmed birds (e.g. ostriches, waterfowl, pheasants, etc.), including an assessment of their role as intermediate hosts for transfer of AI viruses from wild birds to traditionally farmed poultry species, and their potential role for supporting mutation of H5 and H7 LPAI to HPAI viruses.

Session II: Pathogenesis

1. Country authorities should be made aware of different clinical syndromes in different hosts caused by infection by AI viruses as typical disease signs have been seen in infections with recent isolates.
2. Specific genes from virus isolates should be monitored for evidence of reassortments and drift that may contribute to changes in virulence.
3. Surveillance of birds for the presence of H9N2 viruses with the potential to infect mammals should be carried out.
4. Consideration should be given to conduct monitoring of pigs at risk from infections with AI viruses with the potential to transmit to humans.
5. Investigate the pathogenesis and epidemiology of avian influenza viruses in different species of birds and mammals under the coordination of the joint OIE/FAO network with the support of the OIE/FAO Reference Laboratories for AI.
6. Specific research be conducted on AI surveillance and vaccination in farmed ducks.

Session III: Human health implications

1. Further epidemiological studies at the human-animal interface as well as applied and basic research on H5N1 and other AI viruses with potential human health implications should be conducted urgently and by collaboration between the animal OIE/FAO network and the human WHO network.

2 Coordinated research programmes must involve veterinary, public health and industry sectors. Safe and efficacious human and avian vaccines should be developed as a priority.

3 Veterinary and Public health services should work together to improve national, regional and global health security. Public health services should support the agriculture sector/veterinary services in order to control and eliminate the disease at source and to protect farmers and workers from animal infection in the most efficient and efficacious manner.

4 Veterinary and Public health services should strengthen joint activities for surveillance of AI at the human/animal interface. Animal virus isolates and sequence information should be swiftly exchanged between the international reference laboratories of OIE-FAO and those of WHO.

5 FAO, OIE and WHO should collaborate with their Member Countries in the development of appropriate strategies for effective inter-sectoral collaboration during and between crises associated with the emergence of zoonoses.

Session IV: Diagnostics

1. OIE/FAO assist countries in enhancing their veterinary infrastructures to meet the current and future needs for early detection, surveillance and control programmes for avian influenza.
2. OIE/FAO encourage countries/regions to develop a laboratory network that would facilitate the local testing of specimens to decrease turn-around time for diagnostic test results while increasing overall testing capacity. This network should be coordinated through the newly established OIE/FAO network (OFFLU) that could recommend appropriate testing methods, provide training to laboratory personnel, supply quality reagents, and collaborate with OIE/FAO Reference Laboratories.
3. OIE/FAO encourage the development of training programmes for laboratory personnel to ensure that appropriate diagnostic tests are used, that test results are interpreted correctly, and that appropriate quality assurance programmes are being used.
4. OIE/FAO encourage the development of rapid, sensitive, and cost-effective diagnostic tests that have been properly field validated according to OIE guidelines and are appropriate for use in local laboratories involved in the diagnosis of avian influenza.
5. OIE/FAO develop a prototype Material Transfer Agreement (MTA) that could be used by laboratories to facilitate the transfer of viruses to reference laboratories for epidemiologic/research purposes.

Session V: Control of AI (with focus on vaccination)

1. Infections with HPAI viruses be controlled at source, through implementation of risk reduction interventions, including improved biosecurity, stamping out, vaccination, and education awareness programmes.
2. Donors should give priority to reinforcing Veterinary Services and animal health infrastructures in countries infected or threatened by AI.
3. Vaccination should only be used in conjunction with monitoring of vaccinated flocks to ensure efficacy, proper use of the vaccine and absence of virus circulation.
4. Vaccines should comply with OIE standards and vaccination strategies should be consistent with guidelines developed by FAO, and of proven efficacy under experimental and local field conditions.

5. Vaccine delivery systems and vaccination campaigns should be carefully organised and monitored by Veterinary Services.
6. That, wherever appropriate, a surveillance system capable of differentiating infected from vaccinated birds (e.g DIVA) be applied (including use of sentinel birds when possible).
7. That surveillance programmes be defined before vaccination is introduced. Likewise, an exit strategy has to be identified.
8. That strategies be developed and evaluated in statistically based field trials for the appropriate use of vaccination in different epidemiological scenarios which may occur worldwide.

Session VI: Improvement of Management Tools

1. A master plan be prepared for the control and prevention of HPAI in Asia and in other threatened regions, with regional and international coordination.
2. Adequate financial resources be invested to the control of AI in Asia, which is currently estimated at between 100 and 120 million USD over a 3–5 year period.
3. The meeting strongly recommends that OIE and FAO implement activities of the joint global OIE/FAO network of expertise for avian influenza as soon as possible.
4. The existing FAO regional networks for surveillance and diagnosis be sustained in the long term.
5. The FAO/OIE Global Framework for the Progressive Control of Transboundary Animal Diseases (GF-TADs) initiatives be used as a foundation for the regional approach to the control and eradication of AI. The mandates and missions of international and regional organizations be harmonized to avoid gaps and overlapping.
6. Strategies are needed for financing sustainable, concrete action at local level. This is likely to include support for restocking or compensation for losses and should also encompass education on safe poultry keeping and development of appropriate infrastructure and services.
7. National and regional strategies for AI prevention and control should include a careful assessment of the social and economic impact of proposed measures, including the impact on the wider rural economy of changes in the poultry sector. Options for long-term strategies for restructuring of the sectors should be previously considered and the possible negative socio-economic impacts on small and medium holders evaluated as well as the options and cost for mitigation strategies.
8. That, when a decision is made to kill infected or at-risk birds, these should be humanely destroyed and disposed of along with dead poultry, in line with OIE standards. In the case of HP infections, the birds should not be allowed to enter the human food chain or be fed directly or indirectly to other animals including zoo animals.
9. That the OIE International Committee adopts the proposed new surveillance guidelines on AI during the 73rd General Session.

10. That the efficacy of risk reduction and prevention procedures be monitored through targeted surveillance activities, including:
    - post-vaccination surveillance to measure efficacy of vaccination;
    - early identification of virus circulation;
    - monitoring of genetic drift and emergence of new strains;
    - monitoring of reservoirs.
11. That the concept of compartmentalisation be recognised as an additional tool in the control of AI and in the facilitation of safe international trade, subject to the effective implementation of the relevant control measures.
12. That the OIE International Committee adopts the proposed revised Terrestrial Code chapter on AI that incorporates the concept of compartmentalisation and provides risk-based recommendations for trade in live poultry, genetic material and products for human consumption. It also encourages transparency in disease reporting, by limiting trade consequences to situations of significant risk.
13. That the OIE and FAO continue to provide practical advice to Member Countries on the establishment and monitoring of compartments, through additional guidelines.
14. That OIE Member Countries use the new Terrestrial Code chapter and the surveillance appendix as a guide for their national activities and as standards for international trade.
15. That the FAO, World Bank and other multilateral and bilateral donors should continue to provide assistance to further strengthen countries' compliance with international standards, including quality of Veterinary Services.
16. That the OIE develops guidelines for AI virus inactivation in processed products.
17. That strategies be developed for financing sustainable, concrete action at local level, to include support for restocking or compensation for losses, to encompass education on safe poultry keeping and the development of appropriate infrastructure and services.
18. That the OIE designates prescribed tests for international trade where testing is required by the Terrestrial Code.
19. That OIE/FAO Reference Laboratories collaborate to exchange virus isolates and develop internationally agreed standards for diagnostic testing. The exchange of virus isolates and other information such as sequence data between the OIE/FAO network and the WHO laboratory network is urged.
20. Decision making in animal disease control and prevention be based on scientific evidence arising from valid epidemiological data analysis generated from reliable information systems. All efforts should be made to develop such systems even in developing countries.

Adopted by the OIE/FAO International Scientific Conference on Avian Influenza
Paris (France), 7-8 April 2005

General Recommendation for the 73rd OIE General Session

The OIE refers the scientific information generated and discussed at this international conference, as well as this Recommendation to the OIE Regional and relevant Specialist Commissions and request the endorsement by the OIE International Committee during the 73rd General Session in May 2005.

Schudel A, Lombard M (eds): OIE/FAO International Scientific Conference on Avian Influenza.
Dev Biol (Basel). Basel, Karger, 2006, vol 124, p 187.

Poster Session

Schudel A, Lombard M (eds): OIE/FAO International Scientific Conference on Avian Influenza.
Dev Biol (Basel). Basel, Karger, 2006, vol 124, pp 189-199.

Phylogenetic Analyses of Genes from South African LPAI Viruses Isolated in 2004 from Wild Aquatic Birds Suggests Introduction by Eurasian Migrants

C. Abolnik[1], E. Cornelius[2], S.P.R. Bisschop[3], M. Romito[1], D. Verwoerd[4]

[1] Biotechnology Division, Onderstepoort Veterinary Institute, Onderstepoort, South Africa

[2] Department of Veterinary Tropical Diseases, University of Pretoria, Onderstepoort, South Africa

[3] Poultry Reference Laboratory, University of Pretoria, Onderstepoort, South Africa

[4] Pfizer Animal Health, Johannesburg, South Africa

Abstract: In 2004, South Africa experienced its first recorded outbreak of a highly pathogenic notifiable avian influenza (HPNAI) viral strain of the H5N2 subtype in ostriches in the Eastern Cape province. The traditional ostrich-farming areas in the Western Cape province report almost yearly outbreaks of low pathogenicity avian influenza (LPAI) in ostriches, which is attributed to introduction by wild birds and certain climatic patterns. During the winter of 2004, LPAI H3N8, H4N8, H5N2 and H5N1 avian influenza viruses were isolated from wild aquatic birds. All eight genes of the H3N8, H4N8 and H5N1 viruses were analysed. The results show that the H5N1 virus does not belong to the HPAI Z/Z +/V genotype currently circulating in Asia, but that the most recent common ancestors are Russian H5N2 and H5N3 viruses. The N1 gene lacks the stalk deletion associated with virulence. Internal genes probably originate from a pool containing Chinese, Middle Eastern and Italian viruses.

The South African H3N8 and H4N8 viruses appear to have derived their genes from an ecosystem where Asian H5N1, H6N9 and H9N2, Russian H4, and Danish H3N8 viruses have been circulating since 1997. All three viruses share recent nucleoprotein common ancestors with the German and Dutch HPNAI H7N7 viruses from 2003. The diverse pool of genes from which local viruses are derived suggests that reassortment occurred at the Siberian breeding grounds where migratory paths cross, or within the South African ecosystem. This data highlights the importance of surveillance in aquatic migratory birds, particularly members of the Charadriidae, for their potential roles in the introduction of avian diseases to South African poultry and especially ostriches in the case of avian influenza.

INTRODUCTION

South Africa experienced its first recorded outbreak of highly pathogenic notifiable avian influenza (HPNAI) caused by an H5N2 virus, in ostriches during 2004. Outbreaks of low pathogenic avian influenza (LPAI) are generally reported yearly in the ostrich-farming regions in winter; they are attributed to introduction by wild birds and certain climatic patterns. In the past, H7N1 (1991), H5N9 (1994), H9N2 (1995), H10N2, H6N8 (1998) and H10N1 (2001) have been isolated from wild birds and/or ostriches, and an outbreak of LPAI H6N2 affected chickens across the country from 2002 to 2004. LPAI was isolated from wild birds in the ostrich-farming district during a previous survey [1], but it is only recently that molecular epidemiological studies [2,3] have started to unveil the Asian source of South African para- and orthomyxovirus isolates.

The role of waterbirds, particularly ducks, geese and shorebirds in AI ecology is well documented in other countries [4]. The movements of South African indigenous ducks and geese are restricted to sub-Saharan Africa, but at least 18 species of the order *Charadriiformes* (shorebirds or waders) migrate annually from breeding grounds in Siberia [5]. Yet it is indigenous ducks and geese, which inhabit nearby rivers and dams, that are sighted in ostrich camps. Here we report on the isolation and phylogenetic characterisation of three LPAI viruses isolated from indigenous wild ducks culled during the winter months, prior to the HPAI H5N2 outbreak.

MATERIALS AND METHODS

Virus isolation

Fifty three organ samples were collected from yellow-billed ducks (*Anas undulata*), red-billed teals (*Anas erythrorhyncha*), red-knobbed coots (*Fulica cristata*), Cape teals (*Anas capensis*) and Cape shovellers (*Anas smithii*) at Blesbokspruit wetlands (26° 17' S; 28° 30' E) in the Gauteng province. Virus isolation was performed according to OIE guidelines. Three orthomyxoviruses were isolated (Table 1).

Table 1: Avian influenza viruses isolated at Onderstepoort during 2004.

Virus name	Host	Type	H_0 cleavage site amino acid sequence
Duck/South Africa/811/04	Yellow-billed duck	H5N1	RNVPQRETRGLF
Duck/South Africa/1108/04	Cape teal/ Cape shoveller pool	H3N8	RNVPEKQTRGLF
Duck/South Africa/1233A/04	Red-billed teal	H4N8	RNIPEKASRGLF

Genetic and phylogenetic analyses

All eight genes of the three isolates were sequenced so as to determine their genetic relationship with other viruses. Viral RNA was extracted from allantoic fluid with the QIAamp Viral RNA mini kit (Qiagen). Reverse transcription using gene-specific oligonucleotides was performed at 42°C for 90 minutes. Gene-specific primer sets were used to amplify the coding regions. PCR-derived ds-cDNA was used as a template for sequencing on an Applied Biosystems 3100 Genetic Analyzer, using cycle sequencing dye terminator chemistry (Perkin Elmer/Applied Biosystems). Sequences were edited with the Staden software package, Chromas and BioEdit v. 5.0.9 [6], and aligned in ClustalW. Phylip and MEGA version 2.1 [7] were used to construct unrooted phylogenetic trees by the neighbour-joining method and 1000 bootstrap replicates were performed to assign confidence levels to branches.

RESULTS

Surface glycoproteins

Phylogenetic evidence (Fig. 1) shows that the Duck/South Africa/811/04 (H5N1) haemagglutinin gene is phylogenetically separated from the contemporary Asian HPNAI Z/Z +/V H5N1 viruses, furthermore it is also genetically distinct from Italian HPNAI H5N2 viruses and Dutch H5N2/H5N7 viruses. The HPNAI H5N2 virus isolated in South Africa during the 2004 outbreak in ostriches only shares 91 % identities (data not shown). The closest relatives (94 % sequence identities) are the Russian viruses Duck/Primorie/2633/01 (H5N3) and Duck/Primorie/2621/01 (H5N2), which indicates that the original gene pool may be located at waterfowl breeding grounds in Siberia. Protein sequence analysis predicted seven potential N-glycosylation sites in the H protein, but no additional glycosylation site at position 158 (by H3 numbering) was detected, which is in accordance with findings from other non-pathogenic H5 viruses isolated from aquatic birds [8]. The N1 gene is closely-related (96 % identities) to two Italian viruses viz. Chicken/Italy/1067/99 (H7N1) and Turkey/Italy/4580/00 (H7N1) (Fig. 2), however, the Duck/South Africa/811/04 (H5N1) neuraminidase lacks the N-stalk deletion associated with virulence [8], which is present within the Italian N1 genes.

H3-type viruses in Genbank separate into three lineages (Fig. 3): American mallard and seal isolates; American and Eurasian viruses from the 1960s to the 1980s; and Eurasian viruses isolated from 1963 to the present. The Duck/South Africa/1108/04 (H3N8) H3 gene falls within the latter lineage. Within this third lineage, two distinct clades of H3N2 (Korean 2003 viruses) and H3N8 (Far East, Norway, Denmark and South African viruses) are distinguishable. The Duck/South Africa/1108/04 virus H3 gene is most closely related to the Danish virus Mallard/65112/03 (H3N8) (95 % sequence identities).

The phylogenetic distinction between Eurasian and North American H4 viruses is supported by a bootstrap value of 100 (Fig. 4), and within the Eurasian lineage two distinct clades are evident. One of these contains H4N6 viruses isolated between 1956 and 1979, and the other more contemporary H4N6 viruses, including the Duck/South Africa/1233A/04 (H4N8) haemagglutinin gene. This gene shares 98 % sequence identities with those of the Russian viruses isolated in 2002.

The N8-type neuraminidase phylogenetic tree (Fig. 5), which includes N8 genes from both the Duck/South Africa/1108/04 (H3N8) and Duck/South Africa/1233A/04 (H4N8) viruses, demonstrates the Equine, North American and Eurasian lineages previously described for N8 genes [9]. The two South African viruses share 99 % sequence identities, which indicates a common source. Recent common ancestors are shared with the Danish (98 % sequence identities) and Norwegian (97 % sequence identities) H3N8 viruses isolated in 2003.

Internal genes

Figure 6 schematically depicts recent common ancestors of the three South African (SA) viruses, phylogenetic trees are not shown. Matrix protein genes of Duck/South Africa/811/04 (H5N1) and Duck/South Africa/1233A/04 (H4N8) cluster together with viruses from the Far East, Australia and southern Europe (Italy), whereas the Duck/South Africa/1108/04 (H3N8) M gene is genetically unrelated to the other SA viruses, grouping with viruses from the Far East and northern Europe

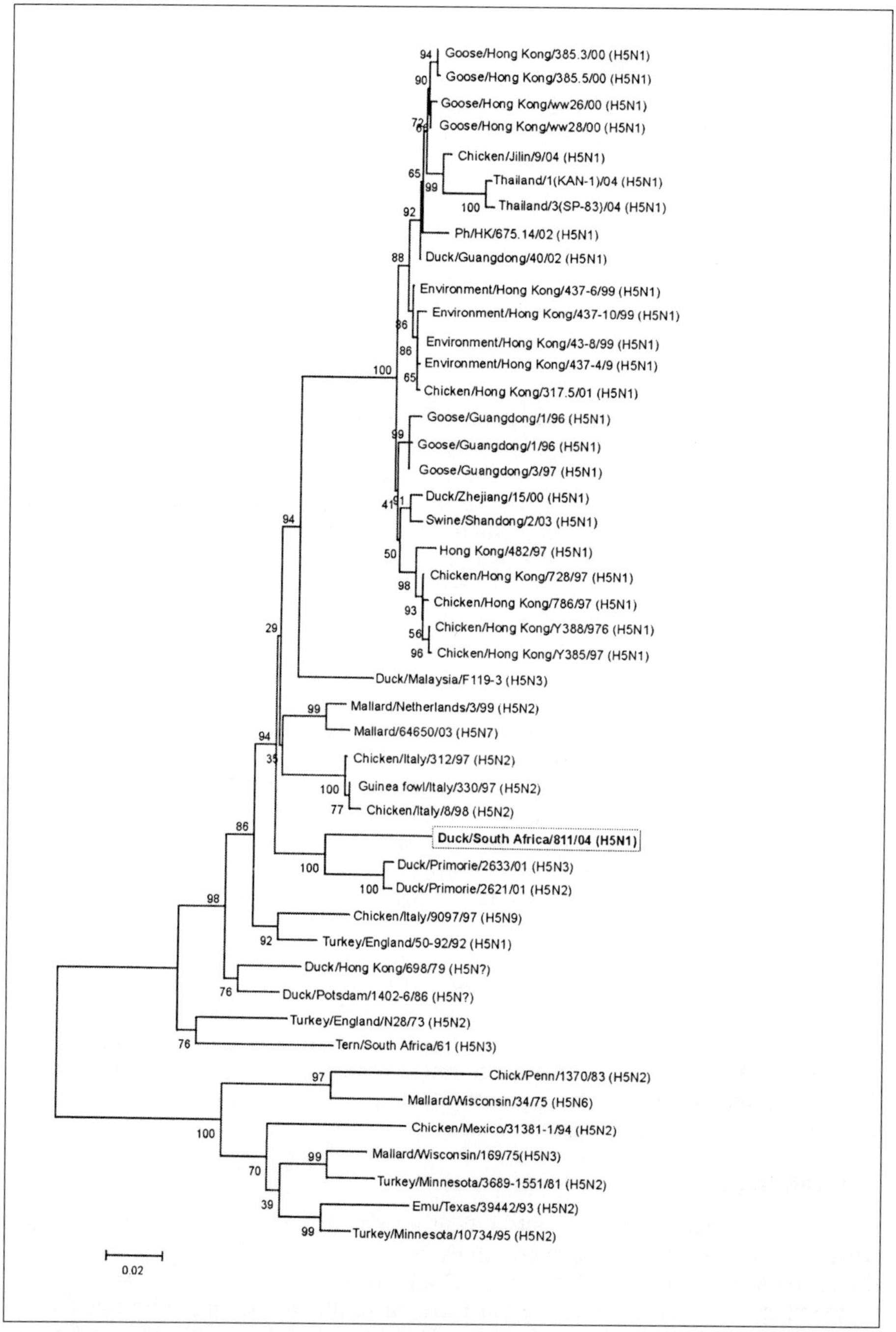

Fig. 1: Phylogenetic tree of the Duck/South Africa/811/04 (H5N1) haemagglutinin gene. The H_0 cleavage site sequences were removed prior to phylogenetic analysis.

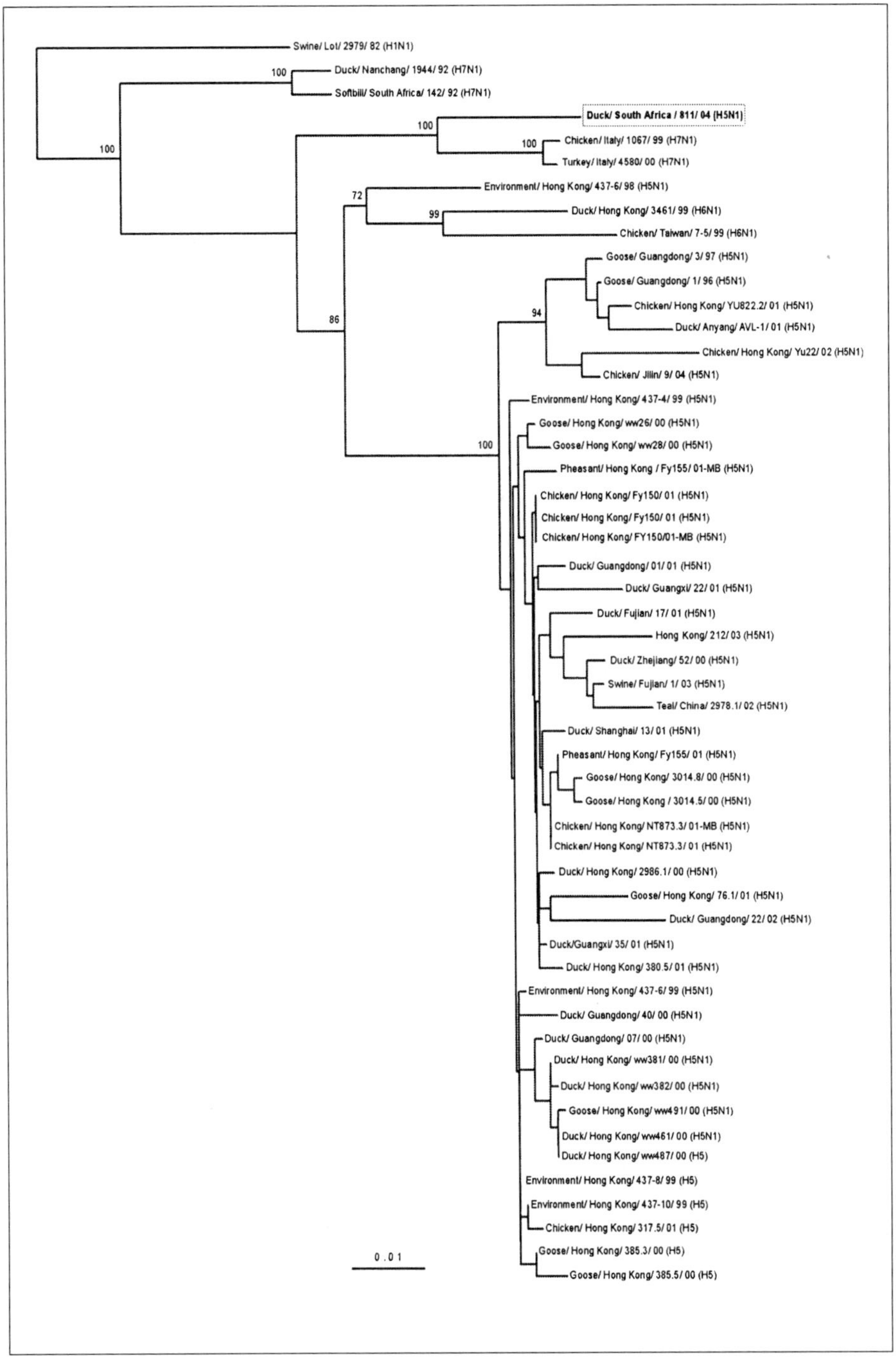

Fig. 2: Phylogenetic tree of the Duck/South Africa/811/04 (H5N1) neuraminidase gene.

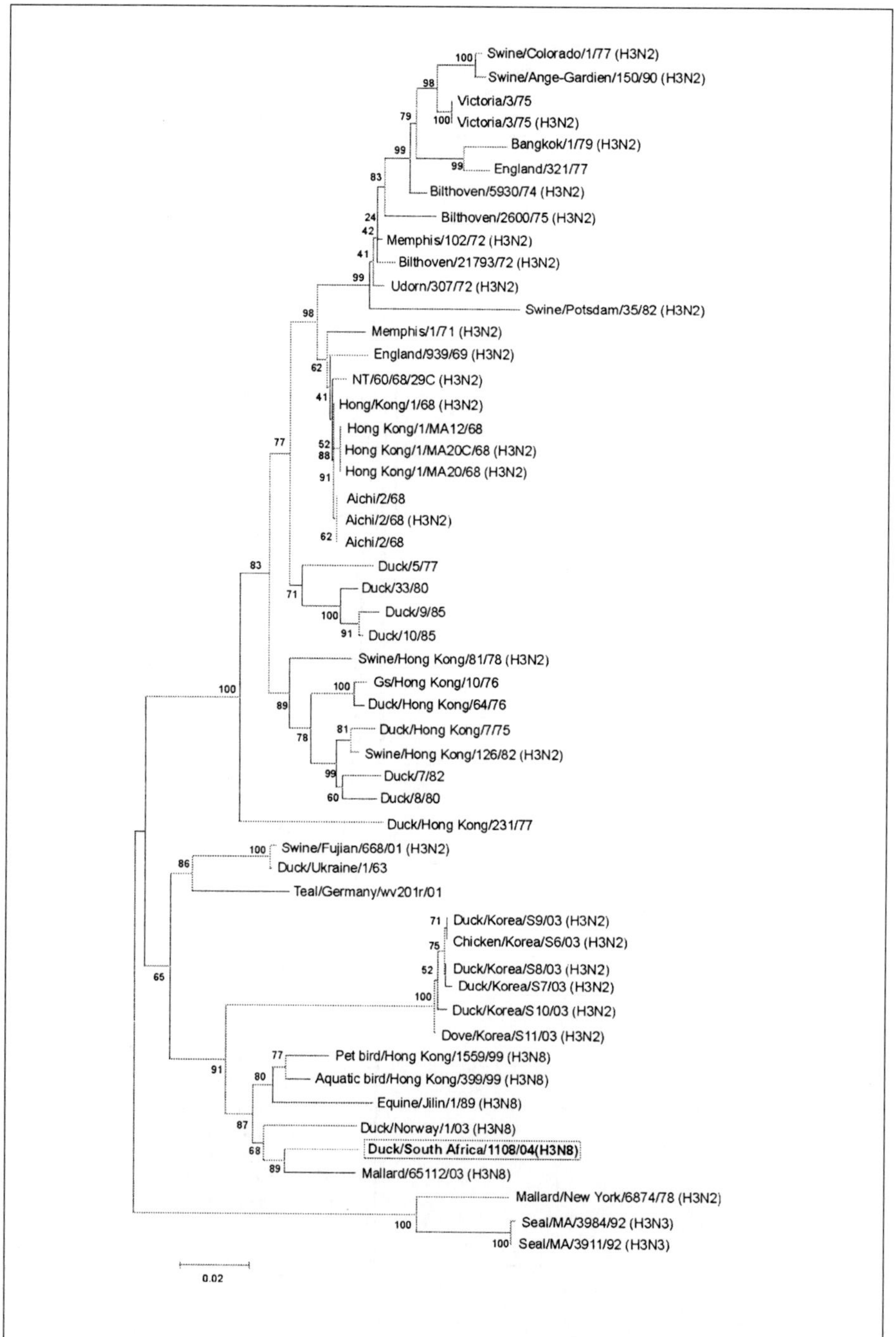

Fig. 3: Phylogenetic tree of the Duck/South Africa/1108/04 (H3N8) haemagglutinin gene.

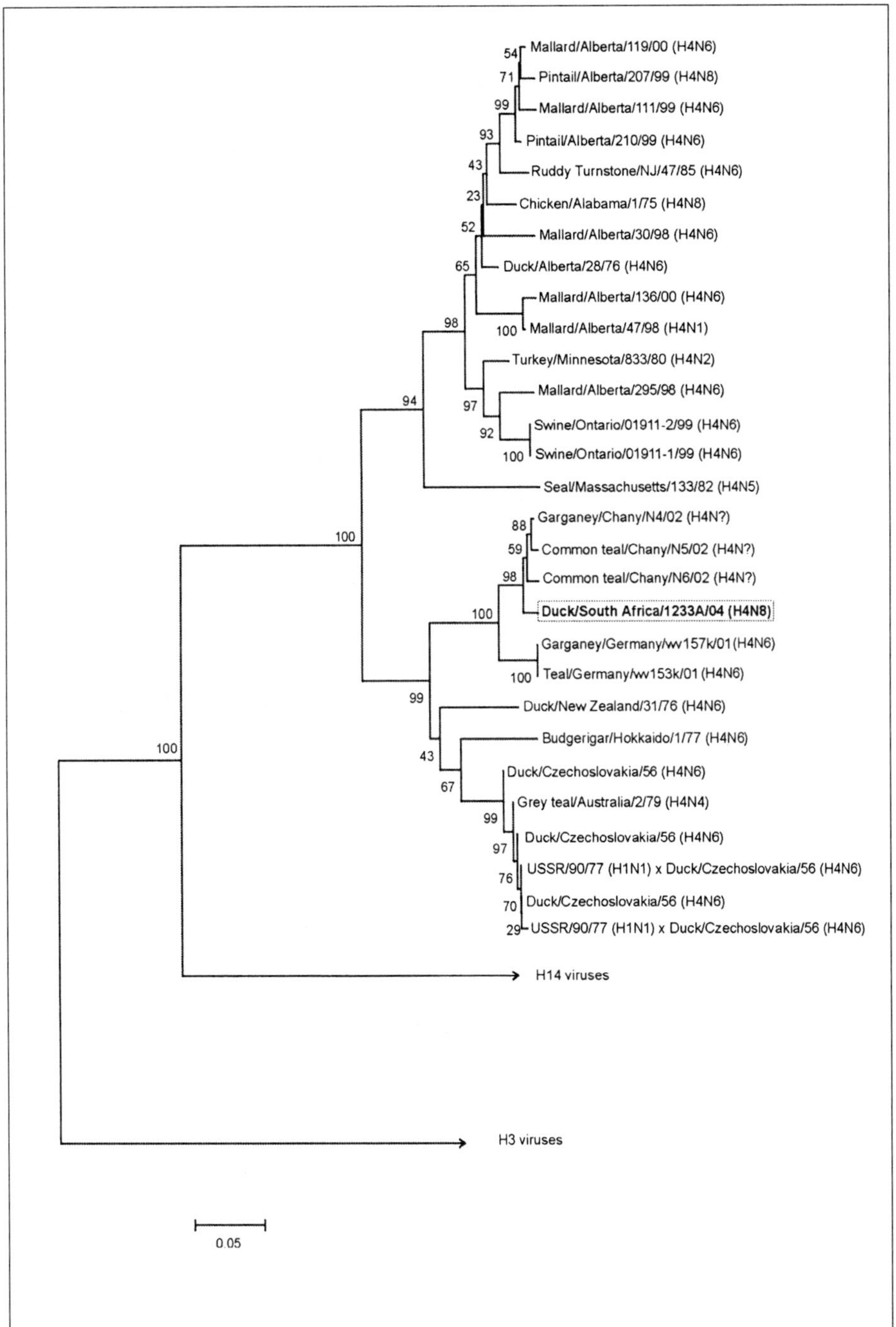

Fig. 4: Phylogenetic tree of the Duck/South Africa/1233A/04 (H4N8) haemagglutinin gene.

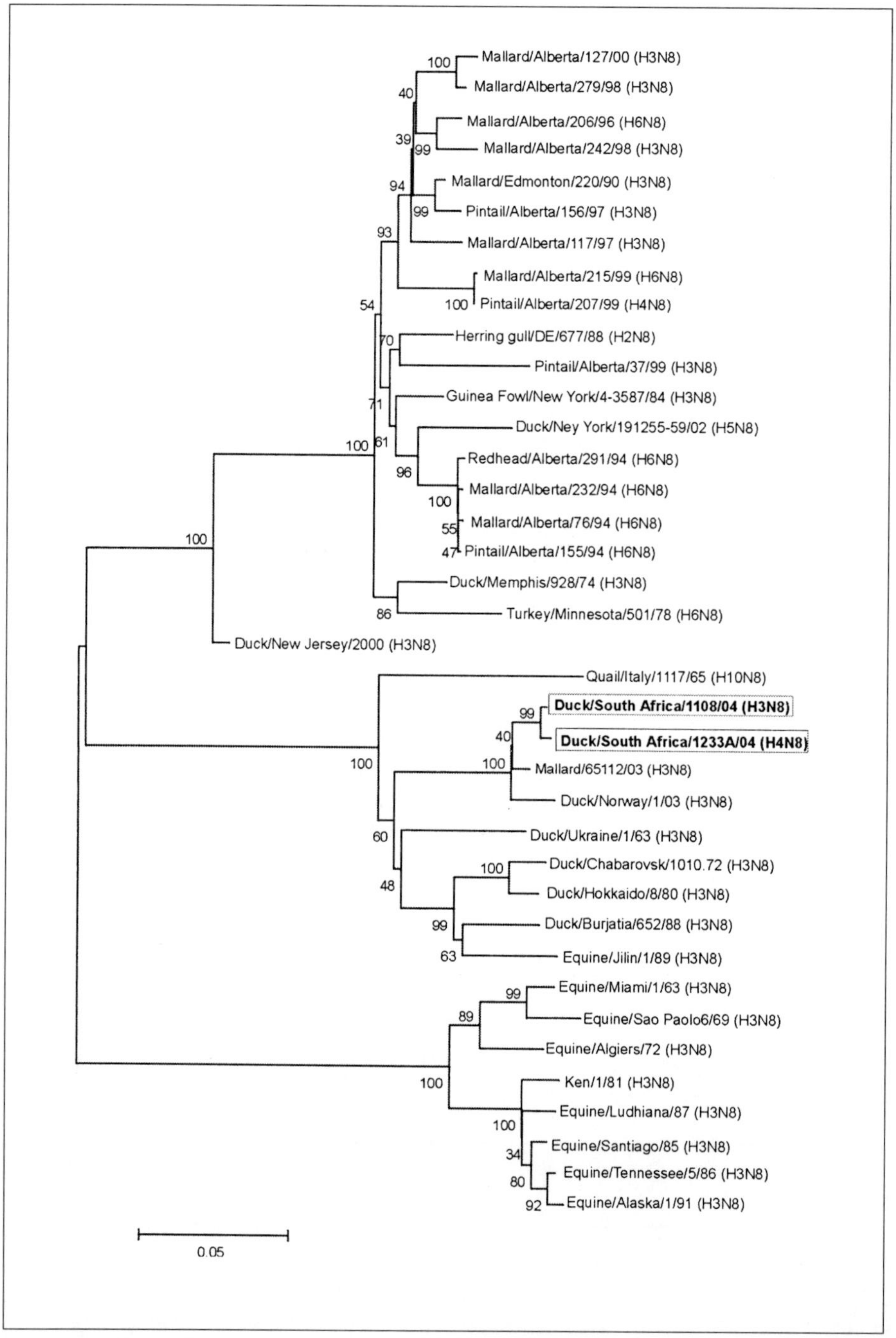

Fig. 5: Phylogenetic tree of the Duck/South Africa/1108/04 (H3N8) and the Duck/South Africa/1233A/04 (H4N8) neuraminidase genes.

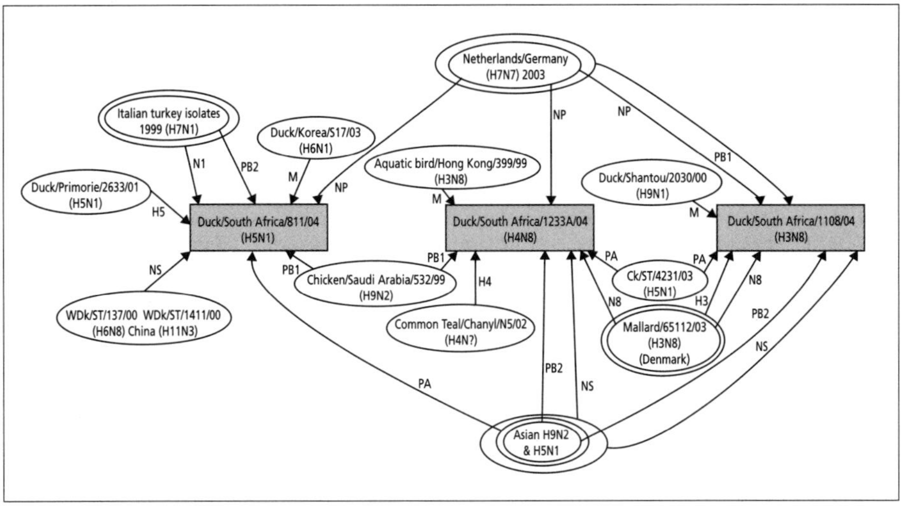

Fig. 6: Recent common ancestors of the Duck/South Africa/811/04 (H5N1), Duck/SouthAfrica/1108/04 (H3N8) and Duck/South Africa/1233A/04 (H4N8) genes.

(Germany, The Netherlands, Ireland). The closest relative of the Duck/South Africa/811/04 (H5N1) M gene is Duck/Korea/S17/03 (H6N1), indicating that the M gene may have co-reassorted with the N1 gene at some time. The Duck/South Africa/1108/04 (H3N8) M gene appears to share a recent common ancestor with highly pathogenic H9N1 viruses isolated in Shantou, China, during 2000.

All nucleoprotein (NP) genes of the three South African LPAI duck viruses are closely related, with 99 % sequence identities shared between Duck/South Africa/1108/04 (H3N8) and Duck/South Africa/1233A/04 (H4N8) viruses and 96 % identities between these two and Duck/South Africa/811/04 (H5N1). Furthermore, the SA viruses share recent common ancestors with the NP genes of the German and Dutch H7N7 viruses.

The Duck/South Africa/811/04 (H5N1) NS gene has close sequence similarity (97 % identities) with those of the Chinese viruses WDk/ST/1737/00 (H6N8) and WDk/ST/1411/00 (H11N3) isolated in 2000. These belong to the A subtype, which contains human, swine, avian and most equine viruses [10]. In contrast, Duck/South Africa/1108/04 (H3N8) and Duck/South Africa/1233A/04 (H4N8) (99 % sequence identities) belong to subtype B, which contains mainly avian viruses.

Phylogenetic analysis of the PA genes reveals that Duck/South Africa/811/04 (H5N1) falls into a cluster that contains mostly Chinese H9N2 viruses isolated from 2000 to 2003 and one H5N1 virus, Duck/Fujian/19/02. The virus Ostrich/South Africa/9508103/95 (H9N2) also belongs to this group, but Duck/South Africa/811/04 (H5N1) is phylogenetically more closely related to the Asian viruses than to the SA ostrich virus, therefore it is likely to be a recent introduction. Duck/South Africa/1108/04 (H3N8) and Duck/South Africa/1233A/04 (H4N8) PA genes are most closely related (97 % sequence identities) to those of highly pathogenic H5N1 viruses from China (Chicken/ST/4231/03) and the Japanese HPNAI H5N1 viruses isolated in 2004 [11].

The Duck/South Africa/811/04 (H5N1) and Duck/South Africa/1233A/04 (H4N8) PB1 genes are very closely related (99 %) but share only 93 % sequence identities with the PB1 gene of Duck/South Africa/1108/04 (H3N8). They do share common ancestors with H9N2 virus PB1 genes isolated during the late 1990s. The Duck/South Africa/1108/04 (H3N8) PB1 gene shares 95 % sequence identities with those of the German and Dutch H7N7 isolates from 2003. This may indicate that reassortment occurred in the South African gene pool.

PB2 genes of Duck/South Africa/1108/04 (H3N8) and Duck/South Africa/1233A/04 (H4N8) share 99 % sequence identities and also share recent common ancestors with those of H5N1 and H9N2 Asian viruses. The Duck/South Africa/811/04 (H5N1) PB2 gene shares a recent common ancestor with Italian virus Turkey/Italy/4603/99 (H7N1) (the N1 gene sequence was also closely related to Italian H7N1 viruses), and a diverse group that includes H9N1, H9N2, H5N1, H7N3 and H7N7 viruses from the Far East, Middle East and Europe (ranging from 95-96 % sequence identities).

Discussion

Phylogenetic analysis revealed that the Duck/South Africa/811/04 (H5N1) virus is neither significantly closely related to the currently circulating HPNAI H5N1 Asian viruses, nor is it the donor of the HPAI H5N2 ostrich haemagglutinin gene. The internal genes of this low pathogenicity H5N1 virus share recent common ancestors with viruses isolated in Korea, Italy, Saudi Arabia and the Far East between 1999 and 2003. We acknowledge that internal gene sequences may not have been published for some of the H and N genes with very high sequence homology to the three SA viruses (particularly the Russian viruses). In those cases, the figures depict more historical ancestral genes. The Duck/South Africa/1108/04 (H3N8) and Duck/South Africa/1233A/04 (H4N8) viruses share common ancestors for most of their internal genes, including isolates from East Asia, Norway, Germany and the Netherlands dating from 1997 to 2004. The sharing of recent common ancestors for the NP gene between all three viruses and the PB1 gene in the case of H5N1 and H4N8 (but not H3N8), suggests that some reassortment may have occurred within the South African environment.

It is unknown whether the differences between the H3/H4N8 viruses and the H5N1 virus are indicative of the utilisation of specific migration routes by particular populations or species. For waders, three main flyways have been defined covering the African region (East Atlantic, Black Sea/Mediterranean, and West Asian/East African). Perhaps the H5N1 virus, with its similarity to Italian viruses, infected its host on the Black Sea/Mediterranean route. One explanation for the close homology of South African avian influenza viruses with viral genes from Germany, Holland, Denmark and Norway, could be that one or more of the species utilise the Wadden sea (coastline of Germany, Holland and Denmark) as a stopover site on their migration route. This theory is supported by the detection of a partial H5 sequence using type-specific primers (data not shown) in the same organ pool from which the H3N8 virus was isolated. This sequence shares 98 % identity with a North American lineage virus, A/Mallard/Wisconsin/169/75 (H5N3). The Wadden sea is an important stopover site for millions of birds migrating from the arctic regions of Siberia, Greenland and North America to the wintering grounds in Europe and Africa and back (Ramsar).

We suggest that waders carry viruses from their breeding and stopover sites, co-inhabited by Eurasian migrants, to South Africa each year. Viruses shed into local wetlands via the faeces are then ingested by sympatric indigenous wild ducks and geese, which then become infected and, in turn, act as reservoir hosts that move extensively throughout the country. These birds are encouraged onto ostrich feed camps by open water sources and feeding points. Under ideal and probably rare conditions (high viral loads, high host densities, cool and moist winter weather) ostriches could ingest infective faeces and become infected with LPAI. Many migrant waders that interact with a greater variety of migrants from an enormous geographical area eventually funnel down to South Africa, which can thus be seen as the end of a 'migratory funnel'. Such birds are limited to a smaller variety and volume of water bodies than is utilised in the northern hemisphere. This maximises the range of AI strains and hosts that could potentially interact. This is the first report of the potential role that migrating water birds (in particular the *Charadriidae*) play in the introduction of avian influenza into South Africa, highlighting the importance of continuing surveillance.

REFERENCES

1 Pfitzer S, Verwoerd DJ, Gerdes GH, Labuschagne AE, Erasmus A, Manvell RJ, Grund C: Newcastle disease and Avian Influenza A virus in wild waterfowl in South Africa. Avian Diseases 2000; 44: 665-660.

2 Abolnik C, Horner RF, Bisschop SPR, Parker ME, Romito R, Viljoen GJ: A phylogenetic study of South African Newcastle disease virus strains isolated between 1990 to 2002 suggests epidemiological origins in the Far East. Arch Virol 2004; 149 (3): 603-619.

3 Abolnik C, Horner RF, Maharaj R, Viljoen GJ: Characterization of a pigeon paramyxovirus (PPMV-1) isolated from chickens in South Africa. Onderstepoort Journal of Veterinary Research 2004; 70: 157-160.

4 Widjaja J, Krauss SL, Webby R, Xie T, RG Webster: Matrix gene of influenza A viruses isolated from wild aquatic birds: ecology and emergence of influenza A viruses. J Virol 2004; Aug: 8771-8779.

5 Underhill LG, Tree AJ, Oschadleus HD, Parker V: Review of ring recoveries of waterbirds in southern Africa 1999. Avian Demography Unit, University of Cape Town.

6 Hall TA: BioEdit: a user-friendly biological sequence alignment editor and analysis program for Windows 95/98/NT. Nucl. Acids Symp 1999; 41: 95-98.

7 Kumar S, Tamura K, Jakobsen IB, Nei M: Molecular Evolutionary Genetics Analysis (MEGA) software, Arizona State University, Tempe, Arizona, USA.

8 Matrosovich M, Zhou N, Kawaoka Y, Webster R: The Surface Glycoproteins of H5 Influenza Viruses Isolated from Humans, Chickens, and Wild Aquatic Birds Have Distinguishable Properties. J Virol 1999; 73 (2): 1146 – 1155.

9 Saito T, Kawaoka Y, Webster RG: Phylogenetic analysis of the N8 neuraminidase gene of influenza A viruses. Virology 1993; 193: 868-876.

10 Suarez DL, Perdue ML: Multiple alignment of the non-structural genes of influenza A viruses. Virus Research 1998; 54: 59-69.

11 Mase M, Tsukamoto K, Imada T, Imai K, Tanimura N, Nakamura K, Yamamoto Y, Hitomi T, Kira T, Nakai T, Kiso M, Horimoto T, Kawaoka Y, Yamaguchi S: Characterization of H5N1 influenza A viruses isolated during the 2003-2004 influenza outbreaks in Japan. Virology 2005; 332: 167-176.

Ms C. Abolnik, Biotechnology Division, Onderstepoort Veterinary Institute, Private Bag X5, Onderstepoort, 0110, South Africa.
E-mail: abolnikc@arc.agric.za

Schudel A, Lombard M (eds): OIE/FAO International Scientific Conference on Avian Influenza.
Dev Biol (Basel). Basel, Karger, 2006, vol 124, pp 201-209.

Ecology and Molecular Epidemiology of H9N2 Avian Influenza Viruses Isolated in Israel during 2000-2004 Epizootic

S. Perk[1], *A. Panshin*[1], *E. Shihmanter*[1], *I. Gissin*[1], *S. Pokamunski*[2], *M. Pirak*[2], *M. Lipkind*[1]

[1] Division of Avian and Aquatic Diseases, Kimron Veterinary Institute, Beit Dagan, Israel

[2] Poultry Veterinary Services, Beit Dagan, Israel

Abstract: The first two isolates of H9N2 influenza virus were picked up from turkey and chicken hosts in May 2000, but the actual epizootic of the low pathogenicity avian influenza (LPAI) H9N2 virus started in December 2001, following a 1.5-year period of silence, during which the H10N7 and H6N3 influenza viruses were isolated sporadically. The outbreak of the H9N2 influenza began in northern Israel, from where the epizootic spread all over the country. Damage was relatively limited because of the widespread use of an inactivated vaccine. Single isolates were recorded in commercial ostrich and goose flocks, and in a wild pigeon. Apart from the routine serological tests, the diagnostics used the RT-PCR (reverse transcription polymerase chain reaction) test with type-specific primers related to the M and nucleoprotein (NP) genes, and a set of subtype-specific primers related to all the haemagglutinin (HA) and neuraminidase (NA) subtypes. All the primers were specially constructed. The part coding for N-terminus of the H_1 chain of the HA gene of 61 out of 400 isolates was sequenced. The isolates showed a high rate of mutability, and differed distinctly from the H9 prototype strain; they belong to the same phylogenetic lineage divided into three sublineages, one of which exhibited a unique cleavage-site motif RSKR. The result indicates that two parallel evolutionary trends originated from the same local " prototype " isolate.

INTRODUCTION

Influenza viruses of serotype H9N2 were recently isolated from outbreaks in poultry in several countries: Germany, Italy, Ireland, Saudi Arabia, Iran, Pakistan, China, Hong Kong, South Africa and the United States [1,2]. The H9N2 viruses isolated from these outbreaks fall into three principal phylogenetic lineages: the first includes viruses from North America and Europe; the second includes viruses from Europe, Eastern Asia and South Africa; and the third includes isolates from Asia (the Middle East, in particular) and Germany [2,3]. Thus, the lineages are not geographically based.

During the last three decades, the Israeli poultry industry has experienced sporadic and limited outbreaks of low pathogenicity avian influenza (LPAI) of various H and N types, that caused relatively limited damage. Since 2000, H9N2 LPAI virus has frequently been isolated from turkey and chicken flocks, and single isolates have been recorded in a commercial ostrich flock and in a wild pigeon. The actual epidemic began in northern Israel, mainly in turkeys. Since 2000, the number of infected flocks has grown steadily, and the virus has spread over almost all the country and affected all the poultry branches. Although the virus has not been eradicated, damage caused by the LPAI H9N2 virus in most branches has been relatively limited by the widespread use of an inactivated vaccine. In fact broiler flocks are the most affected.

Materials and Methods

Viruses

The studies used 61 H9N2 viruses isolated from chickens (30 isolates), turkeys (27 isolates), geese (three isolates) and a domesticated ostrich (one isolate). The isolates were propagated in specific-pathogen-free embryonated chicken eggs. Haemagglutination inhibition (HI) and neuraminidase inhibition (NI) tests were applied for serological identification of the avian influenza virus (AIV) isolates. Subtypes of the viruses were identified by the HI and NI tests, with monospecific polyclonal goat antisera obtained from Dr. R.G. Webster (St. Jude Children's Research Hospital, Memphis, Tennessee). Serological identification was confirmed by reverse transcription polymerase chain reaction (RT-PCR) with type-specific primers related to the M and nucleoprotein (NP) genes, and a set of subtype-specific primers related to the haemagglutinin (HA) and neuraminidase (NA) subtypes [4], which also provided express diagnostics. Viral pathogenicity was estimated according to the OIE Terrestrial Manual [5].

RT-PCR and sequence analysis

The viral RNA was extracted directly from the allantoic fluid with the Ready-Mix Kit (Quiagen). Purified genomic RNA was used to generate cDNA clones by RT-PCR, according to the standard procedure. The sets of HA, NA and NP degenerative primers were used for the RT-PCR reaction and for the subsequent sequence analysis (the sequences of the primers are available in the Avian Diseases Division, Kimron Veterinary Institute).

Analysis of nucleotide and deduced amino acid sequences

The nucleotide and deduced amino acid sequences of the HA gene were edited by using the BioEdit Package, Version 7. Nucleotide and deduced amino acid sequences were aligned with the profile-based progressive alignment procedure (ClustalW, Version 1.4).

Phylogenetic analysis

Nucleotide sequences of the HA gene were used for phylogenetic tree construction. The phylogenetic analysis was performed with the PHYLIP (Phylogeny Inference Package), Version 3.6.

Results

The first two isolates were picked up in May 2000, from a chicken and a turkey, but the actual epizootic started after a 1.5-year period of silence, in December 2001. In the beginning, the cases of H9N2 influenza were registered in two turkey flocks in the central area of Israel and, within about 14 months, the disease had spread throughout the northern and southern parts of Israel, attacking mainly turkeys.

Then, from March 2003 to the present, the disease has predominantly affected chicken flocks. All the isolates were classified as non-pathogenic by the IVPI test. As a rule, the affected birds show mild to severe respiratory signs, oedema of the head and the face (Fig. 1), and decreased egg production. The mortality was generally 0-30 %, depending on the type of secondary infection.

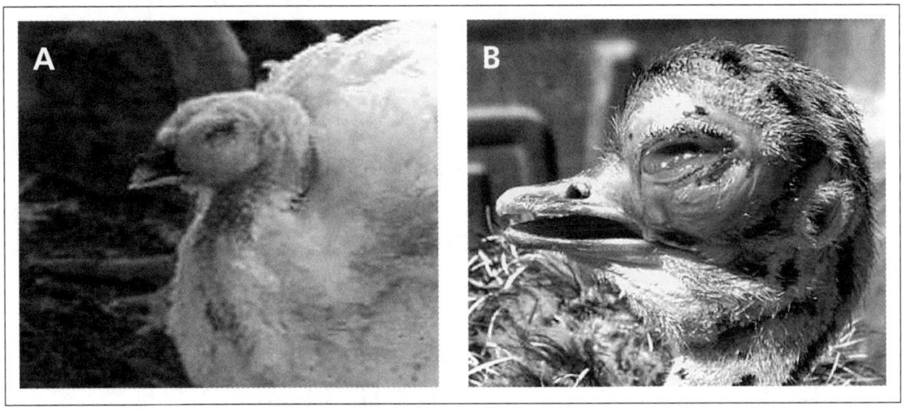

Fig. 1 : **A**- Sinusitis in affected turkey ; **B**- Sinusitis in affected ostrich.

Phylogenetic analysis of the HA protein gene of the Israeli viruses

The phylogenetic relationships among the HA genes of 61 Israeli isolates and 63 H9N2 viruses isolated in other countries were analysed by using the nucleotide sequence of the gene portion between positions 609 and 1039. The data on non-Israeli viruses were taken from the Gene Bank collection. All the Israeli isolates belonged to a single lineage, and three of those from abroad – A/parakeet/Narita/92A/98, A/parakeet/Chiba/1/97, and A/guinea fowl/HongKong/WF10/99 – fell into the same lineage as the Israeli isolates. The Israeli isolates could be divided into three sublineages (Fig. 2). The first sublineage included two viruses, ck/Maale HaHamisha/90658/00 and tk/Neve Ilan/90710/00, isolated in May 2000, i.e., before the massive isolation of H9N2 viruses in Israel that started in December 2001. The second sublineage included the strains isolated between December 2001 and April 2003, together with the virus os/Eshkol/1436/30.10.03, isolated from a domestic ostrich at the end of 2003. The third sublineage comprised the strains isolated from April 2003 until the end of the studies (May 2004).

Analysis of nucleotide and deduced amino acid sequences of HA gene

The complete HA gene was sequenced: the entire length contained 1707 nucleotides. The protein-coding sequence beginning from an ATG start codon and ending with a TAA stop codon consisted of 1683 nucleotides, and the protein HA precursor was 560 amino acid residues long. The Israeli isolates did not exhibit insertions or deletions within the HA gene, whereas rather numerous point mutations were found within the HA protein.

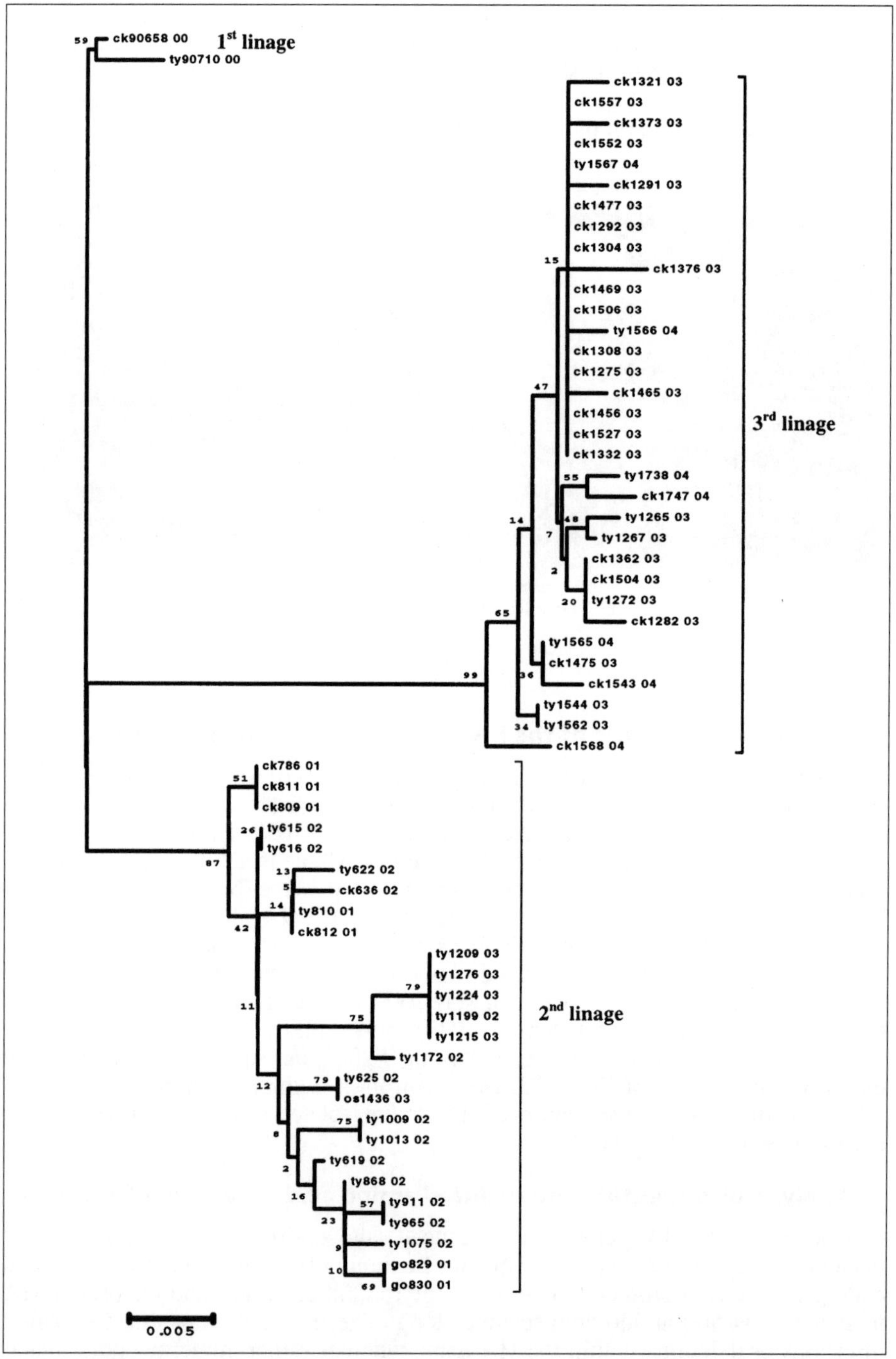

Fig. 2: Phylogenetic tree for the HA gene of the Israeli H9N2 influenza viruses.

Amino acid sequences at the receptor binding site (RBS) of the HA of the H9N2 isolates

It is known that amino acids in the RBS are associated with the receptor binding specificity (for review, see [6]). We studied the nucleotide sequences (189-1039, 851 bp) of 42 H9N2 viruses isolated in Israel. The amino acid sequences (41-323) were deduced from the nucleotide sequences. Five (P^{92}, W^{143}, T^{145}, L^{184}, and Y^{185}) out of seven amino acid residues belonging to the RBS, five (N^{214}, G^{215}, Q^{217}, G^{218}, and R^{219}) out of six belonging to the left edge (LE-RBS) of the receptor-binding pocket, and four (G^{128}, T^{129}, S^{130}, and K^{131}) out of five belonging to the right edge (RE-RBS) of the receptor-binding pocket were highly conservative amongst Israeli isolates. The other four residues – in the positions 173 and 180 in RBS, 216 in LE-RBS, and 132 in RE-RBS – showed variations (Table 1).

Table 1 : Amino acids at the receptor binding sites of HA of H9N2 viruses isolated in Israel.

Sublineage of Israeli isolates	Amino acid residue at the RBS[a]			Number of viruses with following variants of RBS
	I[b]	II[c]	III[d]	
1st sublineage (1)*	PWTHELY[e]	NGQQGR[f]	GTSKA[g]	1
2nd sublineage (16)*	....	......	.....	4
	....	..L...	.....	3
	....A..	..L...	.....	8
	....A..	..L...	....T	1
3rd sublineage (25)*	....	......	.....	1
	....A..	......	.....	5
	....A..	..L...	.....	18
	...QA..	..L...	.....	1

a The number according to H9 HA.
b Receptor binding site.
c Left edge of binding pocket.
d Right edge of binding pocket.
e Amino acid residues at position 92,143, 145, 173, 180, 184, and 185, respectively.
f Amino acid residues at position 214-219.
g Amino acid residues at position 128-132.
* Number isolates belonged to the presented sublineage.
Dots indicate residues identical to those of the first sublineage.

It has been shown that most of the viruses isolated from Israeli chickens contained A^{180} (97 % of isolates) and L^{216} (87 % of isolates). At the same time, amongst the viruses isolated from turkeys, only 50 and 39 % contained A^{180} and L^{216}, respectively. The prevalence of Q^{216} was typical of all the turkey isolates, irrespective of the date of isolation, whereas E^{180} was prevalent only among those turkey viruses that were isolated from May 2000 until February 2003.

Amino acid sequence at the cleavage site of the HA of the H9N2 isolates

We determined the nucleotide sequences (586-1023, 438 bp) of the HA of 61 viruses isolated in Israel. The amino acid sequences (178-323) of the HA were deduced from the nucleotide sequences. According to the cleavage-site amino acid motifs, all the isolates were distributed among three groups. The first group, with the cleavage-site motif RSSR, included the first viruses, which were isolated in 2000, together with those isolated from 24 February 2003 until 17 May 2004. The second group, with the RSNR motif, included only three isolates. The third group, with the RSKR motif, included all the strains isolated from 19 December 2001 until 21 January 2003. The motifs RSNR and RSKR have not been described previously amongst the natural isolates of avian H9N2 influenza viruses.

Phylogenetic analysis of the NP protein gene of the Israeli viruses

The phylogenetic relationships among the NP genes of 33 Israeli isolates were analysed by using the nucleotide sequence of the gene portion between positions 22 and 495. As can be seen in Figure 3, all the viruses fall into two main groups that clearly correspond to the same two groups that were observed for the HA gene, i.e., the first group includes the viruses isolated during 2000-2002 and the second group those isolated during 2003-2004.

Phylogenetic analysis of the NA protein gene of the Israeli viruses

The phylogenetic relationships among the NA genes of 20 Israeli isolates were analysed by using the nucleotide sequence of the gene portion between positions 724 and 1298. As can be seen in Figure 4, the overall pattern was similar to those obtained with the HA and NP genes: the viruses isolated during 2000-2002 differed from those isolated during 2003-2004, with those of the former group showing closer similarity to the "prototype" strain, i.e., the early isolates differed from the "prototype" strain by one change, whereas all the late isolates (2003-2004) differed from the "prototype" strain by four changes.

Discussion

The described characterisation of the Israeli H9N2 influenza viruses was based on 61 viruses isolated systematically during 2000-2004. The first two were isolated in May 2000, after which there was the silent period of about 1.5 years, during which, nevertheless, there were regular observations of various other influenza viruses and paramyxoviruses. Then, from December 2001, there began an actual outbreak, during which many isolates were picked up, which is still continuing (the present studies include the viruses isolated up to May 2004). According to the phylogenetic analysis, all the Israeli isolates fall into a specific lineage, closely related to the Group III described by Liu et al [7], which may indicate that there was a common origin of all the Israeli isolates from a single progenitor, and that the earliest Israeli isolates may be considered to represent such a progenitor.

At the same time, according to the phylogenetic analysis, the Israeli lineage was not homogeneous, so that the viruses may be separated into three sublineages, associated with their times of isolation. Thus, the viruses belonging to these sublineages differ in exhibiting rather large numbers of amino acid substitutions and silent

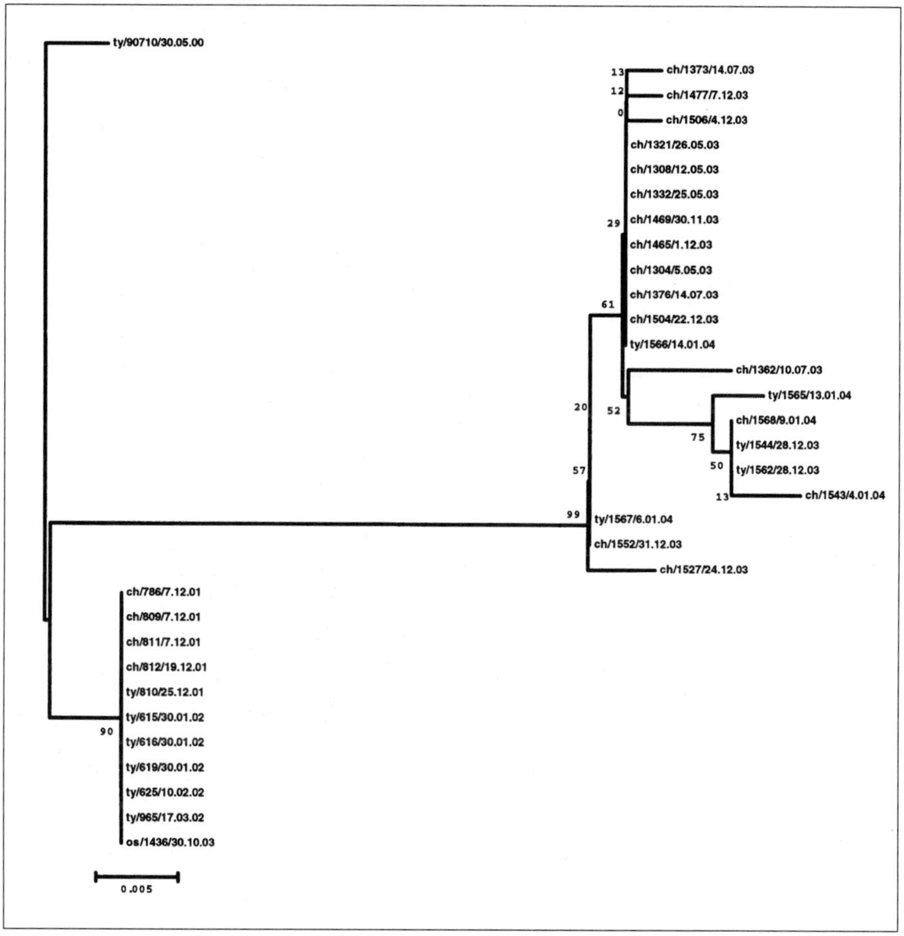

Fig. 3: Phylogenetic tree for the NP gene of the Israeli H9N2 influenza viruses.

mutations. Moreover, there was no indication of a gradual, progressive accumulation of mutations within the sublineages. It seems that the differences appeared suddenly, and not as a result of accumulation of mutations among the viruses circulating within the poultry reservoir.

The data may be attributed to the introduction of new local viruses that circulated beyond the poultry reservoir, probably among feral waterfowl. According to this hypothesis, during the outbreak, there would have been three introductions of the H9N2 AIV into the Israeli population of domestic birds. According to our results, all the Israeli isolates had a common predecessor, which was closely related to the viruses tk/Neve Ilan/90710/00 and ck/Maale HaHamisha/90658/00. The first AIV H9N2 introduction (first sublineage) was registered in 2000 when those viruses were isolated from chickens and turkeys, respectively. However, these viruses did not spread amongst the Israeli poultry.

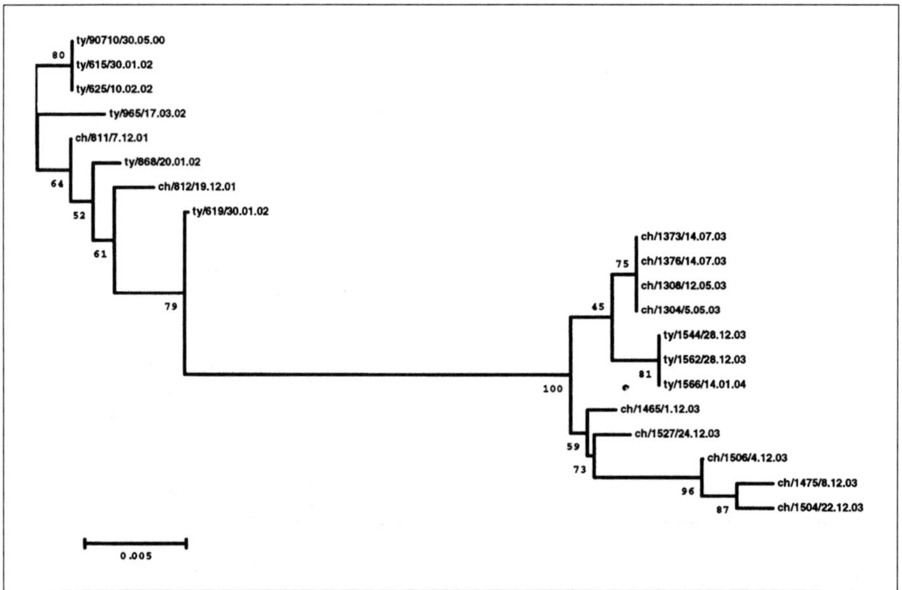

Fig. 4: Phylogenetic tree for the NA gene of the Israeli H9N2 influenza viruses.

The second introduction (second sublineage) of H9N2 AIV occurred 1.5 years later, and turkeys predominated amongst the affected birds. These viruses circulated in Israeli poultry for more than 13 months. The viruses that caused this introduction had more than 98.6 % similarity with the "prototype" strain, tk/Neve Ilan/90710/00. Some peculiarities that characterise these viruses were revealed in the cleavage and receptor binding sites. All the isolates contained either RSNR (three viruses isolated from chickens on 7.12.01 in Tel Adashim) or RSKR (20 viruses isolated from turkeys, two from chickens and two from geese). In receptor binding sites, all the five viruses isolated from chickens contained A^{180} and L^{216}, whereas, among those isolated from turkeys, E^{180} (in 72 % compared with 28 % with A^{180}) and Q^{216} (in 61 % compared with 39 % with L^{216}) were predominant. Thus, amongst the isolates of the second introduction, there was a prevalence of the viruses more adapted to spreading in the turkey population.

The third introduction (third sublineage) of the H9N2 viruses was registered in February 2003; from April 2003 this type of AIV predominated in Israel, and spread predominantly among chickens. The HA genes of these viruses exhibited about 97.0 % similarity with the HA genes of the first sublineage of the Israeli viruses and 96.7 % similarity with those of the second sublineage. The HA protein associated with the third sublineage had the cleavage-site motif RSSR, similar to that of the first sublineage. In the receptor binding site of viruses belonging to the third sublineage, A^{180}, which is more typical of chicken isolates, was found in all nine viruses isolated from turkeys and in 23 (out of 24) of the viruses isolated from chickens. Leucine in position L^{216} was identified in 83 % of the viruses isolated from chickens and in only 44 % of those isolated from turkeys. In contrast, Q^{216}, which is typical of turkeys, was found in 56 % of turkey isolates and in only 17 %

of chicken isolates. Thus, within the third introduction, the isolates more adapted to spreading in the chicken population predominated.

One of the factors in the evolution of low pathogenicity influenza viruses is the immunological pressure, which is increased by the presence of vaccinated birds among poultry. The mass vaccination that started at the end of 2002 was based on the use, as a vaccine strain, of a virus belonging to the second lineage. Since, as mentioned above, a rather rapid evolution of the local viruses proceeded outside the immunised poultry population, the post-vaccinal specific immunity of the population could have been the decisive selecting factor that led to the prevalence of the virus that differed from the vaccinal strain. The finding that the genetic difference between the second and third sublineages was about 3.3 % supports this supposition. However, the corresponding difference in the case of virus os/Eshkol/1436/30.10.03 that was isolated at the same time from the non-vaccinated population of ostriches was only about 0.6-0.7 %.

Acknowledgements

Dr. N. Elkin and Dr. B. Perelman are highly acknowledged for providing pictures. This study was supported by the Kameya fund of the Israel Ministry of Immigration and Absorption and the Israeli Poultry Association grant.

References

1 Alexander DA: Report on avian influenza in the Eastern hemisphere during 1997-2002. Avian Dis 2003; 47: 792-797.

2 Senne DA: Avian influenza in the Western hemisphere including Pacific Islands and Australia. Avian Dis 2003; 47: 798-805.

3 Banks J, Speidel EC, Harris PA, Alexander DJ: Phylogenetic analysis of influenza A viruses of H9 haemagglutinin subtype. Avian Pathol 2000; 29: 353-360.

4 Lee MS, Chang PC, Shien JH, Cheng MC, Shieh HK: Identification and subtyping of avian influenza viruses by reverse transcription-PCR. J Virol Meth 2001; 97: 13-22.

5 OIE Terrestrial Manual. 2004.

6 Skehel JJ, Wiley DC: Receptor binding and membrane fusion in virus entry: The influenza hemagglutinin. Annu Rev Biochem 2000; 69: 531-569.

7 Liu JH, Okazaki K, Mweene A, Shi WM, Wu QM, Su JL, Zhang GZ, Bai GR, Kida H: Genetic conservation of hemagglutinin gene of H9 influenza virus in chicken population in Mainland China. Virus Genes 2004; 29: 329-334.

Dr. S. Perk, Division of Avian and Aquatic Diseases, Kimron Veterinary Institute, P.O. Box 12, Beit Dagan 50251, Israel.
E-mail: shimonpr@moag.gov.il

Schudel A, Lombard M (eds): OIE/FAO International Scientific Conference on Avian Influenza.
Dev Biol (Basel). Basel, Karger, 2006, vol 124, pp 211-224.

HPAI Surveillance Programme in Cambodia: Results and Perspectives

S. Desvaux[1,2], S. Sorn[2], D. Holl[2], D. Chavernac[1], F. Goutard[1], J. Thonnat[3], V. Porphyre[4], C. Ménard[5], E. Cardinale[4], F. Roger[1]

[1] CIRAD, EMVT Department, Epidemiology Unit, France
[2] National Animal Health and Production Investigation Centre, Phnom Penh, Cambodia
[3] CIRAD, EMVT Department, Training Unit, France
[4] CIRAD, EMVT Department, Animal Production Unit, Hanoi, Vietnam
[5] CIRAD, EMVT Department, Integrated Wildlife Management Unit, France

Abstract: Cambodia has faced 15 confirmed highly pathogenic avian influenza (H5N1) outbreaks in different sectors of the poultry industry since January 2004. The country has very limited human and financial resources and, when the outbreak first began, the veterinary services were not equipped with the basic tools to collect accurate epidemiological information or to fight the disease. Therefore, different agencies, under the umbrella of the Food and Agriculture Organisation, are providing support to the Government to strengthen its capacity to diagnose, survey and control the avian influenza (AI) virus. Different surveillance tools are being tested, such as market monitoring and a sentinel villages' network, to offset the weakness of the national passive surveillance network. Several constraints were identified during the implementation of this programme, such as a lack of motivation among provincial staff, the limited capacity of the central team to compile and analyse the data generated, the reluctance of farmers to have their animals sampled, and weak diagnostic capacities. The sustainability of such a surveillance system once international support ends remains to be seen. Participatory epidemiology (PE) may be an appropriate complementary tool to track diseases. PE works on the principle that livestock keepers often possess detailed knowledge of animal diseases and can provide valuable diagnostics that could help in identifying AI outbreaks, particularly in remote areas.

INTRODUCTION

The poultry population in Cambodia is estimated to be approximately 17 million animals [1] distributed across three main sectors: the commercial sector, defined as an industrial system with a high level of bio-security holding over 10,000 animals (covering only two farms in Cambodia); the semi-commercial sector that can be sub-divided into (i) a production system with a moderate to low level of bio-security, holding between 500 and 10,000 animals (covering most of the laying-hen farms and some broiler farms); (ii) a production system with no bio-security, holding between 500 and 3,000 animals (covering most of the duck 'farms'); and (iii) the village poultry sector, which consists of village or backyard production with no bio-security and covers the majority of the poultry population in Cambodia [2].

The first highly pathogenic avian influenza (HPAI) case was confirmed on 23 January 2004 on a semi-commercial laying-hen farm near the capital, Phnom Penh [3]. By the end of April 2004, approximately the end of the first wave, 12 other outbreaks had been detected in both the semi-commercial and village sectors (also one case was confirmed among captive wild birds). Those positive cases were located in five different provinces. By the end of 2004, just one new case was detected in a previously infected province. In 2005, only two cases were detected positive by the end of March [4]. Figures 1 and 2 show the location of outbreak sites and the mapping of the surveillance activities.

The current scanned surveillance system has many weaknesses: a general lack of human resources and a lack of motivation among field staff; a lack of awareness among stakeholders regarding the necessity of declaring an infectious animal disease and the absence of a compulsory obligation to do so; an absence of appropriate information channels; and variable co-operation between official veterinary services and field workers, especially the Village Animal Health Workers (VAHWs). Therefore, given the HPAI crisis, different agencies under the umbrella of the Food and Agriculture Organisation (FAO) [5] provided technical and financial support to the Government to improve its surveillance capabilities, for instance, via farmer awareness campaigns (training and TV spots), field veterinary officer training, and the provision of material support to the provinces (motorbikes, sampling materials, personal protective equipments, etc). Also, assistance was provided to strengthen national control and diagnosis capacities. However, a significant improvement of the surveillance network will require some time and the involvement of large amounts of financial and human resources. Meanwhile, a practical and targeted active surveillance programme is critical to the detection of HPAI outbreaks.

Such a targeted programme was designed and has been progressively implemented since July 2004. It started with the monitoring of markets and the clinical surveillance of semi-commercial poultry farms. Following an initial evaluation in December 2004 [6], changes and modifications were proposed for a second six-month programme. The main objective is to enable the veterinary services to detect new HPAI outbreaks in different sectors without relying solely on the existing and inadequate passive surveillance system. Since the village poultry population represents the main poultry sector in the country, efforts are being made to assess better what is happening within this population. Because of the constraints related to this sector (dispersed information, difficulty of implementing timely laboratory diagnosis), a participatory epidemiology approach was designed using a sentinel villages monitoring system.

A participatory epidemiology approach was also used in a retrospective study aiming to describe the probable spread of the virus beyond the outbreak sites during the first wave of the epizootic. Whenever possible, the programme follows the FAO and OIE recommendation for HPAI surveillance [7].

The specific objectives of the different components of this programme are:

(i) Market monitoring:
   - To assess indirectly the sanitary status of the village poultry sector;
   - To detect possible illegal movement of sick animals.

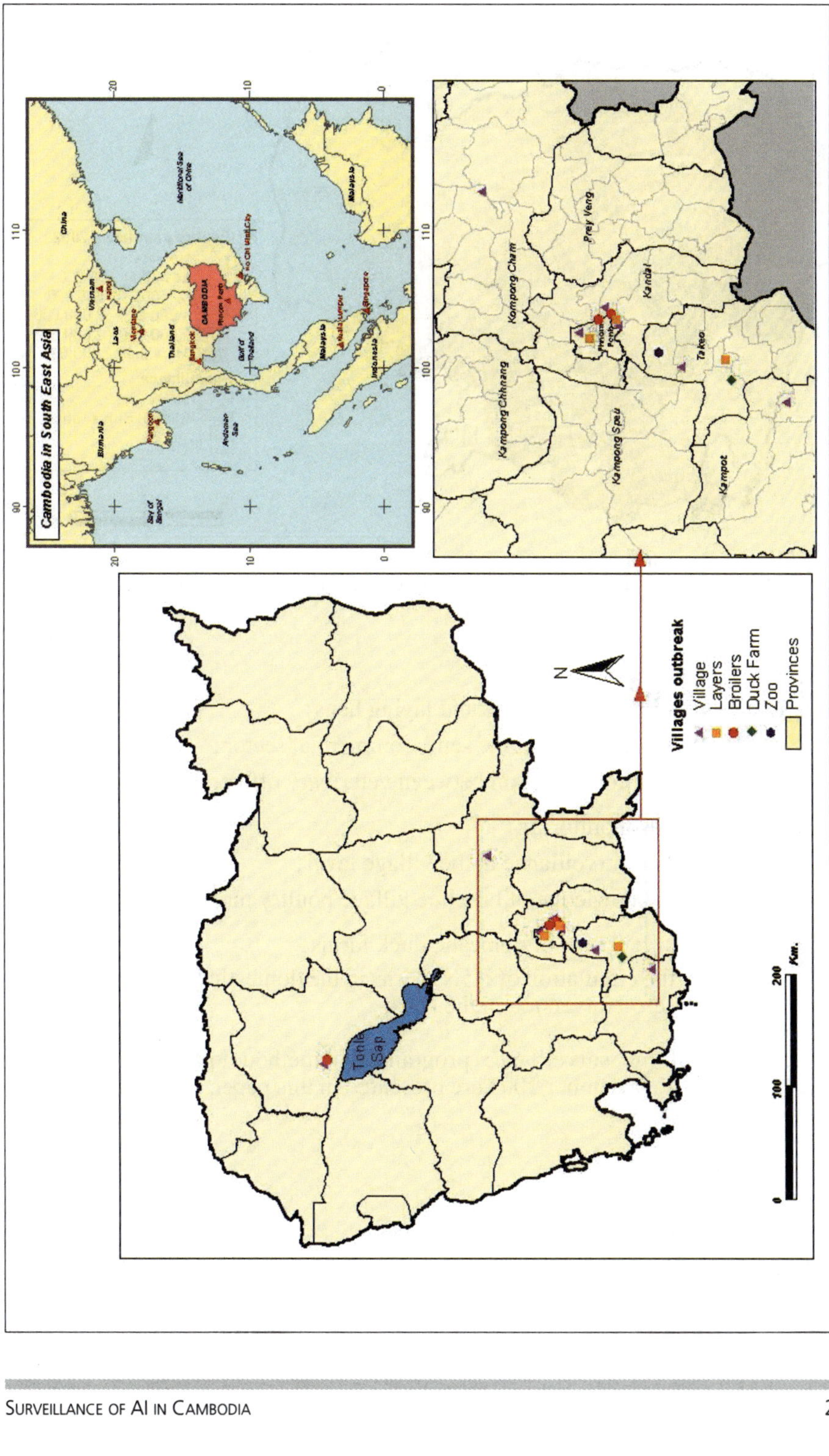

Fig. 1 : Outbreaks detected from January 2004 to end of March 2005.

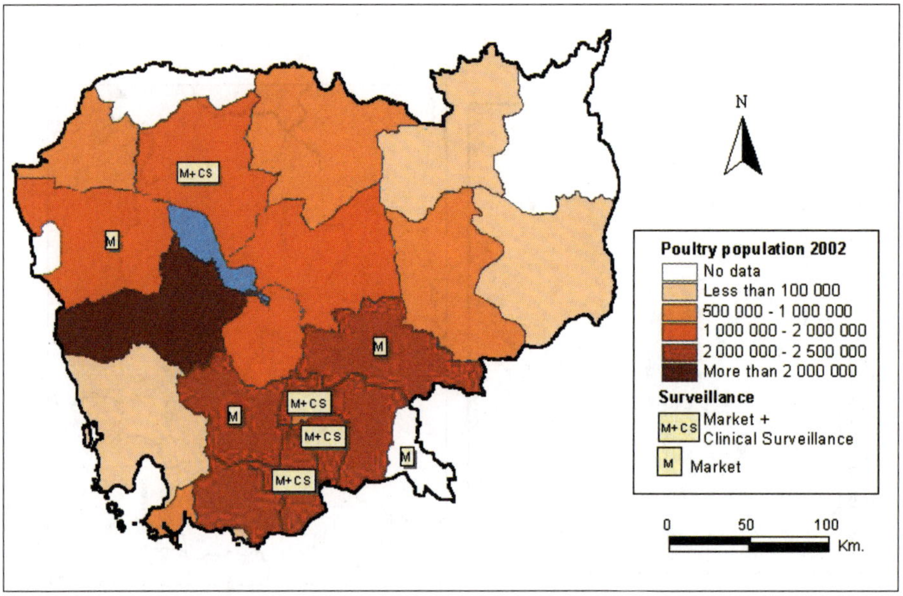

Fig. 2: Mapping of the surveillance activities by province with indication of the total poultry population (DAHP statistic 2002).

(ii) Clinical surveillance of broilers and laying hens:
- To obtain information on the semi-commercial sector;
- To strengthen collaboration between veterinary officers and farmers.

(iii) Sentinel villages monitoring:
- To strengthen surveillance at the village level;
- To improve knowledge of baseline village poultry mortality.

(iv) Serological surveillance of domestic duck farms:
- To assess the circulation of H5N1 virus in the domestic duck population by detecting sero-conversion in the flock.

The details of the surveillance programme's methodology and the results obtained through to December 2004 are presented in this paper, as are the results of the retrospective study.

Materials and Methods

Monitoring and surveillance protocols

Case-definition: In the context of the current surveillance programme, an HPAI case is defined as an animal detected positive by virological analysis for H5N1.

Targeted population: Each component of the surveillance programme targets a specific population. Village poultry are the target of the market monitoring and the sentinel villages monitoring components; layers and broilers in the semi-commercial sectors are the target of the clinical surveillance programme; and ducks in semi-commercial units are the targeted population of the serological surveillance plan.

Sampling methods and sample size: The provinces where surveillance activities have been, and are being, implemented were selected according to three main criteria: their poultry population; their location with regard to neighbouring countries; and the capacity of the provincial team to implement a surveillance programme. To fill gaps in national statistical data on the poultry population, a census of semi-commercial farms was implemented by the national veterinary services. In Phnom Penh, the sampled markets were selected to cover the range of possible origins of the animals.

- Market monitoring: The objective was to adopt an expected prevalence among the live bird population in the markets of 5 % with 95 % confidence. During the first six months of surveillance activities, the expected prevalence was fixed around 12 % to allow the laboratory to adapt its capacity. Samples were taken every two weeks at the provincial level and once a week in Phnom Penh. The minimum number of samples needed varies according to the diagnostic methods used and the types of samples collected (the sensitivity and specificity of the different methods vary).

- Clinical surveillance of broilers and laying hens: The programme was divided into two phases: the first phase, from July to December 2004, involved the clinical surveillance of former outbreak areas (covering a three to ten km radius from the outbreak sites depending on the density of farms); the second phase, which began in January 2005, extended surveillance beyond the former outbreak areas. In this second phase, efforts will be concentrated on the provinces with the highest density of semi-commercial farms. The objective is to have a farm sample, in the selected provinces, to allow the detection of the disease with 95 % confidence if the expected between-farm prevalence is 5 %. If mortality is observed or reported by farmers, the veterinarian has to collect dead animals or samples. During the first phase, a weekly visit was conducted over the course of 30 days, followed by visits every two weeks. In the second phase (from January 2005), a monthly visit is proposed.

- Sentinel villages monitoring: It was proposed that at least one sentinel village should be chosen for each province. They are selected according to several criteria, with a preference for villages where many local chickens and ducks are raised, there are wild birds (villages with big water pounds), and there is a VAHW. The village must be strategically placed; in the concerned provinces, villages are selected where smuggling activities with neighbouring countries are known to occur. The provincial veterinary staff is responsible for organising a meeting and explaining to village stakeholders (e.g. village chief, VAHW, NGOs) what suspect poultry mortality is and how to report it. Suspect mortality means a daily mortality of over 5 % for more than one day (with or without the sudden death of chickens). The district vet is then responsible for visiting the village every month to contact the village chief and the VAHW and to report the poultry mortality events to the province. This activity only began in February 2005.

- Serological surveillance on domestic duck farms: The organisation of monthly sampling on duck farms for H5N1 (and for some H7) antibodies detection using a between-farm expected prevalence of 5 % and a within-farm expected prevalence of 20 % was proposed. Only some provinces will be covered by this programme, selected according to their duck population. In the case of a reported mortality, dead animals are collected and sent for analysis. This activity started in March 2005.

Laboratory analysis: For virological diagnosis, an immunofluorescence test for antigen detection (IFAT) (influenza virus A detection) on tracheal swabs or organ smears was the proposed method (followed by IFAT on cloacal swabs, if the time between sampling and slides fixation could be less than 24 hours). Every suspected and positive sample is confirmed by RT-PCR (polymerase chain reaction) test for RNA detection (H5N1 or H7 virus) at Pasteur Institute of Cambodia using the procedure from the Hong Kong Government virus unit [8]. For serological diagnosis, the haemagglutination inhibition test is used for antibodies detection (against avian influenza sub-type H5N1) [9,10].

Networking organisation: The provincial or district veterinary officers are responsible for the sampling activities and the clinical surveillance in the semi-commercial farms. With regard to village sentinel monitoring, the key persons are the VAHW and the village chief, who collaborate with the district vet to report suspect mortality events. The central epidemiology team is responsible for providing technical support to the field team, in collecting and analysing data, and providing feedback on epidemiological information to the field actors and various stakeholders. The samples were sent by the provincial staff in an ice-box to the laboratory using public transport.

Retrospective study of the 2004 outbreak

The retrospective study of past HPAI outbreaks was designed using participatory methods. Its main objective was to assess the spread of the H5N1 virus around confirmed outbreak places.

Questionnaire: The survey was conducted using semi-structured interviews of key informants (village chiefs, VAHWs or farmers) related to morbidity and mortality events in 2003 and 2004 with a description of symptoms and vaccination status.

Sampling method and sample size: The survey was limited to the area within a three km radius of the outbreak sites. The sampling rate for the villages was chosen with a 95 % confidence of detecting at least one infected village assuming a between-village prevalence of 5 %. All the semi-commercial farms in the area were visited. The animal sampling rate in the village or on the farm was planned to fit with a 95 % confidence of detecting at least one positive bird assuming a within-farm prevalence of 25 %. It was decided to sample animals when a suspect mortality was reported in 2004 or incomplete information was available.

Laboratory analysis: The animals were sampled for both virological and serological tests.

Data analysis: Based on the qualitative and quantitative data of the interviews, criteria were selected to classify the probability that a farm or village faced an outbreak of HPAI from January to May 2004 (Table 1). Those criteria were scored and villages and farms were classified in three categories: low probability; moderate probability and high probability.

Table 1: Criteria and scoring for classification of the villages and the farms.

Criteria	Villages		Farms	
	Yes	No	Yes	No
Outbreak reported in 2004	2	0	2	0
Sudden death reported (health to death within 24 hours without symptoms or with minor symptoms) or symptoms duration less than three days	3 2	0	3 2	0
Cumulative mortality during the outbreak over 40 % for chicken, 30 % for ducks **or** daily mortality over 1 %	2	0	2	0
Case fatality over 60 % for chicken, 20 % for ducks	1	0	1	0
Mortality reported on different species	1	0	1	0
At risk population vaccinated (partly or totally) against NCD and/or fowl cholera	1	0	1	0
Mortality on all age categories	1	0	NA	NA
Total	10 or 11		9 or 10	
Scoring between 2 and 3	Low probability			
Score between 4 and 6	Moderated probability			
Score between 7 and 9 or 11	High probability			

Results

Surveillance programme until December 2004

Market monitoring: from 1 August to 1 December 2004, 712 samples were collected in seven provinces (50 % of the initial objective); none was found positive. The number of samples collected per visit was sometimes below the minimum needed to respect the survey assumptions.

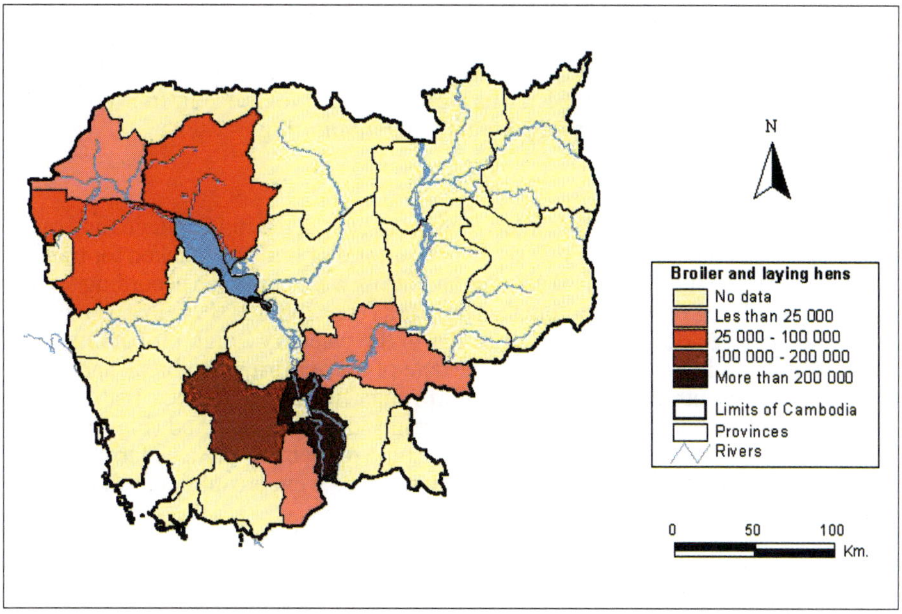

Fig. 3: Broiler and laying-hen semi-commercial farms (Source: Ministry of Agriculture, Forestry and Fisheries, Department of Animal Health and Production 2004 poultry farms census).

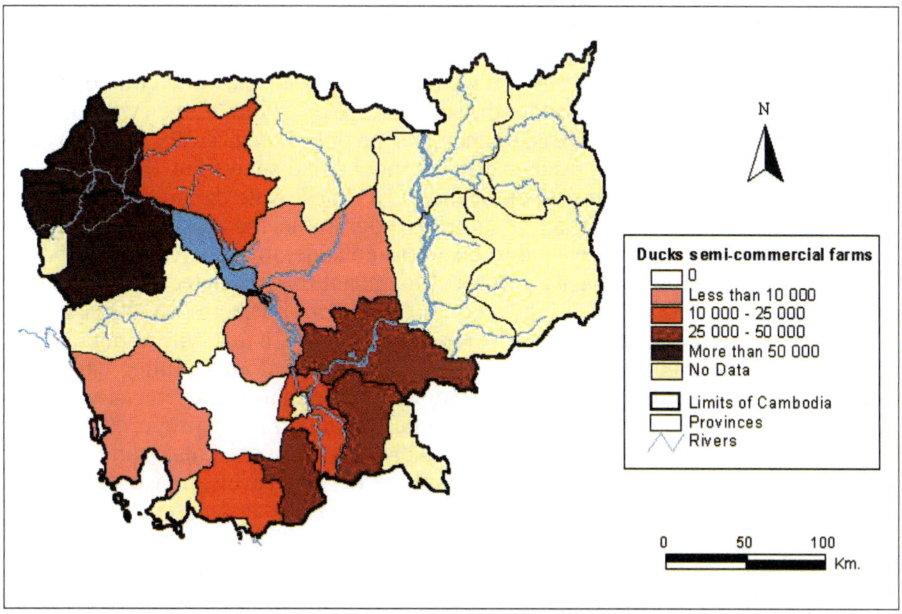

Fig. 4: Ducks semi-commercial farms (Source: Ministry of Agriculture, Forestry and Fisheries, Department of Animal Health and Production 2004 poultry farms census).

Clinical surveillance of broilers and laying hens: The semi-commercial farm census was completed and a Microsoft Access database was developed to enter all the collected information. The results of this census are summarised in Figures 3 and 4. During the first phase, 51 farms were under surveillance in four provinces. No HPAI suspected cases were reported by this monitoring.

Retrospective study

Between May and June 2004, interviews were conducted in 52 villages and on 23 farms selected around the outbreak sites, and samples of birds were taken for triangulation. From those interviews, 70 villages and farms were classified according to their risk of having faced an HPAI outbreak. The results (see Table 2) show that a large percentage of villages or farms were classified in the category "high probability". An analysis of the at-risk period (based on the date of the confirmed outbreak and that of the onset of the outbreak in the village/farm interviewed) confirmed that the high probability villages/farms faced suspect mortality during that period (Figs 5 and 6). The symptoms described by the farmers in the high probability villages/farms are presented in Figure 7. The three main reported symptoms were prostration, sudden death and white diarrhoea.

Discussion

When virological analysis was chosen, the objective was to use the egg inoculation method, which is known for its fine sensitivity. However, this method could not be used under appropriately safe conditions when the first phase of the surveillance programme was implemented. At that time, an alternative method had to be used. This was the IFAT test, which is described as a routine method when used on organ smears [11] and is used routinely for human diagnosis on tracheal swabs. However, it is not validated on cloacal swabs used after having been put in a virus transport medium. Members of the field staff in the surveillance programme, even when trained and asked to collect tracheal swabs, frequently send only cloacal swabs. The sensitivity and specificity of the tests used on poultry should be displayed by the labs and/or studied in close collaboration with epidemiologists to estimate the predictive values.

In the first phase of the market monitoring programme, the assumptions made in the calculation of sample sizes had to take into consideration the constraint posed by the limited diagnosis capacity present; this meant that the detection of positive HPAI animals was not as precise as it could have been. Furthermore, the selection of animals in market places suffered from a bias because, in that type of population, different batches of animals are present and a simple random sampling cannot be representative. Regarding the duck serological surveillance, the precision of the detection of sero-positive animals will also be a problem if the proposed assumptions cannot be respected because of financial or technical constraints. On the whole, the sizes of the samples were below the defined levels, consequently, the representativeness and the precision required were not reached.

The absence of laboratories in the provinces means that the samples collected must be sent to Phnom Penh by public taxi. Because of the distances and the road conditions involved, it is difficult to organise the surveillance of markets in some provinces. In addition to logistical constraints, the motivation of the people working at the provincial level is a problem. They are not always motivated to implement

Table 2: Distribution of the villages and the farms according to the risk of having faced an HPAI outbreak between January and May 2004.

Outbreak number and province	No suspected	Low probability	Moderated probability	High probability	TOTAL
1 Phnom Penh	33.3 % (2/6)		33.3 %	33.3 %	6
2 Takeo/Zoo		14 % (1/7)	0	86 % (6/7)	7
3 Phnom Penh			80 % (4/5)	20 % (1/5)	5
4+9 Kandal/Kien Svay	43 % (3/7)		43 % (3/7)	14 % (1/7)	7
5 + 8 Siem Reap	30 % (7/24)	8 % (2/24)	17 % (4/24)	45 % (11/24)	24
6 Takeo/Daun Keo	25 % (1/4)		1	50 % (2/4)	4
7 Kandal/Takmao	17 % (1/6)		33 % (2/6)	50 % (3/6)	6
10 Takeo/Tramkak			20 % (1/5)	80 % (4/5)	5
11 Takeo/Samrong			17 % (1/6)	83 % (5/6)	6
12 Kompong Cham	NA				
TOTAL	20 % (14/70)	4 % (3/70)	26 % (18/70)	50 % (35/70)	70

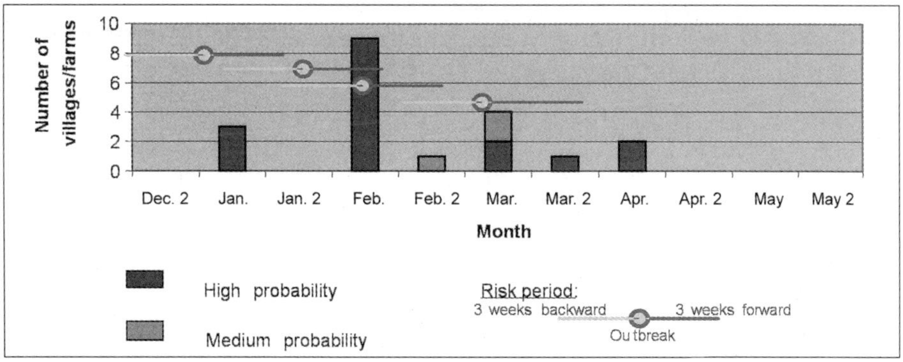

Fig. 5: Takeo Province, four outbreak places, 22 villages/farms visited.

new duties, because they are paid very low salaries and they receive little direction from the central level. Furthermore, in the case of this surveillance programme, the provincial staff received no feedback on their activities from the central team, which probably contributes to their lack of motivation.

Another constraint identified by the teams was that farmers were sometimes very reluctant to see their animals sampled, which would probably have consequences on the serological surveillance of the duck farms. We have to remember that, in Cambodia, there is no regulatory framework for the control of animal diseases, which means that there is no compulsory declaration of an infectious disease. Furthermore, veterinary officers do not have the right to enter farms without the permission of the farmers. In this context, even animal disease workers have no obligation to declare suspicions of animal diseases. For the sentinel villages monitoring

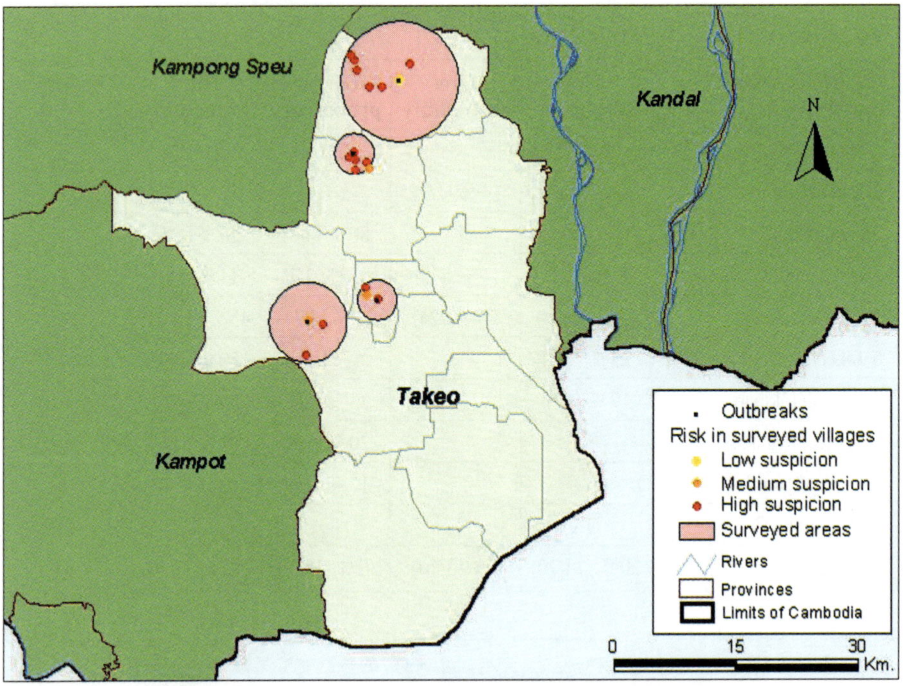

Fig. 6: Mapping of outbreaks and investigated villages in Takeo Province.

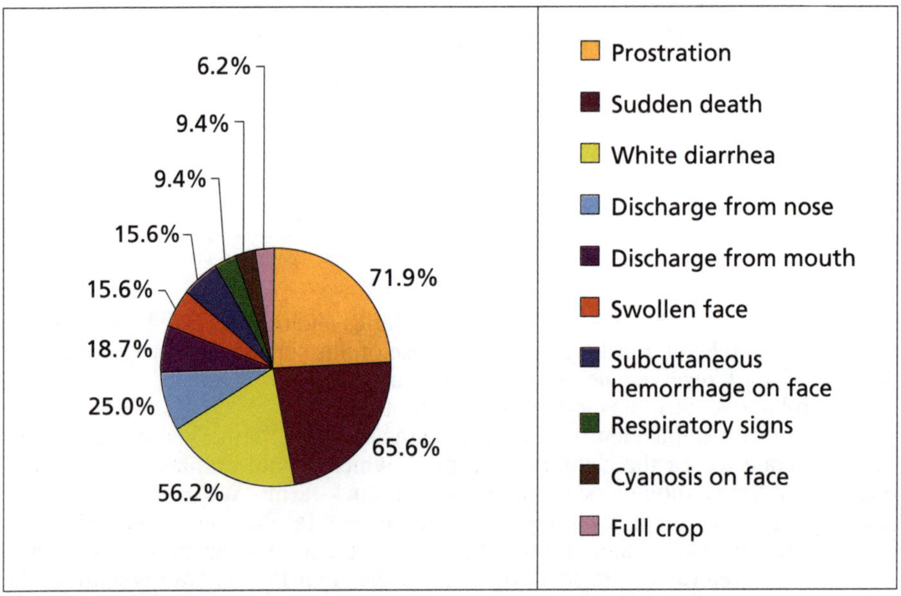

Fig. 7: Symptoms described by the farmers and the village chiefs in the farms and the villages classified in the high risk category.

component, a solution would have to be found to ensure that VAHWs are motivated to declare suspect poultry mortality. Financial incentives were proposed for when the detection of new HPAI cases is confirmed.

The provincial staff also faced different technical problems in the implementation of their activities. One problem was that they were not always able to collect the samples as prescribed. Indeed, they generally are not comfortable doing tracheal swabs, which was the advised sample to collect at that time. Another problem related to the clinical surveillance of semi-commercial farms; staff was not always making a comprehensive analysis and/or report of the situation in the case of a reported mortality or a decrease in the animal population of the farm. The question of competence also is crucial for monitoring sentinel villages: will VAHWs be able to detect a suspect mortality? This question leads to the next point related to the sensitivity and specificity of the detection system. Constraints have been identified at the central level as well, mainly in the team's difficulty in compiling and analysing the data generated by the surveillance activities.

In this context, education and training appear essential and should be applied at each level of a monitoring and surveillance system (MOSS). Indeed, training is a decisive factor in the implementation and functioning of epidemiological surveillance mechanisms. Activity in this domain represents a significant investment. Training programmes must be developed following rigorous methodology to produce satisfactory results. To begin with, the approach must be comprehensive and take into account all the public and private actors who play a strategic role in the surveillance system.

The analysis of training needs, conducted for each category of actors, consists of precisely identifying the skills needed to be built or reinforced in order to obtain the objectives fixed by the framework of the network. This analysis results in the definition of a 'training plan' describing the different training activities to be undertaken and their timing. The plan also identifies the training sites, the structures to be mobilised, and the pedagogical methods to be used. Training programmes must not be developed according to an academic process focused on the contents, but by fixing pedagogical objectives on the competences and capacities to be built [12].

To facilitate the involvement of actors in their training and in the activities that they will later have to conduct, participatory pedagogical techniques should be favoured. Distance learning may also be a useful tool, particularly to harmonise participants' levels when academic differences between them are too great [13]. Finally, the impact of training is assessed by putting into place a complete evaluation mechanism that measures not only how much knowledge participants acquire at the time of the training, but also how participants put this knowledge to work in their professional practice.

Regarding clinical monitoring at the village level, if the VAHW participation is strong, the sensitivity in detecting a new HPAI outbreak can be very good but the monitoring may suffer from a specificity problem if poultry mortality is over reported. Regarding clinical surveillance on semi-commercial farms, the sensitivity of the detection of a new HPAI suspected case will depend mainly on the co-operation of the farmer – is s/he going to declare his/her poultry mortality? – and the capacity of the team to implement an appropriate survey to validate what the farmer says.

In this context, to increase the sensitivity of MOSSs, scanned and targeted surveillance, it is recommended that the vet services, their resources, and the information given by farmers who collaborate with the official structures be reinforced.

In Vietnam RS, where 40 million chickens have been infected or culled during 2004, such recommendations have been implemented during 2005 by the Department of Animal Health; in addition, several small-scale epidemio-surveillance networks try to focus on key points that are supposed to maintain and consolidate long-term motivation of field practitioners and local, officers involved within these networks, i.e. monthly training and discussion sessions to gather information and share experiences; reasonable incentives associated with a clear contractual relationship with veterinary stations at the district level and an informative feedback to network members through a regular newsletter [14,15].

Complementary approaches also need to be implemented, such as participatory epidemiology (PE), the collection of epidemiological data and intelligence relying on widely accepted methods of participatory rural appraisal (PRA). PRA consists of a toolkit of methods for rapid and accurate data collection largely developed for project design, monitoring, and evaluation [16]. PE relies on observation, existing veterinary knowledge of traditional livestock owners, and oral history.

A wide range of PE methods is available, which may be categorised into three main groups: informal interviews of key informants; visualisation methods; and ranking or scoring methods. Information derived from the different methods is cross-checked or 'triangulated' in a similar way that a clinician combines information from different sources to reach a diagnosis. Indeed, the use of conventional veterinary diagnostic tools (observations, livestock keeper interviews, clinical and pathological examinations) is an integral part of, and, in some cases, overlaps with, PE methods. PE methods can be standardised and repeated to improve the reliability of information. The basic requirements for participatory development are a respect for traditional knowledge, a willingness to learn, and an attitude of open-mindedness.

Before using participatory epidemiology, the difficulties or limitations of the method have to be understood: most applications so far have been in sub-Saharan African countries, with pastoral or agro-pastoral informants with strong diagnostic abilities. The method may be less useful with other types of livestock keeper. Indeed, pastoralists seem able to recall disease events accurately over many years and in specific animals (but can other livestock keepers?), and cross-check with timelines and secondary data on disease outbreaks [17]. Although many veterinarians are now using participatory methods, few of them have been trained to do so. Consequently, numerous methods are labelled "participatory" but the principles and most effective practices of participatory inquiry are often overlooked [18].

The development of veterinary-oriented training courses on PE for centrally-based personnel and field staff, therefore, is essential. PE methods could enhance surveillance and control strategies of avian influenza and increase the capacity to identify reservoir species, agro-ecological areas and farming systems likely to maintain the infection. Within PE, participatory disease searching could be used to confirm the absence or presence of disease in a community. Usual validation methods are based on triangulation and frequentist approaches. We suggest the use of Bayesian methods. Indeed, Bayes' theorem is a powerful tool in the rational assessment of diagnostic procedures. For instance, its application in its second alternative form – $P(A|B) = P(B|A)P(A)/ ((P(B|A)P(A) + P(B|Ac)P(Ac))$ – could lead to assessing the probability of having an HPAI true positive by taking into account the events related to the diagnostic made by the farmer (B) and the occurrence of HPAI in the area (A). On the whole, Bayesian inference can update estimates of HPAI rates (posterior probability) based on knowledge (prior probability) and field studies (likelihood function and normalising constant).

Finally, the evaluation of the performance of such a multiple and complex surveillance system, including PE, is needed and should be based on the elaboration of performance indicators. Furthermore, the evaluation of performance could be undertaken using quantitative risk assessment methodologies, e.g. assessing the risk of not detecting new HPAI outbreaks in time.

Conclusion

In 2005, HPAI remains a huge threat in Asian countries. Monitoring and surveillance systems are compulsory tools to improve its control. National MOSS also should be integrated in regional systems to increase the effectiveness of early warning and early reaction processes through data standardisation and information sharing.

References

1 Anon: Annual Report 2002. Ministry of Agriculture, Forestry and Fisheries, Department of Animal Health and Production, Phnom Penh, Cambodia, 2002.

2 Desvaux S: Emergency assistance for the control of avian influenza, Final technical report, CIRAD. Rome, FAO, September 2004.

3 Office International des Epizooties, Paris. Update on avian influenza in animals in Asia (type H5) [update 2004 December 3]. Available at: http://www.oie.int/downld/AVIAN%20INFLUENZA/A_AI-Asia. htm. Accessed December 2004.

4 FAO AIDE news: Update on avian influenza (As of 15/02/2004). Rome, FAO, 2005. news available at http://www.fao.org/ag/againfo/subjects/documents/ai/AVIbull025.pdf.

5 FAO AIDE news: Update on avian influenza (As of 15/06/2004). Rome, FAO, 2004. Available at http://www.fao.org/ag/againfo/subjects/documents/ai/AVIbull016.pdf. Accessed May 2005.

6 Desvaux S: Emergency assistance for the control of avian influenza, Technical report, CIRAD. Rome, FAO, January 2004.

7 FAO: FAO Expert meeting on surveillance and diagnosis of avian influenza in Asia, Bangkok, 21-23 July 2004. Available at: http://www.fao.org/ag/againfo/subjects/en/health/diseases-cards/Guiding%20principles.pdf, accessed February 2005.

8 World Health Organisation: Recommended laboratory tests to identify influenza A/H5 virus in specimens from patients with influenza-like illness. WHO, 2004. Available at http://www.who.int/csr/disease/avian_influenza/guidelines/en/avian_labtests1.pdf, accessed May 2005.

9 Office International des Epizooties: Manual of Diagnosis tests and vaccines for terrestrial animals – 2004. Paris, OIE, chapter 2.1.14.

10 Office International des Epizooties: Proposed new chapter for OIE terrestrial animal health code, chapter 2.1.14. Paris, OIE, 2004. Available at http:/www.oie.int/eng/avian_influenza/proposed%20NEW%20CHAPTER%20Code.pdf, accessed March 2005.

11 Selleck PW, Lowther SL, Russell GM, Hooper PT: Rapid Diagnosis of Highly Pathogenic Avian Influenza Using Pancreatic Impression Smears. Avian Diseases 2003; 47: 1190 – 1195.

12 Roger F, J Thonnat, P Hendrikx, J Domenech: Les systèmes de suivi et de surveillance des maladies et le rôle des acteurs de santé animale publics et privés: l'expérience de l'Afrique – Revue OIE, 2004.

13 Benet JJ, Dufour B, Thonnat J, Weber L, Roger F, Toma B: Surveys concerning the needs for and evaluation of distance learning in veterinary epidemiology. J Vet Med Educ 2005; 32 (1): 68-71.

14 Porphyre V, Nguyen Ngoc S, Ha Minh T, Genewe S, Henry C: Local epidemio-surveillance in swine diseases in Northern Vietnam: description and preliminary results. STVM International Meeting, Hanoi – June 25th-July 1st, 2005. In press.

15 Cardinale E: Le réseau sénégalais d'épidémiosurveillance avaire (RESESAV): presentation et premiers resultants. Epidémiologie et Santé Animale 2000; 37: 105-116.

16 Mariner JC, Catley A, Zepeda C: The role of community-based programmes and participatory epidemiology in disease surveillance and international trade. Community-based Animal Health and Participatory Epidemiology Unit (CAPE), OAU, 2003, in Sones K, Catley A (eds): Primary Animal healthcare in the 21st Century: shaping the rules, policies and institutions. Proceedings of an international conference, 15th -18th October 2003, Mombasa, Kenya. African Union/Interafrican Bureau for Animal Resources, Nairobi – http://www.cape-ibar.org

17 Catley A, Admassu B: Using participatory epidemiology to assess the impact of livestock diseases. FAO-OIE-AU/IBAR-IAEA consultative group meeting on contagious bovine pleuropneumonia in Africa. 2003.

18 Catley A., Mariner JC: Participatory Epidemiology: Lessons Learned and future directions. Proceedings of an international workshop held in Addis Ababa, Ethiopia, 15th to 17th November, 2001. Community-based Animal Health and Participatory Epidemiology Unit, Organization of African Unity/Interafrican Bureau or Animal Resources, Nairobi, 2001, 44 pages.

Dr. F. Roger, Unité Epidémiologie et Ecologie, TA 30/E, Campus International de Baillarguet, F-34398 Montpellier, Cedex 5, France.
E-mail: françois.roger@cirad.fr

Schudel A, Lombard M (eds): OIE/FAO International Scientific Conference on Avian Influenza.
Dev Biol (Basel). Basel, Karger, 2006, vol 124, p 225.

SEPPIC Vaccine Adjuvants for Poultry

L. Dupuis

SEPPIC, Paris, France

Avian influenza and Newcastle disease are the two major diseases of poultry for which inactivated vaccines can be used. To guarantee high levels and long duration of protection, the choice of adjuvant is critical. Aluminium hydroxide adjuvant has been replaced by first generation oil adjuvants based on polysorbate formulations.

The production of the antigen is very specific and the yields of production and the purity of the final antigen is an important step. Once the antigen is defined, it is necessary to vectorise it as a water in oil (W/O) emulsion that needs to respect the following parameters:

Efficacy: to ensure long-term as well as short-term protection; Stability: two years at + 4°C and about one month at 20°C; Viscosity: it must be fluid to permit easy injection of the formulation; Safety: to ensure that the vaccine does not produce adverse reactions in vaccinated poultry or develop blemishes in the carcass.

To get this quality of the vaccine, it is necessary to control the quality of the injectable oils; the quality of the surfactant (purity, oxidation, no residues, chemical definition, stability); and the emulsifying properties – synergy between oil and surfactant and antigenic medium – to get a perfect emulsion. The following table provides a description of the general properties of selected Montanide ISA adjuvants.

Montanide	Oil	Adj/Antig (w/w)	Emulsion	Viscosity (mPa. s)	Efficacy		Safety
					Short term	Long term	
ISA 70	Mineral	70/30	W/O	30	++	+++	++
ISA 775	Mineral and non mineral	70/30	W/O	25	++	++	+++
ISA 763A	Non mineral	70/30	W/O	20	++	++	++++
ISA 206	Mineral	50/50	W/O/W	10	+++	++	+++

Schudel A, Lombard M (eds): OIE/FAO International Scientific Conference on Avian Influenza.
Dev Biol (Basel). Basel, Karger, 2006, vol 124, p 226.

Comparison of Virus Isolation and RT-PCR for Avian Influenza Virus Detection in Iran

R. Toroghi[1], R. Momayez[1], S.M. Tabatabai[2], S. Charkhkar[2], M. Vasfimarandi[2]

[1] Research & Diagnosis of Avian Diseases Department, Razi Vaccine & Serum Research Institute, Tehran, Iran

[2] Iran Veterinary Organisation

Avian influenza (AI) is an economically important viral disease in the Iranian poultry industry because of increased mortality and declines in egg production in affected chicken flocks. Virus isolation in embryonated SPF chicken eggs, a time-consuming method, is the most commonly used diagnostic test. In this study, virus isolation (VI) and RT-PCR for detection of avian influenza virus targeting nucleoprotein of type A avian influenza virus and haemagglutinin (H9) genes were evaluated with trachea samples from 50 clinically affected flocks. Moreover, RT-PCR for detection of H5 and H7 subtypes was applied for the samples. None of the samples was found to be positive for H5 or H7 subtypes. The sensitivity and specificity rates by RT-PCR of the hemagglutinin in comparison with VI, as the conventional method, were 95 % and 93.3 % respectively. The K value between these tests was 0.77. Compared with VI, the sensitivity and specificity of RT-PCR for nucleoprotein was 100 % and 83.3 %, respectively. The K value between VI and RT-PCR of nucleoprotein was 0.66. The results showed substantial agreement for the VI and RT-PCR tests in detection of AI virus. Moreover, RT-PCR for nucleoprotein was found to be more sensitive than RT-PCR for hemagglutinin. In conclusion, RT-PCR is a reliable method for rapid laboratory diagnosis of avian influenza in diseased birds because of its speed and sensitivity. Therefore, it can be used as an alternative to the VI method in surveillance centres where early screening for AI virus is the goal.

Schudel A, Lombard M (eds): OIE/FAO International Scientific Conference on Avian Influenza.
Dev Biol (Basel). Basel, Karger, 2006, vol 124, p 227.

Neutral Evolution of H5N1 Influenza Virus in Birds and Humans

L. Campitelli[1], *M. Ciccozzi*[1], *M. Salemi*[2], *F. Taglia*[1], *S. Boros*[1], *I. Donatelli*[1], *G. Rezza*[1]

[1] Department of Infectious, Istituto Superiore di Sanità, Rome, Italy

[2] Department of Pathology, College of Medicine, University of Florida, Gainesville, FL, USA

In 2004, an epidemic of highly pathogenic avian influenza A (H5N1) virus among domestic poultry affected nine Asian countries, causing human disease in two of these.

To understand better whether there are genetic determinants of transmission of avian influenza strains, we evaluated the mutation rate in H5N1 viral sequences from birds and humans infected during the 1997 and the 2004 (first wave) outbreaks, uploaded from the Influenza Sequence Database. Phylogenetic and positive selection analyses were performed to compare the coding regions of H5N1 isolates. Positive selection analysis was performed by comparing the maximum likelihood estimates of the codon substitution models M7 and M8, implemented in the CODEML program of the PAML package developed by Yang Z. In the 1997 data set, only PB2 was found under positive selection at five positions (82, 318, 334, 727, 355), whereas, in 2004, positions 140, 156 for HA and 204 for NS1 (which is involved, along with PB2, in increase of pathogenicity in mammalian hosts) were under positive selection. Positions 156 and 140 of HA are located within antigenically relevant regions of the molecule, thus positive selection at both of these sites may help the virus to evade the immune response and suggests the existence of an immunological pressure.

The occurrence of adaptive mutation in poultry may be a crucial mechanism by which the virus could improve its transmissibility also among humans. The possibility of this event strengthens the importance of improving surveillance both in humans and poultry.

Schudel A, Lombard M (eds): OIE/FAO International Scientific Conference on Avian Influenza.
Dev Biol (Basel). Basel, Karger, 2006, vol 124, p 228.

Response Policy Options and Compartmentalisation for Avian Influenza Surveillance in New Zealand

S. Cork, D. Geale, R. Thornton, H. Pharo

Biosecurity New Zealand, Ministry of Agriculture & Forestry, Wellington, New Zealand

New Zealand has never recorded a case of highly pathogenic avian influenza (HPAI) in captive or free-flying birds. Low pathogenicity strains (LPAI), including subtype H5N2, have been reported in free-flying waterfowl (mallard ducks) in New Zealand. The risk profile for avian influenza (HPAI) in New Zealand is different from most other countries. New Zealand is distant from other land masses, live-bird markets are uncommon and our waterfowl are not migratory. New Zealand has a number of unique and endangered bird species, therefore diseases and/or disease control measures that may threaten the survival of these birds are of national significance. Response policies to outline the action to be taken in view of surveillance data from wild and captive birds in New Zealand have been developed to take account of the risks associated with different compartments (i.e. commercial poultry, backyard poultry, zoo and other captive birds, wild birds). Recommendations take account of risk to public health, native fauna and the economy. Appropriate control actions would be determined by a Technical Advisory Group (TAG) which will include representation of stakeholders and will be endorsed by an Independent Expert Advisory Panel. Such control actions could include depopulation, vaccination or other options depending on the clinical picture, the virus isolated and the compartment in which the virus was identified. No action would be taken to control LPAI viruses detected in wild birds but the situation would be monitored. Enhanced biosecurity to prevent the interaction of commercial poultry and wild birds is currently recommended.

Schudel A, Lombard M (eds): OIE/FAO International Scientific Conference on Avian Influenza.
Dev Biol (Basel). Basel, Karger, 2006, vol 124, p 229.

Characterisation of H7N3 Influenza Viruses Isolated During the British Columbia Epizootic of 2004

J. Pasick[1], *K. Handel*[1], *J. Copps*[1], *Y. Berhane*[1], *D. Ridd*[1], *K. Hills*[1], *H. Kehler*[1], *C. Cottam-Birt*[1], *J. Neufeld*[1], *S. Czub*[1], *J. Robinson*[2]

[1] Canadian Food Inspection Agency, National Centre for Foreign Animal Disease, Winnipeg, Manitoba, Canada

[2] Animal Health Centre, British Columbia Ministry of Agriculture and Food, Abbotsford, British Columbia, Canada

In February 2004, a highly pathogenic avian influenza (HPAI) outbreak erupted in the Fraser Valley of British Columbia, Canada. Our investigations indicated that the responsible HPAI H7N3 virus emerged suddenly from a low pathogenic avian influenza (LPAI) H7N3 virus precursor. Analysis of the haemagglutinin (HA) genes of the LPAI and HPAI viruses isolated from the index farm revealed the only difference to be the presence of a 21-nucleotide insert at the HA cleavage site of the HPAI virus. We deduced that this insert most likely arose as a result of non-homologous recombination between the HA and matrix (M1) genes of the same virus. Over the course of the outbreak, a total of 37 isolates with, and three isolates without, inserts were characterised. Isolates with inserts could be further categorised into seven variants based on amino acid substitutions that occurred within, or adjacent to, the insert. Intravenous pathogenicity indices ranged from 2.17 to 3.00 depending on the isolate, and the lesions in four- to six-week old and adult layer Leghorn chickens were consistent with those expected for a highly pathogenic virus. The events described here appear very similar to those that occurred in Chile in 2002, where the virulence shift of another H7N3 virus was attributed to non-homologous recombination between the HA and nucleoprotein gene.

Schudel A, Lombard M (eds): OIE/FAO International Scientific Conference on Avian Influenza.
Dev Biol (Basel). Basel, Karger, 2006, vol 124, p 230.

Highly Pathogenic Avian Influenza in Italy: Application of Local Spatial Statistics to Detect Clusters of Infection

A. Mannelli[1], *N. Ferrè*[2], *S. Marangon*[2]

[1] Dipartimento di Produzioni Animali, Epidemiologia ed Ecologia, University of Turin, Italy

[2] Istituto Zooprofilattico Sperimentale delle Venezie, Italy

Local spatial statistics were applied to the highly pathogenic avian influenza (HPAI) epidemic that struck northern Italy during the winter of 1999 – 2000. A function of the number of infected premises (IP's) that were located within discrete distances from each IP, and continuous distance-decay measures of clustering were calculated. Statistical significance of observed results was tested by a Monte Carlo simulation, taking into account the spatial distribution of the population at risk. Significant clusters of HPAI were detected in the province of Brescia and Mantova (Lombardy region), and in the province of Verona (Veneto region). Subsequently, spatio-temporal clustering of HPAI was obtained as the number of new IPs that occurred within a distance of 1.5 km from a previous IP in the temporal risk window (TRW). An IP's TRW is the time interval during which clinical signs of disease can be detected in another flock following transmission from the IP. In this way, we attempted to detect HPAI cases that most likely originated from viral transmission from neighbouring IPs. Maximum spatio-temporal clustering was observed in the Lombardy region, where up to 80 % of flocks that were located within 1.5 km from certain IPs in TRW subsequently became infected by HPAI. Our results suggest that pre-emptive slaughter and depopulation of at-risk flocks, which were mostly carried out in Veneto, were effective in controlling the epidemic.

Schudel A, Lombard M (eds): OIE/FAO International Scientific Conference on Avian Influenza.
Dev Biol (Basel). Basel, Karger, 2006, vol 124, p 231.

Variability of the NS1 Protein Obtained from Italian AI Isolates of the H7 Subtype

W.G. Dundon, A. Milani, G. Cattoli, I. Capua

OIE and National Reference Laboratory for Newcastle Disease and Avian Influenza
Istituto Zooprofilattico Sperimentale delle Venezie, Legnaro, Padova, Italy

To verify the homogeneity of the non-structural 1 (NS1) protein of representative avian influenza (AI) viruses of the H7 subtype isolated in Italy during 1999-2004, the gene encoding the NS1 protein from a collection of isolates obtained since 1999 in Northern Italy was analysed by sequencing. The complete sequence of the NS1 gene of 40 AI viruses (28 LPAI and 12 HPAI) isolated from a spectrum of bird species was determined and compared phylogenetically. The isolates were separated into two previously described clades designated A and B. Group A isolates were made up of H7N3 (n = 11), H7N7 (n = 3), H7N4 (n = 1) subtypes while group B consisted of H7N1 (n = 24) and H10N4 (n = 1) subtypes. In addition, analysis of the amino acid sequence of the NS1 protein from the 12 HPAI isolates revealed a previously unreported isoleucine residue at position 136 in addition to a novel C-terminal truncation.

The data presented reveals that NS1 proteins of AI viruses are not as conserved as originally believed. In addition, the novel primary structure of the NS1 protein of HPAI isolates that have circulated in northern Italy indicate that a diagnostic test to be used in the framework of a "DIVA" (differentiating infected from vaccinated animals) strategy based on the detection of antibodies to the NS1 protein may encounter some difficulties in field validation. Work in progress is focusing on whether the variability identified confers functional or immunogenic advantages on those viruses that posses them and on the antigenic profile of the NS1 protein of a wider selection of AI viruses.

Schudel A, Lombard M (eds): OIE/FAO International Scientific Conference on Avian Influenza.
Dev Biol (Basel). Basel, Karger, 2006, vol 124, pp 232-233.

Descriptive Analysis of the Avian Influenza Virus (H5N1) Epidemic in Thailand in 2004

T. Tiensin[1,2], *P. Chaithaweesup*[1], *T. Songserm*[3], *A. Chaisingh*[4], *W. Hoonsuwan*[1], *O. Pasavorakul*[1], *C. Buranathai*[1], *T. Parakamawongsa*[1], *S. Premashthira*[1], *M. Nielen*[2], *J.A. Stegeman*[2]

1 Department of Livestock Development, Bangkok, Thailand

2 Department of Farm Animal Health, Faculty of Veterinary Medicine, Utrecht University, the Netherlands

3 Department of Pathology, Faculty of Veterinary Medicine, Kasetsart University, Nakhon Pathom, Thailand

4 National Institute of Animal Health, Department of Livestock Development, Thailand

Key-words: Avian influenza, epidemiology, control measures, Thailand.

In January 2004, laboratory diagnosis confirmed the presence of highly pathogenic avian influenza (H5N1) virus in poultry and humans in Thailand. Control measures such as stamping-out, movement restrictions, and hygienic measures were implemented. In 2004, 1,417 villages in 60 of 76 provinces throughout Thailand were affected. Over 62 million birds were destroyed to control the disease and for animal welfare reasons. H5N1 viruses transmitted from poultry to humans led to hospitalisation of 17 people; 12 of them died. Additionally, domestic cats, tigers and leopards were killed by H5N1 viruses. About 83 % of infected flocks were backyard chickens and ducks. Outbreaks were concentrated in the central, the lower part of the northern, and the eastern regions of Thailand, which are wetlands, water reservoirs and areas densely populated with poultry. The relative risks (RR) of infection of poultry flocks, based on cumulative incidences over 2004, were around four times higher in the central region and 1.5 times higher for the eastern region, compared to the northern region. Based on RRs, the risk of HPAI infection seemed five times higher in layers and broilers and 1.5 times higher in ducks, compared to backyard chickens. However, in these observations, size of flock was considered as a confounder in relation to HPAI infection. As a result of various factors, including the extent of the period between introduction of the virus into the country and its conclusive diagnosis of the initial outbreak, lack of biosecurity in certain production sectors, difficulty in detecting HPAI clinical signs in ducks, seasonal weather conditions, and lack of public participation and awareness, HPAI viruses disseminated widely in large areas throughout Thailand, resulting in a complex situation for tracing and controlling the disease. In early 2005, the epidemic is still continuing in Thailand.

Schudel A, Lombard M (eds): OIE/FAO International Scientific Conference on Avian Influenza.
Dev Biol (Basel). Basel, Karger, 2006, vol 124, p 234.

H5 Avian Influenza Antibodies in Rural Poultry of Thai-Binh Province-Vietnam

D.Q. Phuong[1], *N.T. Dung*[2], *J.P. Christensen*[1]

[1] Department of Veterinary Pathobiology, the Royal Veterinary and Agricultural University Frederiksberg, Denmark

[2] Department of Virology, National Institute of Veterinary Research (NIVR), Dong Da, Hanoi, Vietnam

Avian influenza (AI) caused by a highly pathogenic H5N1 virus was recognised in Vietnam in late December 2004. Since then, the disease has had enormous impact on poultry production and also the public health implications have been dramatic.

The disease appeared in Thai Binh province in the North of Vietnam in January 2004. Approximately one month after the last recognised outbreak in that province, a seroprevalence study primarily for H5 virus antibodies was conducted to elucidate basic aspects of the post-epidemic epidemiology of AI in rural poultry in Vietnam. In addition, virus isolation was attempted.

Blood samples and cloacal swab samples were obtained from 587 birds including 379 chickens, 76 ducks and 132 muscovy ducks from five districts of the province and representing 106 households. High levels of antibodies to H5 virus were observed in birds belonging to the three species sampled. However, a significant difference in prevalence of H5 antibodies between the three species of birds was demonstrated. A high percentage of the ducks were seropositive (78 %), in contrast to the chickens of which only 6 % showed seroconversion. The observation that few ducks died and only at the beginning of the outbreak in Thai Binh, coupled with the fact that a very high percentage of the ducks were positive for antibodies against H5 virus, demonstrate the potential of domestic ducks to act as a reservoir for AIV, including HPAI.

Schudel A, Lombard M (eds): OIE/FAO International Scientific Conference on Avian Influenza.
Dev Biol (Basel). Basel, Karger, 2006, vol 124, pp 235-236.

Isolation of Influenza A Viruses Belonging to the H7N7 and H7N4 Subtypes from Wild and Domestic Waterfowl in Italy

C. Terregino[1], G. Cattoli[1], V. Guberti[2], R. De Nardi[1], M. Scremin[2], M.S. Beato[1], I. Capua[1]

[1] OIE and National Reference Laboratory for Newcastle Disease and Avian Influenza, Istituto Zooprofilattico Sperimentale delle Venezie, Italy

[2] Istituto Nazionale per la Fauna Selvatica "A. Ghigi ", Bologna, Italy

Following the outbreaks of avian influenza (AI) in Italy between 1997 and 2004, a surveillance programme, funded by the Italian Ministry of Health was carried out on wild birds captured in wetlands in northern Italy. Between November 2003 and March 2005, 1512 cloacal swabs and 350 tracheal swabs were collected from wild birds captured in wetlands in northern Italy, from game-fowl and from backyard flocks including waterfowl.

Cloacal and tracheal swabs were screened by real time reverse transcription polymerase chain reaction (RT-PCR) [1] and, when positive, virus isolation was attempted as described in EU Directive 92/40/EC.

Eight isolates were identified as influenza viruses belonging to the H7N7 subtype, four of which were isolated from wild mallard ducks, two from teal, one from a domestic duck and one from a domestic goose. Another isolate obtained from a mallard was subtyped as H7N4. Sequence analysis of the cleavage site of the haemagglutinin gene showed that all nine isolates are low pathogenicity avian influenza viruses. Interestingly, the H7N7 isolates from wild birds and the ones from the domestic waterfowl share a haemagglutinin sequence homology of 99.3 %.

The results of this surveillance programme support the theory that backyard flocks, particularly those that include domestic ducks and geese, might act as a link between the natural reservoir and poultry. The evidence reported herein also indicates that Italy is continuously at risk of the introduction of H7 viruses, and supports the application of prophylactic vaccination in densely populated poultry areas (DPPA) of northern Italy [2]. Continuing surveillance programmes in areas at risk, including both wild birds and poultry, will improve our knowledge of the ecology, epidemiology and prevention of AI infections.

REFERENCES

1 Cattoli G, Drago A, Maniero S, Toffan A, Bertoli E, Fassina S, Terregino C, Robbi C, Vicenzoni G, Capua I: Comparison of three rapid detection systems for type A influenza virus on tracheal swabs of experimentally and naturally infected birds. Avian Pathology 2004; 33 (4): 432-437.

2 CEC: Commission Decision 2004/666/EC of 29 September 2004 on introducing vaccination to supplement the measures to control infections with low pathogenic avian influenza in Italy and on specific movement control measures and repealing Decision 2002/975/EC. Official Journal of the European Commission 2004; L303: 35-44.

Schudel A, Lombard M (eds): OIE/FAO International Scientific Conference on Avian Influenza.
Dev Biol (Basel). Basel, Karger, 2006, vol 124, p 237.

Fighting Avian Influenza Needs a Step Forward Now

H. Kiezebrink

Herman Kiezebrink Institute, Epe, The Netherlands

Herman Kiezebrink Institute (HKI) was responsible for culling 15 million birds on 900 farms during the AI epidemic in Europe. Animal welfare has always been most important in our approach.

Non-commercial poultry in Asia

Non-commercial poultry in rural areas are a high risk to human health with the potential to cause a pandemic outbreak. Addressing this is the biggest challenge to the global community. HKI has produced cheap, effective and safe systems to eradicate AI in rural areas.

European model

The cost of the recent outbreaks in Europe was crippling to the poultry industry. HKI developed a risk-management model to limit the consequential losses by 60 % both to the industry and the EC, based on AI insurance for farmers. A partnership is created between veterinary services and farmers' organisations. HKI provides the equipment, training and planning to enable the disease outbreak to be attacked within 48 hours.

New techniques

We have employed all the techniques described by the **OIE**. We have developed these techniques to improve animal welfare, biosecurity, cost effectiveness and to reduce the risk to human health, for example:

- fast and effective culling of 10,000 adult turkeys per hour;
- culling techniques for non-commercial poultry in rural areas in Asia for a capital cost of only 25 euros per device;
- revolutionary disinfecting technique using only water salt and electricity at a cost of only 250 euros per unit.

Schudel A, Lombard M (eds): OIE/FAO International Scientific Conference on Avian Influenza.
Dev Biol (Basel). Basel, Karger, 2006, vol 124, pp 238-239.

TAQMAN-MGB Probe One-Step Quantitative Real-Time PCR with Internal Positive Control for Avian Influenza Virus RNA Detection

L. Di Trani[1], *B. Bedini*[1], *E. Falcone*[1], *I. Donatelli*[2], *L. Campitelli*[2], *B. Chiappini*[1], *M.A. De Marco*[3], *M. Delogu*[4], *A. Camarda*[5], *G. Vaccari*[1], *C. Buonavoglia*[5]

[1] Department of Food and Animal Health, Istituto Superiore di Sanità, Italy

[2] Department of Parasitic, Immune-Mediated and Infectious Diseases, Istituto Superiore di Sanità, Italy

[3] National Wildlife Institute, Italy

[4] Department of Veterinary Public Health and Animal Pathology, University of Bologna, Italy

[5] Department of Animal Health and Well-Being, Faculty of Veterinary Medicine of Bari, Italy

Development of rapid, highly specific and sensitive assays for the prompt identification of avian influenza viruses (AIVs) circulating in the field to survey the emergence of potentially pandemic viruses, is one of the primary objectives of the research-management on AIV.

Though being sensitive and specific for AIV detection, conventional reverse transcription polymerase chain reaction (RT-PCR) is time-consuming, it does not allow for quantification of viral load and requires a number of manipulations of samples, thus increasing the risk of carry-over contamination.

Recently, quantitative, fluorescence-based real-time RT-PCR (RRT-PCR) assays have been proposed in different formats for AIV detection. In this study, a one-step RRT-PCR with Minor Groove Binder (MGB) probe was developed. A DNA probe with conjugated MGB group forms a stable duplex with single-stranded DNA target; moreover, the use of MGB probe has demonstrated low background fluorescence and improved assay specificity and sensitivity in comparison to the common non-MGB probes. Addition of an internal positive control to each sample before the processing allowed monitoring of the reliability of RNA extraction and subsequent PCR amplification, eliminating the occurrence of false negative results.

A panel of avian, equine, swine and human Influenza A reference viruses was first assayed by the test. After optimisation of the RRT-PCR, 1152 cloacal swabs collected from hunted wild birds were tested and 15 samples were found positive for AIV. These results were further confirmed by a conventional RT-PCR targeting a different gene segment.

Schudel A, Lombard M (eds): OIE/FAO International Scientific Conference on Avian Influenza. Dev Biol (Basel). Basel, Karger, 2006, vol 124, p 240.

Swedish Guillemots Harbouring Influenza A Virus with a Mix of American and Eurasian Gene Segments

A. Wallensten[1,2], V.J. Munster[3], R.A.M. Fouchier[3], B. Olsen[4,5]

1 Smedby Health Centre, Kalmar County Council, Kalmar, Sweden

2 Division of Medical Microbiology Department of Molecular and Clinical Medicine (IMK) Faculty of Health Sciences, Linköpings Universitet, Linköping, Sweden

3 Department of Virology and National Influenza Centre, Erasmus Medical Centre, Rotterdam, The Netherlands

4 Department of Infectious Diseases, Umeå University, Umeå, Sweden

5 Department of Biology and Environmental Science, Section for Zoonotic Ecology and Epidemiology, University of Kalmar, Kalmar, Sweden

As part of our continuing influenza A virus surveillance in wild birds in Northern Europe, guillemots on the island of Bonden in the northern Baltic Sea, were screened. Three out of 26 sampled birds tested positive by reverse transcription polymerase chain reaction (RT-PCR). Two of these were characterised as subtype H6N2. Phylogenetic analyses showed that the PB2, PB1, HA, M and NS gene segments belonged to the American lineage of influenza A viruses, whereas the PA, NP and NA gene segments belonged to the Eurasian lineage. This is the first report of a recombinant avian influenza A virus isolated in Europe with genes of American and Eurasian origin and also the first report of an avian influenza A virus isolation from European guillemots.

Schudel A, Lombard M (eds): OIE/FAO International Scientific Conference on Avian Influenza.
Dev Biol (Basel). Basel, Karger, 2006, vol 124, pp 241-242.

Highly Pathogenic Avian Influenza Epidemic in Italy: Study of the Risk Factors by Survival Analysis

E. Rossi[1], *A. Mannelli*[2], *M. Toson*[1], *M. Dalla Pozza*[1], *L. Busani*[1], *S. Marangon*[1]

[1] Centro Regionale di Epidemiologia Veterinaria (CREV) – Istituto Zooprofilattico Sperimentale delle Venezie, Legnaro (PD), Italy

[2] Dipartimento di Produzioni Animali, Epidemiologia ed Ecologia – Università di Torino, Grugliasco (TO), Italy

Background

From December 1999 to April 2000, a large epidemic of highly pathogenic avian influenza affected Lombardia and Veneto regions (north-east Italy). More than 400 outbreaks were observed, causing death or culling of 16,000,000 birds and severe economic losses. Control measures indicated in the Directive 92/40/CE were applied. In addition, pre-emptive slaughter of at-risk farms was implemented mainly in one region.

The aim of the work was to evaluate the contribution of several risk factors to the spread of the infection and the efficacy of the pre-emptive slaughter in controlling the epidemic.

Methods

Data on animal species and production, size and location of the infected farms were collected. The time of virus introduction in the farm was estimated.

A case was defined as a farm that, during the observation period, became infected. In the same period, uninfected or slaughtered farms were considered as censored. Cox multivariate regression model was applied for the hazard ratio (HR) evaluation.

Results

The model showed significant correlation with the animal species involved (HR = 3.2 for turkey and HR = 2.2 for hens), the size of the farm (HR = 1.5 for larger farms) and the presence of other infected farms in a radius of 1500 and 3000 metres (HR = 1.5 and HR = 1.4 respectively). Comparing the two regions, the pre-emptive slaughter was protective against the infection (HR = 0.4).

Discussion

Raising turkeys and hens, particularly in large holdings, and proximity to previously infected farms were the most relevant risk factors for a farm to be infected. The efficacy of pre-emptive slaughter was confirmed.

Schudel A, Lombard M (eds): OIE/FAO International Scientific Conference on Avian Influenza.
Dev Biol (Basel). Basel, Karger, 2006, vol 124, p 243.

Efficacy of the Vaccination During the H7N3 Low Pathogenicity Avian Influenza Epidemic in Italy in 2002-2003

M. Toson, M. Dalla Pozza, E. Rossi, L. Busani, S. Marangon

Centro Regionale di Epidemiologia Veterinaria (CREV), Istituto Zooprofilattico Sperimentale delle Venezie, Legnaro (PD), Italy

Introduction

From 1997 to date, avian influenza (AI) viruses caused four epidemics in the densely populated poultry area (DPPA) in northern Italy. In 2002-2003 an epidemic resulting from a low pathogenicity (LPAI) virus subtype H7N3 occurred. No measures to control LPAI are provided for in the current European Union legislation, but the previously experienced epidemics moved Italian authorities to put in force measures to prevent the spread of LPAI and avoid possible re-emergence of highly pathogenic AI (HPAI). Restriction measures were immediately implemented, followed after 2.5 months by a vaccination programme. A heterologous vaccine that allowed the distinction between vaccinated and infected animals (DIVA) was used in turkey and layer flocks. The virus infected 388 farms, 86 % of them were meat-type turkey farms. About 7.6 millions of birds were involved. Among the vaccinated, 88 turkey flocks were infected.

The aim of this paper is to describe the efficacy of the vaccination strategy by the estimate of the reproduction rate (R) in vaccinated and non-vaccinated poultry populations.

Methods

Data on the total poultry population during the epidemic, on the time of infection and on the vaccination status were collected and entered in a stochastic model to estimate R.

Results

The estimates of R for the global poultry population at risk before and after the vaccination campaign were 2.9 (IC 95 % = 2.3-3.9) and 0.6 (IC 95 % = 0.5-0.7), respectively.

Discussion

The vaccination, together with restrictive measures, reduced significantly the diffusion of the virus among the poultry farms, allowing the control of the epidemic in DPPA.

Schudel A, Lombard M (eds): OIE/FAO International Scientific Conference on Avian Influenza.
Dev Biol (Basel). Basel, Karger, 2006, vol 124, p 244.

Influenza Virus Circulation in Wild Ducks and Coots in Italy During H5N2 and H7N1 Poultry Epidemic Periods (1998-1999)

M.A. De Marco[1], E. Foni[2], L. Campitelli[3], M. Delogu[4], E. Raffini[2], C. Chiapponi[2], G. Barigazzi[2], P. Cordioli[2], L. Di Trani[5], I. Donatelli[3]

[1] Istituto Nazionale per la Fauna Selvatica " A. Ghigi ", Ozzano E. (BO), Italy

[2] Istituto Zooprofilattico Sperimentale della Lombardia e dell'Emilia-Romagna, Units of Parma, Lugo (RA) and Brescia, Italy

[3] Department of Infectious, Parasitic and Immune-Mediated Diseases, and Department of Food Safety and Veterinary Public Heath, Istituto Superiore di Sanità, Rome, Italy

[4] Department of Veterinary Public Health and Animal Pathology, University of Bologna, Italy

Two epidemics of avian influenza because of H5 and H7 highly pathogenic viruses occurred in poultry in Italy in 1997/98 and 1999/2000, respectively. The circulation of these serotypes in wild aquatic birds was investigated, examining 488 cloacal swabs and 488 sera collected from 162 coots and 326 ducks trapped in Italian wetlands during three wintering periods, from 1998 to 1999. Seroprevalences against influenza A viruses, detected by a double antibody sandwich blocking ELISA were 16 % in coots, and 44.5 % in ducks. Among the *Anatidae* group, duck species wintering in Mediterranean areas (DWMA) showed significantly higher values than ducks wintering in South-Saharan areas (DWSSA) of Africa. To detect H5 and H7 antibodies, the haemagglutination-inhibition (HI) assay and two competitive ELISA tests (H5-ELISA and H7-ELISA) using monoclonal antibodies (MAbs) specific for H5 and H7 subtypes, were performed. None of the aquatic bird species were found seropositive to H7 subtype, whereas H5 positive sera were found by both HI and ELISA assays in ducks only. The highest H5 seroprevalences were detected by H5-ELISA ; overall, 5 % (10/201) of DWMA tested H5-seropositive by this assay, with annual seroprevalences ranging from 1.6 % (2/123) to 11.8 % (6/51), in 1998 and 1999 respectively. In the present study, only five viruses belonging to H1N1, H11N6, and H2N3 subtypes were isolated from ducks. However, the H5 seroconversion observed in one mallard duck at the beginning of 1998 indicates that H5 virus circulation also occurred in the study area.

Schudel A, Lombard M (eds): OIE/FAO International Scientific Conference on Avian Influenza.
Dev Biol (Basel). Basel, Karger, 2006, vol 124, p 245.

Isolation and Characterisation of a Highly Pathogenic H5N1 Influenza Virus from Eagles Smuggled from Thailand into Europe

S. Van Borm, B. Lambrecht, M. Boschmans, M. Decaestecker, D. Morales, M. Gonze, M. Vandenbroeck, T. Van Den Berg

Avian Virology & Immunology Unit, Veterinary & Agrochemical Research Centre (VAR), Brussels, Belgium

The 2003-2004 highly pathogenic avian influenza epidemic caused by A/H5N1 viruses is now believed to be endemic in at least six south-eastern Asian countries and it not only affects birds. Its host range includes several mammals, including 69 laboratory-confirmed human cases to date, with 46 fatal cases, after direct transmission of the virus. On 18 October 2004, two *Spizaetus nipalensis* crested hawk eagles smuggled into Europe from Thailand were seized and sacrificed at Brussels International Airport. Both eagles showed enteritis and one presented bilateral pneumonia. Samples were taken from lungs and inoculated into embryonating eggs, which died in less than two days. The isolated virus was denominated A/crested eagle/Belgium/01/2004. The antigenic sub-typing as H5N1 was made by haemagglutination inhibition using 12 monospecific polysera, and the diagnosis was confirmed by nucleoprotein gene (general for type A influenza) and H5-specific reverse transcription polymerase chain reaction (RT-PCR). Over 600 contact birds were euthanised but all tested negative. The high pathogenicity of the virus was demonstrated by measuring the intravenous pathogenicity index in six-week old specific-pathogen-free (SPF) chickens (IVPI = 2.94) and confirmed in 12-week old layers. The partial sequencing of the haemagglutinin (HA) gene indicated six basic amino acid residues in the cleavage site and a close relationship within the Z genotype cluster to currently circulating strains in Thailand, although some mutations were evident, among which one resulted in a unique arginine (R) > lysine (K) replacement at the cleavage site. This study demonstrates that international air travel and smuggling represent significant threats for the introduction and worldwide dissemination of H5N1 viruses.

Schudel A, Lombard M (eds): OIE/FAO International Scientific Conference on Avian Influenza.
Dev Biol (Basel). Basel, Karger, 2006, vol 124, p 246.

Avian Influenza in Asia – The Challenges Ahead

L.D. Sims

Asia Pacific Veterinary Information Services Pty Ltd, Manunda Qld, Australia

Highly pathogenic avian influenza (HPAI) H5N1 viruses are still circulating in a number of Asian countries. A major challenge facing many of the infected countries is inadequate surveillance capacity, which can lead to cases of infection and disease remaining undiagnosed. This structural problem will not be overcome in the short to medium term. Therefore, it will be necessary to build HPAI control strategies around imperfect information. Data from elsewhere in the region will assist this process but may not be entirely applicable because of the marked regional differences in the various poultry production sectors and marketing systems among infected countries.

Infected countries have largely addressed HPAI as an animal health emergency. They should now design and implement integrated, long-term control programmes for HPAI based on reviews of likely infection pathways for each sector of the poultry industry. A suite of appropriate interventions should then be developed for those sectors considered to be playing a key role in the spread of H5N1 HPAI viruses. All available management options must be considered, covering technical, socio-economic and political factors of the proposed interventions, before measures suited to the local situation are adopted. These pathways and measures need to be reviewed regularly.

Two countries are using vaccination widely to control HPAI as a response to endemic disease and infection. This is a valid response that appears to have significantly reduced the levels of disease, virus shedding and potential for spread. However, unless there is a significant change in the nature of circulating viruses or major structural changes in the smallholder sector in these countries, it is unlikely that vaccination can be withdrawn for a considerable period of time. Managing the move towards reduced dependence on vaccination in these countries will be a major challenge.

Schudel A, Lombard M (eds): OIE/FAO International Scientific Conference on Avian Influenza.
Dev Biol (Basel). Basel, Karger, 2006, vol 124, p 247.

Ancestors of H5 and H7 Highly Pathogenic Avian Influenza Outbreaks Found in Wild Birds in Northern Europe

V.J. Munster[1], A. Wallensten[2], C. Baas[1], M. Stervander[2], G.F. Rimmelzwaan[1], B. Olsen[2], A.D.M.E. Osterhaus[1], R.A.M. Fouchier[1]

[1] Department of Virology and WHO National Influenza Centre, ErasmusMC, Rotterdam, The Netherlands

[2] Kalmar County hospital, Department of Microbiology, Kalmar, Sweden

Wild birds, in particular waterfowl, represent the natural reservoir of avian influenza A viruses (AIV). AIVs usually cause no disease signs in their natural host, but problems may arise upon introduction in non-natural host species. AIVs are occasionally transmitted to other species, such as horses, pigs, marine mammals, ostriches, chickens, turkeys and humans, leading to influenza outbreaks among these animals.

In contrast with North America, information about AIVs in Eurasia is limited. However, AIVs found in Eurasian birds are of particular interest, because of their genetic differences from AIVs in the Americas, and the zoonotic potential of certain Eurasian strains is currently the cause of serious problems.

Between 1999 and 2002, we isolated 17 H5 AIVs with various NA subtypes (N2, N3, N6 and N9) and 16 H7 AIVs with various neuraminidase (NA) subtypes (N3, N7 and N9) from migrating mallards. Sequence analysis revealed high homology with recent fowl plague viruses that caused the outbreaks in Italy in 1997 (H5N2), 1999 (H7N1), 2001 (H7N3) and in the Netherlands, Belgium and Germany in 2003 (H7N7). Phylogenetic analysis confirms the relationship of these viruses to those that caused the fowl plague outbreaks, indicating the ancestral relationship of these viruses towards the fowl plague viruses. Interestingly, the majority of the H7 viruses were isolated before the 2003 H7N7 in The Netherlands during the fall migration of the mallards to their wintering grounds.

Our data indicate that AIV surveillance in wild birds provides an opportunity to develop reagents for diagnostic purposes and vaccine development before influenza outbreaks.

Schudel A, Lombard M (eds): OIE/FAO International Scientific Conference on Avian Influenza.
Dev Biol (Basel). Basel, Karger, 2006, vol 124, pp 248-249.

TROVAC AI H5, an Avian Influenza Fowlpox Vector Vaccine, as an Alternative Vaccine for Hatcheries

M. Bublot[1], D.E. Swayne[2], P. Selleck[3], E. Montiel[4], N. Pritchard[5], M. Lee[6], T.R. Mickle[4]

1 Merial SAS, Lyon, France

2 Southeastern Regional Poultry Laboratory, Agricultural Research Service, U.S. Department of Agriculture, Athens, GA, USA

3 Commonwealth Scientific and Industrial Research Organisation, Geelong, Australia

4 Merial Avian Global Enterprise, Gainesville, GA, USA

5 Merial Select, Inc. Gainesville, GA, USA

6 Merial Avian Global Enterprise, Kuala Lumpur, Malaysia

Inactivated vaccines are the most widely used vaccines in avian influenza (AI) controlled vaccination programmes, but there is currently no serology test commercially available that can differentiate infected from vaccinated birds (DIVA test). TROVAC AI H5, a fowlpox recombinant expressing the haemagglutinin of an H5 isolate, received a conditional license in U.S.A in 1998 and then was registered in Mexico, Guatemala and El Salvador. More than one billion doses of TROVAC AI H5 have been used so far with no reported adverse reactions. This vaccine protects chickens against mortality and morbidity and decreases shedding after challenge with a wide panel of H5-subtype AI strains. It provided 100 % protection against mortality/morbidity induced by challenge with recent Asian HP H5N1 isolates and reduced the challenge virus shedding from respiratory and gastrointestinal tracts by 2.5-4.5 log 10 of virus. TROVAC AI H5 is fully active in maternal antibody positive broiler chickens from breeder hens vaccinated with killed AI and/or fowlpox. However, after placement of chickens in the field, fowlpox vaccination or natural infection interferes with TROVAC AI-induced immunity. Birds vaccinated with TROVAC AI H5 will develop antibodies detectable by the haemagglutination inhibition (HI) test using the appropriate antigen. However, they will not produce antibodies against matrix/nucleoprotein detectable by common serological tests such as AGP and ELISA, which therefore can be used as DIVA tests. Another advantage of TROVAC AI H5 over inactivated vaccine is that it is fully efficacious when administered once in one-day old birds, and it is compatible with Marek's disease vaccination. These features make TROVAC AI H5 an ideal vaccine to be used in hatcheries.

Schudel A, Lombard M (eds): OIE/FAO International Scientific Conference on Avian Influenza.
Dev Biol (Basel). Basel, Karger, 2006, vol 124, p 250.

The Use of Vaccination as a Primary Eradication Tool of HPAI Outbreak in Indonesia

T.S.P. Naipospos

Directorate General of Livestock Services, Jakarta, Indonesia

Key words: Vaccination, avian influenza, Indonesia.

An outbreak of highly pathogenic avian influenza (HPAI) was detected in Indonesia in August 2003. The epidemic continues as disease moves into new areas and less vulnerable flocks in infected areas become infected. The peak intensity of losses has passed, with reduced numbers of outbreaks since major losses began in November/December 2003. The disease has most probably spread rapidly because of movements of live birds to most of the larger islands in Indonesia.

The primary eradication tool used has been vaccination. There are eight different inactivated vaccines available (three locally manufactured; one from China; and four from Mexico). These are either H5N1 subtypes or, in the case of Mexican vaccines, H2N2 subtypes.

Vaccination has been proved to be effective in preventing local losses and in reducing the "virus load" in the environment. The vaccination has taken effect, since the epidemic has been slowed and the vulnerable flocks have decrease in number from April 2004 up to present.

Pathogenicity and challenge testing was used to measure the vaccine efficacy. A challenge test was used to measure the level of protection of local vaccine against field strains collected from three different locations. The result showed that the local vaccine could give a 90 % protection rate. The result of a haemagglutination inhibition (HI) test showed that the mean antibody titres of vaccinated chicken at two weeks post-challenge has been increased significantly.

Various field studies to monitor the antibody titres post-vaccination in layer, broiler and local chicken at different ages were conducted to assess the duration of immunity and the effectiveness of vaccination for both local and import vaccines. The variation of protective antibody titres in the vaccinated chicken population were shown to be satisfactory and booster application has given a high antibody titre in farms adopting a high level of biosecurity.

A molecular characterisation of the isolates of AI viruses from different times and locations has been conducted continuously up to the present to be able to identify the most appropriate LP virus selected for replacing the existing master seed of local vaccine.

Schudel A, Lombard M (eds): OIE/FAO International Scientific Conference on Avian Influenza.
Dev Biol (Basel). Basel, Karger, 2006, vol 124, p 251.

Study of Avian Influenza in Indonesia: Molecular Characterisation of the Virus Collected from Outbreaks

N.L.P.I. Dharmayanti, R. Damayanti, R. Indriani, A. Wiyono, R.M.A. Adjid

Indonesian Research Institute for Veterinary Science, Bogor, West Java, Indonesia

Key words: Avian influenza virus, characterisation, poultry, Indonesia.

Avian influenza outbreaks in poultry have been reported in Java Island since October 2003. More than 30 isolates of avian influenza virus had been isolated during October 2003 to February 2005. The virus has been identified as HPAI H5N1 subtype. Sixteen of them were then characterised further at genetic level and also for their pathogenicity. The phylogenetic analysis revealed that all avian influenza virus isolates were closely related to avian influenza virus from China (A/Duck/China/E319-2/03 (H5N1). The molecular basis of pathogenicity in the haemagglutinin (HA) cleavage site showed that the isolates of avian influenza virus have multiple basic amino acid (B-X-B-R) indicating that all the isolates were still virulent forms of avian influenza virus (highly pathogenic avian influenza virus). It is concluded that there was not much change in the virus characteristics, since it was first identified from an outbreak of avian influenza in poultry in Indonesia.

Schudel A, Lombard M (eds): OIE/FAO International Scientific Conference on Avian Influenza. Dev Biol (Basel). Basel, Karger, 2006, vol 124, p 252.

Molecular Characteristic of H5N1 Avian Influenza A Virus in Thailand, 2004

C. Buranathai[1], A. Chaisigh[1], B. Nuansrichay[1], S. Damrongwattanapokin[1], Y. Limlamthong[1], S. Payungporn[2], S. Chutinimitkul[2], A. Amonsin[3], J. Keawcharoen[3], A. Theamboonlers[2], P. Phakdeewirot[2], K. Oraveerakul[3], N. Viseshakul[3], R. Thanawongnuwech[3], S. Suradhat[3], Y. Poovorawan[2]

[1] Department of Livestock Development, Rajathevi, Bangkok, Thailand

[2] Centre of Excellence in Viral Hepatitis Research Unit, Faculty of Medicine, Chulalongkorn University, Bangkok, Thailand

[3] Faculty of Veterinary Science, Chulalongkorn University, Bangkok, Thailand

Influenza A virus subtype H5N1 caused a rapidly fatal systemic disease in domestic chicken, duck and other avian species, and was transmitted directly from poultry to humans. The virus also extended its host range to *Felidae*, causing fatal pneumonia in cats, tigers and leopards. We have sequenced the whole genome of the Thai influenza A (H5N1) viruses: A/Chicken/Nakorn-Pathom/Thailand/CU-K2/04, isolated during early 2004. H5N1 isolated from different avian species from a different outbreak between January 2004 and January 2005 was also characterised. Phylogenetic analysis was performed in comparison to AI viruses from the Hong Kong 1997 and other H5N1 isolates reported during 2001 to 2004. Molecular characterisation of the haemagglutinin (HA) gene of the Thai H5N1 revealed a common characteristic of a highly pathogenic AI (HPAI), with polybasic amino acid in the HA cleavage site, a 20-codon deletion in the neuraminidase gene, a five-codon deletion in the non-structural (NS) gene and polymorphisms of the M2 and PB2 genes. We also evaluated an outbreak of AI in tiger and showed evidence of probable tiger-to-tiger transmission in the tiger zoo. Sequencing and phylogenetic analysis of those viruses showed no difference from the first isolate obtained in January 2004. There was no mutation of histidine to tyrosine at position 274 of the neuraminidase molecule after Oseltamivir treatment. In both isolates, a single amino acid substitution, Glu to Lys, at the position 627 (E627K) in the PB2 protein responsible for H5N1 pathogenicity in mammals and five codon deletion in the NS gene were similar to the H5N1 viruses isolated in the same epidemic. Molecular characterisation of H5N1 viruses from the following continuous outbreaks showed that there were no significant point mutations in critical regions.

Schudel A, Lombard M (eds): OIE/FAO International Scientific Conference on Avian Influenza.
Dev Biol (Basel). Basel, Karger, 2006, vol 124, p 253.

Novel Diagnostic Tests for the Surveillance of Avian Influenza

C.M. Lamichhane[1], D. Perez[3], V. Vakharia[3], E. Deshaies[2], S. Leterme[2], E. Yeh[1], R. Sanders[1], B. Glidewell[1], C. George[1]

1 Synbiotics Corporation, San Diego CA, USA
2 Synbiotics Europe, Lyon, France
3 VA-MD Regional College of Veterinary Medicine, University of Maryland, College Park, USA

Novel diagnostic assays are developed for the rapid and efficient large-scale screening of avian influenza (AI) virus and associated antibodies. One of these tests is a rapid antigen capture assay that will detect all 15 haemagglutinin sub-types of Type A Flu in 15 minutes. The product can be used farm-side or in the laboratory for the detection of Type A Flu, including South East and East Asian H5N1 isolates. This study examines the sensitivity and specificity of the assays as they compare with that of the standard Agar-Gel immuno-Precipitin (AGP) antibody test, virus isolation (VI), and other commercial products. The efficacy of the above assays for the surveillance of AI antibodies and antigens is reviewed.

Schudel A, Lombard M (eds): OIE/FAO International Scientific Conference on Avian Influenza.
Dev Biol (Basel). Basel, Karger, 2006, vol 124, p 254.

Survival and Stability of HPAI H5N1 in Different Environments and Susceptibility to Disinfectants

T. Songserm[1], *R. Jam-on*[1], *N. Sae-Heng*[1], *N. Meemak*[2]

[1] Faculty of Veterinary Medicine, Kasetsart University, Nakornpathom, Thailand

[2] Centre of Veterinary Research and Development, Department of Livestock Development, Rachaburi, Thailand

We studied the survival and stability of highly pathogenic avian influenza (HPAI) H5N1 isolated from affected chickens in Central Thailand. The study was done by determining the survival of HPAI H5N1 in allantoic fluid, chicken faeces, cooked meat or eggs tested under local temperature in Central Thailand, including sunlight, shadow, water, and different cooking methods. Susceptibility of HPAI H5N1 to different disinfectants was also studied. The dose of HPAI H5N1 used in the experiment was 0.2 ml $10^{6.3}EID_{50}$/ml in 0.8 ml allantoic fluid, chicken faeces, one cubic inch of meat or eggs. After testing under different environments/conditions, virus re-isolation from the residue in samples was done by chicken embryoinjection, haemagglutination and haemagglutination inhibition test. The results showed that the virus in allantoic fluid or faeces was completely killed within 30 minutes after placing the sample in sunlight at 32-35 °C. The virus could survive for ten days in allantoic fluid and four days in chicken faeces when placed in shade at 25-32 °C. The same amount of the virus in water obtained from a rice field where HPAI H5N1-affected ducks were raised, survived for three days. By cooking meat and eggs injected with the HPAI H5N1 virus to 70 °C, for more than three minutes, the virus was completely killed. The HPAI H5N1 in faeces was completely killed within five minutes with glutaraldehyde, ammonium chloride, peracetic acid, and sodium hypochloride.

Schudel A, Lombard M (eds): OIE/FAO International Scientific Conference on Avian Influenza.
Dev Biol (Basel). Basel, Karger, 2006, vol 124, p 255.

Clinical, Gross-Histopathologic and Immunohistochemical Findings of Grazing Ducks Affected with HPAI H5N1 in Thailand

T. Songserm[1], N. Sae-Heng[1], R. Jam-on[1], K. Witoonsatient[1], N. Meemak[2]

[1] Faculty of Veterinary Medicine, Kasetsart University, Nakornpathom, Thailand

[2] Centre of Veterinary Research and Development, Department of Livestock Development, Rachaburi, Thailand

During an outbreak of highly pathogenic avian influenza (HPAI) H5N1 in Thailand, ducks, especially grazing ducks raised in rice fields, were also affected. We followed and observed 11 flocks of grazing ducks, containing about 2,000-3,000 ducks in each flock, in central and western Thailand. The grazing ducks observed were mixed-breed native-khaki Campbell-cross laying ducks. Clinical signs, virus shedding, pathology and immunohistochemistry were studied in the ducks. Virus shedding was studied by virus isolation from cloacal swabs. Gross- and histopathology was studied in ducks found dead or moribund. Immunohistochemistry for detecting the virus antigen was done in formalin-fixed tissues routinely processed for histopathology. It was found that ducks at three weeks old, reared in houses had no clinical sign of HPAI H5N1 infection, or virus shedding. After being moved to the post-harvested rice field in contaminated areas, virus shedding was found for seven to ten days before the affected ducks showed clinical signs, including depression, circling, convulsion, dyspnea and blindness. Gross- and histopathological findings included severe pneumonia, pulmonary oedema, necrotising pancreatitis, encephalitis, keratitis, conjunctivitis, nephritis, enteritis, lymphoid depletion/necrosis and haemorrhage in serous membranes. By immunohistochemistry, viral antigen was detected in several organs including brain, trachea, lung, kidney, intestine, pancreas and liver. Our findings show that the affected grazing ducks have high potential for spreading H5N1 HPAI viruses in Thailand.

Schudel A, Lombard M (eds): OIE/FAO International Scientific Conference on Avian Influenza.
Dev Biol (Basel). Basel, Karger, 2006, vol 124, pp 256-257.

Assessment of the Efficacy of a Commercial Inactivated H5N2 Vaccine to Prevent the Experimental Infection of Ducks by a European LP H5N3

M. Cherbonnel, K. Louboutin, V. Jestin

French Agency for Food Safety (AFSSA), French Reference Laboratory for Avian Influenza and Newcastle Disease, Unit of Avian and Rabbit Virology, Immunology and Parasitology, Ploufragan, France

Free-range domestic ducks may have direct or indirect contacts with wild bird species known as a reservoir of low pathogenic (LP) avian influenza viruses (AIV). As such, they may become infected with a wide range of LP AIV subtypes without any clinical signs. (In Asia they can also carry H5N1 highly pathogenic avian influenza virus (HPAIV) asymptomatically.) However, the asymptomatic infection of domestic ducks with LP H5/H7 AIV has been more or less occasionally reported in Europe. It is a matter of concern, since H5/H7 infected domestic ducks may be a source of infection for other poultry species. To prevent such an event, the prophylactic vaccination of domestic ducks at high risk of infection could be considered, provided data are established to suggest its effectiveness. Since no data are available in the vaccine files concerning the protection afforded in ducks, the first step was to determine whether commercially available vaccines can prevent the infection of ducks by recent European AIV strains.

In the present study, the efficacy of a commercial inactivated H5N2 vaccine to prevent the infection of mule ducks by a French LP H5N3 isolate (A/dk/France/02166/2002) was experimentally assessed. This vaccine is prepared with the LPAIV A/Ty/MN/3689-1751/1981 as a water in oil emulsion and given subcutaneously.

Fifty AI seronegative five-week old conventional mule ducks maintained in quarantine from one day old were allotted in five groups and maintained in BL3 facilities during the study: (i) one control group, (ii) one group vaccinated once with twice the chicken vaccine dose (ck dose) recommended by the supplier, and challenged with $10^{6,4}$ DIE_{50} by combined eye drop, intranasal and intratracheal, three weeks later, (iii) one group vaccinated with twice the ck dose, boosted two weeks later with one ck dose and challenged similarly to group 2 but two weeks after the boost, (iv) and (v) the two other groups remained unvaccinated but were challenged as previously described at eight and ten weeks old, together with group 2 and group 3 respectively. The same schedule was followed using 50 AI seronegative one-day old conventional mule ducks, except that a unique ck dose was administrated irrespective of the group. So, depending on whether ducks received one vaccination or a prime-boost, they were challenged at three weeks old or five weeks old, respectively.

The serological response was monitored before each vaccine administration, using a haemagglutination inhibition (HI) test and H5N3 antigen (homologous with the challenge strain); cloacal and tracheal shedding was monitored three and five days after challenge, using M-based real time reverse transcription polymerase chain reaction (RT-PCR) (correlated with virus isolation using egg inoculation).

Five-week old vaccinated ducks displayed a higher (statistically significant) HI response in comparison with one-day old vaccinated ducks. The highest HI response (7.4 $\log_2 \pm 1.9$) was observed two weeks after the boost of five-week old vaccinated ducks. However, irrespective of the vaccination scheme and the age, no statistic differences were observed between vaccinated and unvaccinated ducks with respect to (i) the ratio of ducks shedding virus and (ii) quantities of shed virus. Several hypotheses are considered to explain this failure, among them the phylogenetic distance between the vaccine strain and the challenge strain, the insufficient haemagglutinin (HA) content of the vaccine. So, to check the first hypothesis, further trials are in progress in our laboratory using Eurasian strain-based vaccines.

Schudel A, Lombard M (eds): OIE/FAO International Scientific Conference on Avian Influenza.
Dev Biol (Basel). Basel, Karger, 2006, vol 124, p 258.

Phylogenetic Analysis of Avian Influenza Subtype H6 Viruses Isolated in France Between 2000 and 2004

G. Le Gall-Reculé, J. Rousset, K. Louboutin, J. Lamandé, C. Allée, V. Jestin

French Agency for Food Safety (AFSSA), French Reference Laboratory for Avian Influenza and Newcastle Disease, Unit of Avian and Rabbit Virology, Immunology and Parasitology, Ploufragan, France

The complete sequence of the HA1 gene of 12 H6N2 and H6N8 isolates was compared. Nine isolates (seven H6N2 and two H6N8) were obtained from meat turkeys and turkey breeders reared in the west part of France between 2001 and 2004. They exhibited respiratory signs, decreased food consumption, increased mortality and, for breeders, egg drop production. Another H6N2 isolate was obtained from breeder ducks exhibiting mucosal nasal discharge without mortality, their holding being located close to one of the previous H6N2-infected meat-turkey holdings. In addition, two H6N2 isolates obtained in 2000 from sentinel ducks sharing the same environment as wild birds at a bird sanctuary located in the west part of France, were analysed. The 12 sequences were compared to some published sequences from American and Eurasian viruses isolated in the 1970s, and from contemporary aquatic and terrestrial birds, to determine molecular evolution among H6 viruses. The sequences of the French viruses were very similar to each other, although one H6N2 isolate from turkey showed a deletion of one amino acid. Six isolates possessed the amino sequence PQVETR/G at the cleavage site and six isolates, among them the two H6N2 isolates obtained in 2000 from sentinel ducks, the amino sequence PQIETR/G. The phylogenetic tree revealed that viruses isolated from France clustered in a group including German viruses isolated in the last few years. Phylogenetic relationships are discussed particularly according to the migratory routes from northern Europe.

Schudel A, Lombard M (eds): OIE/FAO International Scientific Conference on Avian Influenza.
Dev Biol (Basel). Basel, Karger, 2006, vol 124, p 259.

A New Neurokinin 1 Receptor Agonist as Potential Treatment and Prophylactic Measure in Poultry and Humans for Avian Influenza (AI)

M.L. Witten[1], *S.S. Wong*[1], *N.N. Sun*[1], *P.J. Munzel*[2]

[1] Joan B. and Donald R. Diamond Lung Injury Laboratory, Dept. of Pediatrics, University of Arizona College of Medicine, USA

[2] ImmuneRegen Biosciences Asia Pte. Ltd., Singapore

A/HongKong 8/68 influenza virus (HKV) was used in a murine model of occupational toxicology inducing acute respiratory distress syndrome (ARDS). C57BL/6 mice were exposed to JP-8 jet fuel inhalation one hour/day over seven days to wipe out pulmonary immune response, as shown previously. At day seven, mice received HKV by nasal inoculation. They were divided into two groups; HKV only (HKV-) and mice receiving [Sar^9, Met $(O_2)^{11}$]- Substance P (SP+), 1 μM/15 minutes/day via nebuliser (HKVHS). HKV-mice developed influenza symptoms; decreased body weight, fever, dehydration, nasal discharge after five days and at day +7 began to die from ARDS. Remaining mice were sacrificed according to protocol. HKVHS mice did not develop influenza symptoms, however, were sacrificed at day +7 to compare lung tissues vs HKV-. HKVHS showed leukotriene B4 levels at 33 % of HKV- and normal lung cell counts after broncho-alveolar lavage. HKV- had very high lung cell counts and pathological lung injury evidence. Electron micrographs (EM) of HKV- showed absence of airway cilia, swollen airway epithelial cells, large numbers of mitochondria, and colonies of HKV. 200 EM of HKVHS did not show any lung injury evidence neither did any HKV- colonies.

Farmers, the poultry industry, health-care workers are at great risk of acquiring avian influenza (AI) through infected poultry. We suggest collaborative community models of SP + intervention; SP + prophylaxis in large poultry farms and SP + as vaccination replacement or adjuvant.

SP+ is a potential AI treatment and prophylactic agent against all AI strains, as the mechanism is strong general immunomodulation, not vaccination.

Schudel A, Lombard M (eds): OIE/FAO International Scientific Conference on Avian Influenza.
Dev Biol (Basel). Basel, Karger, 2006, vol 124, p 260.

Avian Influenza Situation in Poland

Z. Minta[1], *K. Śmietanka*[1], *K. Domańska-Blicharz*[1], *G. Tomczyk*[1], *B. Szewczyk*[2]

[1] National Reference Laboratory for Avian Influenza and Newcastle Disease, Department of Poultry Diseases, National Veterinary Research Institute, Pulawy, Poland

[2] Division of Molecular Virology, Intercollegiate Faculty of Biotechnology, University of Gdańsk- Medical University of Gdańsk, Gdańsk, Poland

Poland has never experienced highly pathogenic avian influenza. However, in 1995, an epidemic of low pathogenic avian influenza caused by avian influenza virus (AIV) H7 occurred in turkey flocks. A survey conducted between 1997 and 2002 in poultry, revealed a lack of active infections but two AIVs H5 were isolated in 2002 from robin and seagull. The pathogenicity of four AIVs isolated from turkeys and wild birds assessed by sequencing of the haemagglutinin (HA) cleavage site confirmed that the strains were low pathogenic (absence of multiple basic amino acids). These results showed concordance with in vivo studies (IVPI = 0,0).

Since 2003, a national survey programme for AIV infections in poultry and wild birds has been conducted in Poland according to the guidelines provided in the Commission Decisions 2002/649/EC (2003 and 2004) and 2004/615/EC (2004). In 2003, 8260 samples of sera or faeces from poultry and 363 samples of faeces from free-living birds were tested serologically in haemagglutination inhibition (HI) test (H5 and H7 antigens) or virologically on specific-pathogen-free (SPF) embryonated eggs. In 2004, 11,103 sera/faeces samples (poultry) and 514 faeces samples (wild birds) were tested.

Antibodies to AIV H5 were detected in four samples from three geese flocks: one serum from one flock in 2003 and three sera from one flock (tested twice) in 2004. Antibodies to AIV H7 were found in two samples of sera from two chicken flocks in 2003. Positive flocks were retrospectively investigated at the holding with no further suspicion of AIV infection. No virus was isolated from poultry flocks, including seropositive flocks, and free-living birds.

List of Participants

ABOLNIK Celia, ARC-Onderstepoort Veterinary Institute, Old Soutpan Road, Onderstepoort, Pretoria 0118, South Africa.

AKOL George, Veterinary Services, Provincial Department of Agriculture, Private Bag X 0040, Bisho 5605, South Africa.

ALEXANDER Dennis, Veterinary Laboratories Agency, Weybridge New Haw, Addlestone Surrey KT15 3NB, United Kingdom.

ANGOT Jean-Luc, Administrative Department, World Organisation for Animal Health (OIE), 12 rue de Prony, FR-75017 Paris, France.

ARREOLA Jose Manuel, Bachoco, Maíz No. 18, Col. Granjas Esmeralda, Mexico 09810, Mexico.

AUVIGNE Vincent, Agronomes et Véterinaires Sans Frontières, 4 allée Charles Gounod, FR-35760 Saint-Grégoire, France.

AZIZ AIDAROS Hassan Andel, Regional Commission for the Middle East, OIE Revsc M.E. 19, Almessaha St., 12311 Dokki-Cairo, Egypt.

BALDANTI Fausto, Servizio di Virologia, IRCCS Policlinico San Matteo, IT-27100 Pavia, Italy.

BANKS Jill, Veterinary Laboratories Agency, Woodham Lane, Surrey KT15 3NB, United Kingdom.

BANKS Rhona, Fort Dodge Animal Health, Flanders Road, Hedge End, Southampton SO30 4QH, United Kingdom.

BARCOS Luis, OIE Representation for the Americas, Cerviño 3101, 2ª floor, Buenos Aires 1425, Argentina.

BEATO Maria Serena, Istituto Zooprofillatico delle Venezie, Viale dell'università 10, IT-35020 Legnaro, Italy.

BELEV Nikola, OIE Representation for Eastern Europe, President of the OIE Regional Commission for Europe, Bld Wasil Lewski 110, BG-1527 Sofia, Bulgaria.

BEN JEBARA Karim, Animal Health Information Department, World Organisation for Animal Health (OIE), 12 rue de Prony, FR-75017 Paris, France.

BENZERRAK Saadi, Agronomes and Veterinaires sans Frontieres, 58, rue Raulin, FR-69361 Lyon, France.

BERGES Jean-Michel, Aid-Sponsored Programmes, World Organisation for Animal Health (OIE), 12 rue de Prony, FR-75017 Paris, France.

BERLAUD Stéphane, Administrative Department, World Organisation for Animal Health (OIE), 12 rue de Prony, FR-75017 Paris, France.

BERLINGIERI Francesco, International Trade Department, World Organisation for Animal Health (OIE), 12 rue de Prony, FR-75017 Paris, France.

BERNARDI Zeno, Poultry Technical Service, Veronesi-Aia, Corte la Pellegrina, IT-37036 San Martino Buon Albergo VR, Italy.

BIN Chua Sin, Agri-Food and Veterinary Authority of Singapore, 5 Maxwell Road #04-00, Tower Block, MND Complex, Singapore 069110, Singapore.

BIN MANGKAT Abdul Aziz, Epidemiology & Veterinary Medicine, 8th floor, Wisma Chase Perdana, Off Jalan Semantan, Bukit Damansara, 50630 Kuala Lumpur, Malaysia.

BISGAARD Magne, The Royal Veterinary and Agricultural University, Dept. of Pathobiology, Stigbøjlen 4, DK-1870 Frederiksber C, Denmark.

BLAHA Thomas, Institute for Epidemiology, University of Veterinary Medicine, Buescheler Strasse 9, DE-48456 Bakum, Germany.

BOISSIEU Cyril, 10 Allée du Dr Zamenhof, Bat. Carlotta, FR-31100 Toulouse, France.

BÓNÉ Barbara, Ministry of Agriculture and Rural Development, Kossuth tér 9-11, HU-1055 Budapest, Hungary.

BONMARIN Isabelle, Institut de Veille Sanitaire, 12 rue du Val D'Osne, FR-94415 Saint Maurice Cedex, France.

BOONPROM Enkvetchakul, Bird Health Quality Assurance, Sun Valley Thailand, 23/1 Moo 2 Khowwong, Praputthabat, TH-18120 Saraburi, Thailand.

BOUGUEDOUR Rachid, Ministry of Agriculture and Rural Development, 12 Blvd Colonel, Amirouche, Algiers 16000, Algeria.

BOYAZOGLU Jean, Regional Activities Department, World Organisation for Animal Health (OIE), 12 rue de Prony, FR-75017 Paris, France.

BROWN Ian, Avian Virology, FAO/OIE/EU Reference Laboratory for AI, Veterinary Laboratories Agency, Weybridge New Haw, Addlestone, Surrey KT15 3NB, United Kingdom.

BRÜCKNER Gideon K., Agriculture Western Cape, Private Bag X1, Elsenburg 7607, South Africa.

BRUGERE-PICOUX Jeanne, Ecole nationale vétérinaire d'Alfort, 7 av Général de Gaulle, FR-94704 Maisons-Alfort Cedex, France.

BUBLOT Michel, Virology Research Projects, Merial, BP 39H - Virology 254 Rue Marcel Mérieux, FR-69007 Lyon, France.

BUCK Peter, Public Health Agecy of Canada, Centre for infectious disease, Prevention and Control, Tunney's Pasture Bulding #6 PL 0602C 2nd Floor, Room 2375, Ontario K1A 0L2, Canada.

BURANATHAI Chantanee, Emerging Diseases Veterinary Epidemiology, Department of Livestock Development, 69/1 Phaya Thai Road, Bangkok 10400, Thailand.

BUSANI Luca, Istituto Zooprofilattico delle Venezie, Viale dell'Università 10, IT-35020 Legnaro (Padova), Italy.

CALDERÓN Julio Ernesto, Control y Erradicación de Enfermedades Aviares OIRSA, Calle Ramón Belloso, final Pje. Isolde. Colonia Escalón, San Salvador (01) 61, El Salvador.

CAMPITELLI Laura, Italian WHO National Influenza Centre, Istituto Superiore di Sanità, Viale Regina Elena 299, IT-00161 Roma, Italy.

CAPORALE Vincenzo, Istituto Zooprofilattico Sperimentale, dell'Abruzzo e del Molise "G. Caporale", Via Campo Boario, IT-64100 Teramo, Italy.

CAPUA Ilaria, Istituto Zooprofilattico Sperimentale delle Venezie, Laboratorio de Virologia, Viale dell'Universita 10, IT-35020 Legnaro-Padova, Italy.

CARLSSON Ulla, National Veterinary Institute, Ulls vag 2 B, SE-751 89 Uppsala, Sweden.

CATTOLI Giovanni, Research & Development Unit, Istituto Zooprofilattico Sperimentale delle Venezie, Viale dell'Universita 10, IT-35020 Legnaro-PD, Italy.

CHAISEMARTIN Daniel, Information Systems, World Organisation for Animal Health (OIE), 12 rue de Prony, FR-75017 Paris, France.

CHÁVEZ GONZÁLEZ Sergio, Unión Nacional de Avicultores, Medellin 325, Col. Roma Sur 06760 D.F., Mexico.

CHEN Hualan, National Avian Influenza Reference Laboratory, Harbin Veterinary Research Institute, CAAS, 427 Maduan Street, Harbin 15000ce, P.R. of China.

CHRISTENSEN Jens Peter, The Royal Veterinary & Agricultural University, Dept. of Pathobiology, Stigbøjlen 4, DK-1870 Frederiksberg, Denmark.

CHUNG-HWEI Yao, Bureau of Animal and Plant Health Inspection and Quarantine, 3F, 51, Chung Ching S. RD., Sec.2 Taipei,Taiwan 100, Taipei China.

CLARK James, Foreign Animal Diseases, Canadian Food Inspection Agency, 59 Camelot, Nepean, Ontario K1A 0Y9, Canada.

COBANOV Darko, State Veterinary Office of Bosnia & Herzegovina, Radićeva 8/II, Sarajevo 71000, Bosnia & Herzegovina.

COLLEEN Annett, Alberta Agriculture, Food and Rural Development, 909 Irricana Rd.N.E., Airdrie, Alberta T4A 2G6, Canada.

CORK Susan, MAF Biosecurity New Zealand, P.O.Box 2526, Wellington, New Zealand.

COX Nancy, WHO Collaborating Centre for Surveillance, Epidemiology and Control of influenza, Influenza Branch, Viral Disease Division, National Ceters for Infectious Diseases and Prevention, 1600 Clifton Road, Mailstop G16, Bldg 7, Room 111, Atlanta, GA 30333, USA.

CROIZIERS DE LACVIVIER Jean-Pierre, Administrative Department, World Organisation for Animal Health (OIE), 12 rue de Prony, FR-75017 Paris, France.

CURRIE Richard, Poultry Business Unit, Fort Dodge Animal Health, Flanders Road Hedge End, Southampton SO30 4QH, United Kingdom.

CZIFRA Georg, The National Veterinary Institute, Travvägen 12, SE 75 189 Uppsala, Sweden.

DAHM Carlo, Administration des Services Vétérinaires, Résidence St. Louis 211, rte d'Esch, LU-1471 Luxembourg – City L, Luxembourg.

DAMOSER Johann, CVO Austria, Ministry of Health and Women, Radetzkystraße 2, AT-1031 Vienna 1031, Austria.

DE CALUWÉ Denis, Herman Kiezebrink Institute, Kerkstraat 2, BE-9160 Lokeren, Belgium.

DE FOUCAULD Jean-Cassien, Biological Registration, CEVA-Phyalxia Co. Ltd., Szállás u. 5, HU-1107 Budapest, Hungary.

DE MARCO Maria Alessandra, Istituto Nazionale per la Fauna Selvatica, Via Ca' Fornacetta 9, IT-40064 Ozzano Emilia (BO), Italy.

DEL REAL Gustavo, Centro de Investigacion en Sanidad Animal (CISA), Valdeolmos, ES-28130Madrid, Spain.

DELOGU Mauro, Università degli Studi di Bologna, Department of Veterinary Public Health and Animal Pathology, Via Tolara di Sopra 50, IT-40064 Ozzano Emilia (BO), Italy.

DESHAIES Eric, Synbiotics Europe, 2 rue Alexander Fleming, FR-69007 Lyon, France.

DI TRANI Livia, Dept.of Food Safety and Veterinary Public Health, Istituto Superiore di Sanità, Viale Regina Elena, 299, IT-00161 Rome, Italy.

DIAZ François, Recognition procedures for diagnostic, Scientific and Technical Department, World Organisation for Animal Health (OIE), 12 rue de Prony, FR-75017 Paris, France.

DOCTRINAL Delphine, Ecole Nationale Vétérinaire de Lyon, 1 avenue Bourgelat, FR-69280 Marcy l'Etoile, France.

DOLE Natalie, Public Safety & Emergency Preparedness Canada, 122 Bank Street, Ottawa Ontario K1A 0P8, Canada.

DOMENECH Joseph, Animal Health Service, Animal Production and Health Division, Agriculture Department, FAO, Viale delle Terme di Caracalla, IT-00100 Roma, Italy.

DONATELLI Isabella, Italian WHO National Influenza centre, Istituto Superiore di Sanità, Viale Regina Elena 299, IT-00161 Roma, Italy.

DORETTO Luciano Jr., Brasilian Reference Laboratory, Agriculture Ministry, Rua Raul Ferrari s/n°, Campinas/Sâo Paulo 13100-105, Brazil.

DROPPERS Willem, Veterinary Public Health, World Organisation for Animal Health (OIE), 12 rue de Prony, FR-75017 Paris, France.

DUGAS Raymond, Publications Department, World Organisation for Animal Health (OIE), 12 rue de Prony, FR-75017 Paris, France.

DUNBAR Sandra, Department of Agriculture and Rural Development, Room 723 Dundonald House, Upper Newtownards Road, Belfast BT4 3SB, Ireland.

DUNDON William, Istituto Zooprofilattico delle Venezie, Via dell'Università 10, IT-35020 Legnaro (PD), Italy.

DUPUIS Laurent, SEPPIC, 75 Quai d'Orsay, FR-75007 Paris, France.

DUVAL Vincent, UFR Sciences et techniques de la côte basque, appt 7- bât 1- résidence Zaldiska, 1 rue Salvat Hardoy, FR-64990 Saint Pierre d'Irube, France.

DYRTING Kitman, Veterinary Laboratory, Agriculture Fisheries and Conservation Department, HKSAR, Tai Lung Veterinary Laboratory, Lin Tong Mei, Sheung Shui, Hong Kong SAR 999999, China (PR).

EDWARDS Steven, VLA Weybridge, New Haw. Addlestone, Surrey KT15 3NB, United Kingdom.

ELGAR Kerri, Ambassade d'Australie, 4 rue Jean Rey, FR-75015 Paris, France.

ELLIS Trevor, Veterinary Laboratory, Tai Lung Vet Laboratory, Agriculture Fisheries & Conservation Department, Lin Tong Mei, Sheung Shui, New Territories, Hong-Kong SAR.

ESPINOZA Cora María, Servicio Nacional de Sanidad y Calidad, Agroalimentaria, Paseo Colón 367, Buenos Aires 1063, Argentina.

FARBOS Jacques, Conseil Général Vétérinaire, Ministère de l'Agriculture de l'Alimentation de la Pêche et de la Ruralité, 251 rue de Vaugirard, FR-75732 Paris Cedex 15, France.

FORGE Frédéric, Library of Parliament, 151 Parks Street, Room 430, Ottawa K1A 0A9, Canada.

FRANCART Joel, General Food Directorate, 251 rue de Vaugirard, FR-75732 Paris Cedex 15, France.

FUJITA Teruhide, OIE Representation for Asia and the Pacific, East 311, Shin-Aoyama Bldg, 1-1-1 Minami-Aoyama, Minato-ku, Tokyo 107-0062, Japan.

GASPARYAN Tigran, Department of Veterinary Numerating, Ministry of Agriculture of the Republic of Armenia, Nalbandiana 48, 375010 Yerevan, Armenia.

GAYNOR Sally, Department of Agriculture & Food, Kildare Street, Dublin 2, Ireland.

GERSTENBERG Cornelia, Disease Control, Department of Agriculture, Private Bag X 138, Pretoria 0001, South Africa.

GHAZAL Mohammed, Animal Wealth Department, Ministry of Agriculture and Fisheries of United Arab Emirates, P.O.Box 1509, Dubai 5556, United Arab Emirates.

GILBERT Jeffrey, World Health Organization, 401 Dongwai Diplomatic Building, 23 Dongzhimenwai Ave, Chaoyang, CN-100600 Beijing, P.R. of China.

GROMADZKA Beata, Department of Molecular Virology, Intercollegiate Faculty of Biotechnology, Gdansk University and Medical University of Gdansk, Kladki 24, PL-80-822 Gdansk, Poland.

GUERIN Jean-Luc, École Nationale Vétérinaire de Toulouse, 23 Chemin des Capelles, BP 87614, FR-31076 Toulouse Cedex 3, France.

GULLY Paul, Public Health Agency of Canada, 130 Colonnade Road, Room 166B, A.L. 6501C, Ottawa, Ontario K1A 0K9, Canada.

GUSTAFSSON Pia, Vet. insp at the Animal Disease Control Division, Swedish Board of Agriculture, Vallgatan 8, SE-551 82 Jönköping, Sweden.

HAGOP Isbentchian, Avimex, Maiz 18, Col. Granjas Esmeralda, Mexico 09810, Mexico.

HAMDAN ALNAQABI Mohammed Ali, Animal Health of Animal Wealth Department, Ministry of Agriculture and Fisheries of United Arab Emirates, P.O. Box 1509, Dubai 5555, United Arab Emirates.

HARDER Timm, Friedrich-Loeffler Institute, Boddenblick 5a, DE-17493 Greifswald-Insel Riems, Germany.

HARI Aleksandra, Veterinary Administration of the Republic of Slovenia, Parmova 53, SI-1000 Ljubljana, Slovenia.

HARM Kiezebrink, Herman Kiezebrink Institute, Binnenhaven 1, NL-6709 PD Wageningen, The Netherlands.

HENDRIKSEN Birgit, Division of animal diseases, Danish Veterinary and Food Administration, Mørkhøj Bygade 19, DK-2860 Søborg, Denmark.

HOEFLECHNER Andrea, Division for Animal Health, Bundesministerium für Gesundhelt und Frauen, Radetzkystrasse 2, AT-1030 Wien, Austria

HORNER Roger Françis, Veterinary Laboratory, Provincial Department of Agriculture, P.O. Box X2 Cascades, Pietermaritzburg 3201, South Africa.

IKEDA Kazuyuki, Ministry of Agriculture, Forestry and Fisheries, 1-2-1 Kasumigaseki, Chiyoda-ku, JP-100-8950 Tokyo, Japan.

IRZA Victor, FGI Federal Centre for Animal Health, RU-600901 Yur'evets, Vladimir, Russia.

ISHIBASHI Tomoko, International Trade Department, World Organisation for Animal Health (OIE), 12 rue de Prony, FR-75017 Paris, France.

ISHIKAWA Kiyoyasu, Ministry of Agriculture,Forestry and Fisheries, 1-2-1 Kasumigaseki, Chiyoda-ku, JP-100-8951 Tokyo, Japan.

JESTIN Véronique, Avian Virology and Imunology, Agence Française de Sécurité Sanitaire des Aliments, Zoopôle Les Croix B.P. 53, FR-22440 Ploufragan, France.

JORGENSEN Poul Henrik, Danish Institute for Food and Veterinary Research, Hangovej 2, DK-8200 Aarhus, Denmark.

JUTZI Samuel, Animal Production & Health Division, FAO, Viale delle Terme di Caracalla, IT-00100 Roma, Italy.

KAMAKAWA Hiroyuki, Animal Health and Animal Products Safety Division, Food Safety and Consumer Affairs Bureau, Ministry of Agriculture, Forestry and Fisheries of Japan, 1-2-1, Kasumigaseki, Chiyoda-ku, Tokyo, Japan.

KAUTA Nicholas, Livestock Health and Entomology, Ministry of Agriculture, Animal Industry and Fisheries, P.O. Box 513, Entebbe 256, Uganda

KEONG Leong Hon, Inspection Services and Epidemiology, Agri-Food and Veterinary Authority, Veterinary Public Health Centre, 10 Perahu Road, SG-718837Singapore, Singapore.

KIDA Hiroshi, Hokkaido University, School of Veterinary Medicine, Department of Disease Control, Kita 18, Nishi-9 Kita-ku, JP-060-0818 Sapporo, Japan.

KIVIRUUSU Sirpa, Ministry of Agriculture and Forestry, PO Box 30, FI-00023 Helsinki, Finland.

KOCH Guus, Central Institute for Animal Disease Control, Lelystad (CIDC-Lelystad), Department of Virology, Post Box 2004m, NL-8203 AA Lelystad, The Netherlands.

KOEN Pieter, Animal Health, Department of Agriculture, Private Bag X 1, Elsenburg, Stellenbosch 7607, South Africa.

KOHUT Peter, Walsh Engineers Europe, 5, place du Champ de Mars, Bastion Tower 20-21, BE-1050 Brussels, Belgium.

KUMAR BANDYOPADHYAY Santanu, Government of India, Dept of Animal Husbandry & Dairyng, Ministry of Agriculture, Krishibhavan, IN-110001 New Delhi, India.

LABROVIC Ankica, Veterinary Administration, Ulica Grada Vukovara 78, Zagreb 10000, Croatia.

LADDOMADA Alberto, European Commission, DG Health and consumer protection, Rue Froissart 101, Room 3/60, BE-1049 Brussels, Belgium.

LAGUNA Natalia Moreno, Ministerio de Agricultura, Pesca y Alimentación, Subdirección General de Sanidad Animal, c/Alfonso XII, 62, 1ªPlanta, ES-28014 Madrid, Spain.

LAMICHHANE Chinta, Research & Dev, Synbiotics Corporation, 11011Via Frontera, San Diego, CA 92127, USA.

LANY Petr, University of Veterinary and, Pharmaceutical Sciences, Palackeho 1/3, CZ-612 42 Brno, Czech Republic.

LE GALL Ghislaine, French Agency for Food Safety, BP 53, FR-22440 Ploufragan, France.

LEAL Simón, Universidad Central de Venezuela, Facultad de Ciencias Veterinarias, Avenida Universidad, El Limón- Maracay, Estado Aragua, Venezuela.

LEFORBAN Yves, World Organisation for Animal Health (OIE), 12 rue de Prony, FR-75017 Paris, France.

LELLI Rossella, Istituto Zooprofilattico Sperimentale Abruzzo-Molise, Campo Boario, IT-64100 Teramo, Italy.

LETERME Serge, Research & Developpment, Synbiotics Europe, FR-69007 Lyon, France.

LINDSTROM Tina, Ministry of Agriculture Food and Consumer Affairs, Fredsgatan 8, SE-103 33 Stockholm, Sweden.

LOMBARD Michel, International Association for Biologicals (IABs), 22, rue Crillon, FR-69006 Lyon, France.

LOZANO DUBERNARD Bernardo, Avimex, Maiz 18, Colonia Granjas Esmeralda, Mexico 09810, Mexico.

LUBROTH Juan, Infectious Disease Group, Animal Health Service, FAO, Viale delle Terme di Caracalla, IT-00100 Roma, Italy.

MACIULSKIS Petras, State Food and Veterinary Service, Siesiku 19, Vilnius 07170, Lithuania.

MANDOLA Maria Lucia, Istituto Zooprofilattico Sperimentale del Piemonte, Liguria e Valle d'Aosta, Via Bologna 148, IT-10148 Torino, Italy.

MANNELLI Alessandro, Dipartimento di Produzioni Animali Epidemiologia Ecologia, Università di Torino, Via Leonardo da Vinci 44, IT-10095 Grugliasco, Italy.

MANUGUERRA Jean Claude, 28 rue du Docteur Roux, FR-75724 Paris Cedex 15, France.

MARANDI Mehdi Vasfi, D.G.Poultry Health Dept, Iran Veterinary Organization, S.J.Asad abadi St., P.O. Box, 14155/6349, Theran, Iran.

MARANGON Stefano, Istituto Zooprofilattico Sperimentale delle Venezie, Via Romea 14/A, IT-35020 Legnaro-Padova, Italy.

MARGERIT Pascal, Respiratory Protection, Bacou Dalloz, Paris Nord 33 Rue des Vanesses, FR-95958 Roissy, France.

MARIE Brigitte, Direction des Services vétérinaires du Morbihan, 6, avenue Edgar Degas, FR-56000 Vannes, France.

MARQUEZ Miguel, Intervet International, Azahares No. 242 Rancho Contento, Zapopan, Jalisco 45222, Mexico.

MARSHALL Pablo, ABEF - Associação Brasileira dos Produtores e Exportadores de Frango, Av. Brigadeiro Faria Lima, 1912, 12° andar - Conjunto 12-A, São Paulo/SP 01452-922, Brazil.

MARTANO Manuela Giulia, Istituto Zooprofilattico Sperimentale del Piemonte, Liguria e Valle d'Aosta, Via Bologna 148, IT-10154 Torino, Italy.

MARTIN Ana Moreno, IZS Lombardia ed emilia romagna, Via Bianchi 9, IT-25100 Brescia, Italy.

MARTIN Pedro Rosado, Ministerio de Agricultura, Pesca y Alimentación, Subdirección General de Sanidad Animal, calle Alfonso XII número 62, ES-28071 Madrid, Spain.

MARTIN Vincent, Animal Health Serivce, FAO, Viale delle Terme di Caracalla, IT-00100 Roma, Italy.

MARTYN Jeggo, CSIRO, Australian Animal Health Laboratory, PMB 24, Geelong Victoria 3220, Australia.

MASSI Paola, Animal Health Institute of Forlì, Istituto Zooprofilattico Sperimentale della Lombardia e dell'Emilia, Via Marchini 1, IT-47100 Forlì, Italy.

MATTER Hans C., Swiss Federal Office of Public Health, Schwarztorstrasse 96, CH-3003 Berne, Switzerland.

McLEOD Anni, FAO, Viale delle Terme di Caracalla, IT-00100 Roma, Italy.

McNAMEE Perpetua, Department of Agriculture and Rural Development, CPED Unit Room 534, Dundonald House Upper Newtownards Road, Belfast BT4 3SB, Ireland.

MEROZ Michael, Biovac, P.O. Box 300, IL-30600 Or Akiva, Israel.

MESLIN François-Xavier, WHO, 20 Avenue Appia, CH-1211 Genève 27, Switzerland.

MICHEL Virginie, Research Unit, AFSSA (French Agency for food Safety), BP 53 – Zoopole, FR-22440 Ploufragan, France.

MICKLE Tom, Business Development and Strategic Marketing, Merial, 1112 Airport Parkway S.E., Gainesville, GA 30503, USA.

MINGARDO Maurizio, Poultry Technical Service, Fancon-Ilta, Via Donanzola 43, IT-36020 Campiglia dei Berici VI, Italy.

MINGUEZ TUDELA Isabel, European Commission, DG RTD, 200 rue de la Loi, BE-1049 Brussels, Belgium.

MODISANE Botlhe, Disease Control, Department of Agriculture, Private Bag X 138, Pretoria 0001, South Africa.

MOERANE Rabone, Veterinary Services, Northern Cape, Provincial Department of Agriculture, Private Bag X 5018, Kimberley 8300, South Africa.

MOERK Tina, Danish Veterinary and Food Administration, Mørkhøj Bygade 19, DK-2860 Søborg, Denmark.

MOJZIS Miroslav, State Veterinary Institute Zvolen, Pod Drahami 918, Zvolen 960 86, Slovakia.

MOLFESE J. Isidro, Asociación Latinoamericana de Avicultura, Arce 441 – 3 F, (C1426BSE) Buenos Aires, Argentina.

MOLINA Jose Q., Bureau of Animal Industry, Department of Agriculture, Visayas Avenue, Diliman, Quezon City, Philippines.

MOUSSY Patrice, European Commission, Rue de la Loi 200, AIDCO/E6 L41 03/09, BE-1049 Brussel, Belgium.

MRWEBI Lubabalo, Veterinary Services, Provincial Department of Agriculture, Private Bag X 0040, Bisho 5605, South Africa.

MUNSTER Vincent, ErasmusMC, Burg. van walsumweg 312, NL-3011 MZ Rotterdam, The Netherlands.

MUNZEL Peter, ImmuneRegen BioSciences Asia Pte Ltd, 528 East Coast Rd. #17-04, SG-458969 Singapore, Singapore.

NAEEM Khalid, National Reference Laboratory for Poultry Diseases, Animal Science Institute, National Agricultural Research Center, Park Rd, Islamabad 44000, Pakistan.

NGUYEN Thi Hai Chi, Ecole nationale vétérinaire d'Alfort, 7 av Général de Gaulle, FR-94704 Maisons-Alfort Cedex, France.

NORTHOFF Erwin, FAO, Viale delle Terme di Caracalla, IT-00100 Roma, Italy.

NUNN Mike, Animal Health Science, Office of the Chief Veterinary Officer, Department of Agriculture, Fisheries and Forestry, PO Box 858, Canberra ACT 2601, Australia.

OKANE Peter, O'Kane Poultry, 170 Larne Road Ballymena, County Antrim BT42 3HA, Ireland.

OLIVIER Adriaan, Klein Karoo Group, PO Box 241, Oudtshoorn 6620, South Africa.

OLSEVSKIS Edvins, Epizootic Diseases Surveillance Unit, Food and Veterinary Service, Republikas laukums 2, Riga LV – 1010, Latvia.

ONITA Iuliana, Institute for Diagnosis and Animal Health, Dr. Staicovici street, 63 number, 3 sector, 050557 Bucharest, Romania.

OREAMUNO TOLEDO José Joaquin, Ministerio de Agricultura y Ganadería, Del Cementerio de Jardines del Recuerdo, 1Km 1/2 al Oeste, De la entrada de Ciencias del Deporte, 300 m al Norte, Cenada Apdo.3-3006. Heredia, Costa Rica.

ORESHKOVA Nadia, NRL for NDV and AI, CVO - National Diagnostic and Research Veterinary Medical Institute, BG-1606 Sofia, Bulgaria.

ORSI Maria Angela, Sector of Pouthry Disease, Ministery of Agriculture, Rua Raul Ferrari s/n° – Jardim Santa Marcelina, Campinas/Sâo Paulo 13.100-105, Brazil.

ORTALI Giovanni, Poultry Technical Service, Veronesi-Aia, Corte la Pellegrina, IT-37036 San Martino Buon Albergo VR, Italy.

ORUSA Riccardo, Istituto Zooprofilattico Sperimentale Piemonte, Liguria, Valle d'Aosta, Centro di Referenza per le Malattie degli Animali Selvatici, Via G. Rey 5, IT-11020 Aosta, Italy.

PALYA Vilmos, Ceva-Phylaxia Veterinary Co. Ltd., Szallas u. 5., HU-1107 Budapest, Hungary.

PANIN Alexander, The All Russian State Centre for Quality and Standartisation of Veterinary Drugs, 5, Zvenigorodskoe shosse, RU-123022 Moscow, Russia.

PAPPAIOANOU Marguerite, Infectious Disease Epidemiology, School of Public Health, University of Minnesota, 1300 S. 2nd. St., Suite 300, Minneapolis, MN 55404, USA.

PASICK John, Classical Swine Fever & Avian Diseses Section National Centre for Foreign Animal Disease, 1015 Arlington Street, Winnipeg, Manitoba R3E 3M4, Canada.

PAVLIK Ivo, OIE Ref. Laboratory for Paratuberculosis, Veterinary Research Institute, Hudcova 70, CZ-621 32 Brno, Czech Republic.

PERK Shimon, Division of Avian Diseases Laboratories, Kimron Veterinary Institute, P.O. Box 12, IL-50251 Bet-Dagan, Israel.

PERLMAN Benny, ABIC Biological Laboratories Teva Ltd., PO Box 489 West Industrial Zone, IL-99100 Beit Shemesh, Israel.

PETRINI Antonio, International Trade Department, World Organisation for Animal Health (OIE), 12 rue de Prony, FR-75017 Paris, France.

PICAULT Jean Paul, AFSSA Ploufragan, BP 53, FR-22440 Ploufragan, France.

PICKETT Heather, Compassion in World Farming Trust, 5a Charles Street, Petersfield, Hampshire GU32 3EH, United Kingdom.

PIENAAR Anna Catharina Elizabeth, Department of Agriculture, Private Bag X 138, Pretoria 0001, South Africa.

PINTO Julio, Animal Health Information Department, World Organisation for Animal Health (OIE), 12 rue de Prony, FR-75017 Paris, France.

PITTMAN Maria, EFSA, Rue de Genève 10, BE-1140 Evere, Belgium.

POKAMUNSKI Simon, Ministry of Agriculture and Rural Development, 36/5 Golombl St., IL-42247 Natanya, Israel.

PRANDINI Francesco, Merial Animal Health, Milanofiori-Strada 6-Palazzo E5, IT-20090 Assago (MI), Italy.

RALEIGH Patrick, Department of Agriculture and Food, Central Veterinary Research Laboratory, Abbotstown, Castleknock, Dublin 15, Ireland.

RAULT Paul, Sanitary service, SYSAAF, SYSAAF, SRA, INRA, FR-37380 Nouzilly, France.

REIERSEN Jarle, Poultry Diseases, Icelandic Veterinary Services, Keldur v/Vesturlandsveg, Reykjavik 112, Iceland.

RIGGI Alain, Maïsadour Division Animale, BP 21 route de Tartas, FR-40500Saint Sever, France.

ROBERTON Jacues, 116, rue Pierre et Marie Curie, BP 7251, FR-37072 Tours Cedex, France.

RODRIGUES DA COSTA DUARTE Luciano, Ministério da Agricultura Pescas e Florestas, Quinta de S. José, São Pedro de Merelim, PT-4710-859 Braga, Portugal.

ROGER Francois, Epidemiology Unit CIRAD, CIRAD, EMVT Department, TA 30/E, Campus International de Baillarguet, FR-34398 Montpellier Cedex, France.

ROMLAMDUAN Narin, Animal Health and Tecnical Service Office, C.P. Group of Company, 29/2 M.9 Suwintawong Rd. Lumpackchee Nongjok, TH-10530 Bangkok, Thailand.

ROWE Bernard, Tesco Stores Ltd, PO Box 44, Cirrus Building A, Shire Park Welwyn Garden City, Hertfordshire AL7 1ZR, United Kingdom.

SABIROVIC Mirzet, Defra, Area 405, 1A Page Street, London SW1P 4PQ, United Kingdom.

SAKAMOTO Kenichi, National Institute of Animal Health, Diagnostic Laboratory, Department of Exotic Diseases Research, 6-20-1 Josui-honcho, Kodaira, JP-187-0022 Tokyo, Japan.

SAMOREK-SALAMONOWICZ Elzbieta, National Veterinary Research Institute, Al. Partyzantow 57, PL-24-100 Pulawy, Poland.

SANCHEZ Azucena, Laboratorio Central de Veterinaria, Ministerio de Agricultura, Pesca y Alimentación, Cta. Algete Km 28110 Algete-Madrid, ES-28110Madrid, Spain.

SANGUANSERMSRI Donruedee, Naresuan University, Department of Microbiology and Parasitology, Faculty of Medical Science, TH-65000 Phitsanulok, Thailand.

SANGUANSERMSRI Phanchana, Naresuan University, Department of Biochemistry, Faculty of Medical Science, TH-65001 Phitsanulok, Thailand.

SANTIWATTANATAM Boonpeng, Quality Standard System Centre, Charoen Pokphand Foods Public Co., Ltd., 313 C.P. Tower 18th Fl., Silom Rd., Bangrak, Bankok 10500, Thailand.

SCHUDUEL Alejandro, Scientific and Technical Department, World Organisation for Animal Health (OIE), 12 rue de Prony, FR-75017 Paris, France.

SCHOUSTRA Willem, Ministry of Agriculture, Nature and Food Quality, Bezuidenhoutseweg 73, PO Box 20401, NL-2500 EK Den Haag, The Netherlands.

SCHUMACHER Caroline, Dept. des Grandes Prophylaxies, Mérial, 29 Av. Tony Garnier BP 7123, FR-69348 Lyon Cedex 07, France.

SELLECK Paul, Australian Animal Health Laboratory, Division of Animal Health, Institute of Animal Production & Processing, Private Bag 24, Geelong Victoria 3220, Australia.

SENNE Dennis, Diagnostic Virology Laboratory, National Veterinary Services Laboratories, P.O. Box 844, Ames, Iowa 50010, USA.

SIBARTIE Dewan, Scientific and Technical Department, World Organisation for Animal Health (OIE), 12 rue de Prony, FR-75017 Paris, France.

SIDIBE Amadou Samba, OIE Representation for Africa, BP 2954, Bamako, Mali.

SIHVONEN Liisa, National Veterinary and Food Research Institute (EELA), PO Box 57, FI-00581 Helsinki, Finland.

SIMS Les, Asia Pacific Veterinary Information Services, P.O. Box 353 Manunda, Queensland 4870, Australia.

SINCLAIR Marna, State Veterinarian Epidemiology, Department of Agriculture, Private Bag X1 / Muldersvlei Road, Elsenburg 7607, South Africa.

SINDHUNANSKUL Surachai, Bangkok Agro-Industrail Products Public Co.,Ltd., 29/2 Moo 9 Suwintawong Rd.,Lumpackchee, Nongjok, TH-10530 Bangkok, Thailand.

SMIETANKA Krzysztof, National Veterinary Research Institute, Al. Partyzantow 57, PL-24-100 Pulawy, Poland.

SONCINI Ricardo Alfredo, Sadia S.A., Rua Senador Attilio Fontana #86, Concordia SC 89700-000, Brazil.

SONGSIVILAI Sirirurg, National Center for Genetic Engineering and Biotechnology, National Science and Technology Development Agency, 113 Thailand Science Park Paholyothin Road, TH-12120 Pathumthani, Thailand.

SOTGIA Stefano, European Commission Food & Veterinary Office, Grange, Office 1/124, Dunsany Co. Meat, Ireland.

SOUILLARD Rozenn, AFSSA, Unité EBEAC Site de Beaucemaine BP 53, FR-22440 Ploufragan, France.

STEENSELS Mieke, Veterinary and Agrochemical Research Centre, Avian Virology and Immunology Unit, Groeselenberg 99, BE-1180 Brussels, Belgium.

STOEHR Klaus, WHO Global Influenza Programme, WHO/CDS/CSR/GIP, Department for Communicable Disease, Surveillance and Response, CH-1211 Geneve 27, Switzerland.

STONFER Maurizio, Bayer Health Care - Animal Health Division, Viale Certosa 130, IT-20156 Milano, Italy.

SUAREZ David, Southeast Poultry Research Laboratory, 934 College Station Road, Athens, GA 30605, USA.

SUAREZ Sarai, Scientific and Technical Department, World Organisation for Animal Health (OIE), 12 rue de Prony, FR-75017 Paris, France.

SUMMERFIELD Artur, Institute of Virology and Immunoprophylaxis, Sensemattstrasse 293, CH-3147 Mittelhäusern, Switzerland.

SWAYNE David, Southeast Poultry Research Laboratory, 934 College Station Road, Athens, Georgia 30605, USA.

TEGNELL Anders, The National Board of Health and Welfare, Smittskyddsenheten Socialstyrelsen, SE-106 30 Stockholm, Sweden.

THIERMANN Alejandro, OIE Terrestrial Code Commission, World Organisation for Animal Health (OIE), 12 rue de Prony, FR-75017 Paris, France.

THUER Barbara, Institute of Virology and Immunoprophylaxis, Sensemattstrasse 293, CH-3147 Mittelhäusern, Switzerland.

TIEN-JYE Chang, College of Veterinary Medicine, National Chung Hsing University, 9Fl., No. 51, Sec. 2, Chungching S. Rd., Jungjeng Chiu, Taipei 100, Tapei China.

TIENSIN Thanawat, Department of Farm Animal Health, Faculty of Veterinary Medicine, Utrecht Univesity Yalelaan 7, NL-3584 CL Utrecht, The Netherlands.

TOSCANI Tonino, Poultry Technical Service, Amadori, Via del Rio 400, IT-47020 San Vittore di Cesena FC, Italy.

VALDER Wolf-Arno, European Commission - Sanco E2, Rue Froissart 101-3/72, BE-1049 Bruxelles, Belgium.

VALLAT Bernard, World Organisation for Animal Health (OIE), 12 rue de Prony, FR-75017 Paris, France.

VAN AARLE Paul, Intervet International, P.O. Box 31, NL-5830 AA Boxmeer, The Netherlands.

VAN BORM Steven, Veterinary and Agricultural Research Centre, Avian Virology and Immunology Unit, Groeselenberg 99, BE-1180 Brussels, Belgium.

VAN DEN BERG Thierry, Avian Virology & Immunology Unit, Veterinary & Agrochemical, Research Centre (VAR), 99, Groeselenberg, BE-1180 Brussels, Belgium.

VAN HAVERBEKE Georges, 16 Av. du Lac, FR-31320 Vigoulet-Auzil, France.

VAN NAM Hoang, Department of Animal Health, Ministry of Agriculture and Rural Development, Phuong Mai, Dong Da, Hanoi, Vietnam.

VANNIER Philippe, Laboratoire d'Etudes et de Recherches, Avicoles et Porcines, Zoopole B.P. 53, FR-22440 Ploufragan, France.

VIGOUROUX André, Coinseil Général Vétérinaire, Ministère de l'Agriculture de l'Alimentation de la Pêche et de la Ruralité, 251 rue de Vaugirard, FR-75732 Paris, France.

VILLAREAL-CHAVEZ Cesar, Animal Health Emergency Programs, Exotic Animal Disease Commission, Km 15.5 Carr. Mexico Toluca palo Alto, Cuajimalpa, Mexico 05110, Mexico.

VINCO Leonardo James, Poultry Technical Service, Bignami, Via Amendola 2/1, IT-40011 Anzola Emilia BO, Italy.

VITASEK Josef, Department of Animal Health and Welfare, State Veterinary Administration of the Czech Republic, Slezská 7, CZ-120 56 Prague 2, Czech Republic.

VLADIMIR Borisov, Laboratory for poultry vaccine preparations, FGI Federal Centre for Animal Health, RU-600901 Yur'evets, Vladimir, Russia.

VLASOV Nikolay, Federal Service for Veterinary and Phytosanitary Control, Orlikov per.,1/11, RU-107139Moscow, Russia.

VOLFORD Zsolt, Ministry of Agriculure and Rural Development, Kossuth tér 9-11, HU-1055 Budapest, Hungary.

VOSS Matthias, Veterinary Specialist for Poultry Diseases, Diagnostic Laboratory, Lohmann Tierzucht GmbH, Abschnede 64, P.O. Box 460, DE-27454 Cuxhaven, Germany.

WAELEN Susanne, Ministry of Agriculture, Nature and Food Quality, PO Box: 20401, Bezuidenhoutseweg 73, NL-2500 EK The Hague, The Netherlands.

WALLENSTEN Anders, The National Board of Health and Welfare, Smittskyddsenheten Socialstyrelsen, SE-106 30 Stockholm, Sweden.

WEIJTENS Martijn, Ministry of Agriculture, Nature and Food Quality, P.O.Box 20401, NL-2500 EK The Hague, The Netherlands.

WEINANDY Herbert, Bundesministerium für Verbraucherschutz, Ernähung und Landwirtschaft, Rochusstraße 1, DE-53123 Bonn, Germany.

WILLEBERG Preben, Danish Food and Veterinary Administration, Mørkhøj Bygade 19, DK-2860 Søborg, Denmark.

WILSON David, International Trade Department, World Organisation for Animal Health (OIE), 12 rue de Prony, FR-75017 Paris, France.

WITTEN Mark, Dept. of Pediatrics, University of Arizona, 1501 N. Campbell Ave, P.O. Box 245073, Tucson, AZ 85724, USA.

YEHIA Ghazi, OIE Representation for the Middle East, World Organisation for Animal Health (OIE), Kfarchima, Old Road of Saida, Beirut 6220, Lebanon.

YOUNUS Israt Ara, Renata Agro Industries Ltd., House # 450, Road # 31, New DOHS, Mohakhali, Dhaka 1206, Bangladesh.

ZAMBERG Yehuda, Shafit Biological Laboratories Ltd., IL-60990 Kibbutz-Shefayim, Israel.

ZAMPAGLIONE Maria, World Organisation for Animal Health (OIE), 12 rue de Prony, FR-75017 Paris, France.

ZANELLA Antonio, University of Milano, Via Gioberti 19, IT-25128 Brescia, Italy.

ZEPEDA Cristobal, Centers for Epidemiology & Animal Health, OIE Collaborating Center for Animal Disease, Surveillance Systems and Risk Analysis, 2150 Centre Ave Building B, Fort Collins, CO 80526-8117, USA.

ZGONNYK Nataliya, State Department of Veterinary Medicine, Ministry of Agricultural Policy of Ukraine, 24 Kreshchatik str., Kiev 01001, Ukraine.

ZRELLI Malek, Services Vétérinaires, Ministère de l'Agriculture, 30 rue Alain Savary, TN-1002 Tunis, Tunisia.

Index of Authors

Abolnik C.: 189
Alexander D.J.: 45, 77

Banks J.: 45
Bisschop S.P.R.: 189
Brown I.H.: 45, 93

Capua I.: 15, 99, 109
Cardinale E.: 211
Cattoli G.: 99
Chavernac D.: 211
Chen H.: 73, 127
Chow K.W.: 133
Cornelius E.: 189

Desvaux S.: 211
Domenech J.: 23
Dyrting K.C.: 133

Edwards S.: 159
Ellis T.M.: 133
Essen S.C.: 45

Gissin I.: 201
Goutard F.: 211
Guerne-Bleich E.: 171

Holl D.: 211

Jiang Y.: 127
Jutzi S.C.: 5

Kida H.: 69

Lee C.W.: 117
Leung C.: 133
Li C.: 127
Li H.: 73
Lipkind M.: 201
Londt B.: 45
Lubroth J.: 23

Manvell R.J.: 45
Marangon S.: 109
Martin V.: 23
McLeod A.: 171
Ménard C.: 211
Meslin F.-X.: 3

Naeem K.: 145

Olivier A.J.: 51

Panigrahy B.: 37
Panshin A.: 201
Pantin-Jackwood M.: 61
Pedersen J.C.: 37
Peiris J.S.M.: 133
Perk S.: 201
Pfeiffer D.: 23
Pirak M.: 201
Pokamunski S.: 201
Porphyre V.: 211

Qiao C.: 73, 127

Roger F.: 211
Romito M.: 189

Sakoda Y.: 69
Senne D.A.: 37
Shell W.: 45
Shihmanter E.: 201
Siddique N.: 145
Sims L.D.: 23, 133
Slingenbergh J.: 23
Slomka M.: 45
Sorn S.: 211
Stallnecht D.E.: 37
Suarez D.L.: 37, 117
Swayne D.E.: 61, 85, 117

Thonnat J.: 211
Tian G.: 127

Vallat B.: 11
Van Aarle P.: 151
Verwoerd D.: 189
Villareal C.L.: 125

Wang X.: 127
Wong C.W.: 133
Wong H.K.H.: 133

Yang H.: 73
Yu K.: 73, 127

Zepeda C.: 163

•••••••••••••••••

Developments in Biological Standardization

Vol. 23: Madrid 1973	Sterilization and sterility testing of biological substances
Vol. 24: San Francisco 1973	Preservatives in biological products
Vol. 25: Lyon 1973	Requirements for poultry virus vaccines
Vol. 26: Budapest 1973	Selected veterinary vaccines
Vol. 27: Budapest 1973	Purity of human plasma proteins
Vol. 28: London 1974	Immunity to infections of the respiratory system in man and animals
46th Symp., London 1974	Breeding of simians and their uses in developmental biology. Ed. Lab. Animals Ltd. (6)
Vol. 29: Geneva 1974 (WHO/IABS)	Standardization and control of allergens administered to man
Vol. 30: Milan 1974	Viral hepatitis
Vol. 31: Rabat 1975	Brucellosis (II)
Vol. 32: Paris 1975 (OIE/IABS)	Colstridial sera and vaccines for veterinary use
Vol. 33: Douglas 1975	Vaccination by the non-parenteral route
Vol. 34: Budapest 1976	Pyrogenicity, innocuity and toxicity test systems for biological products
Vol. 35: Lyon 1976	Foot-and-mouth disease vaccines
Vol. 36: Lyon Washington D.C. 1976	Freeze-drying of biological products
Vol. 37: Geneva 1976	Standardization of cell substrates for the production of virus vaccines
Vol. 38: London 1977	Biological preparations in the treatment of cancer
Vol. 39: Geneva 1977	Influenza immunization (II)
Vol. 40: Marburg 1977	Standardization of rabies vaccines (III) (WHO/IABS)
Vol. 41: Guadeloupe 1978	Vaccinations in the developing countries
Vol. 42: Paris 1978	Second General Meeting of European Society of Animal Cell Technology
Vol. 43: Brussels 1978	Immunization: Benefit versus risk factors
Vol. 44: Villars 1979	Test methods for the quality control of plasma proteins
Vol. 45: San Antonio 1979	The Standardization of animals to improve biomedical research, production and control
Vol. 46: Oxford 1979	Third General Meeting of European Society of Animal Cell Technology
Vol. 47: Bilthoven 1980	Reassessment of inactivated poliomyelitis vaccine
Vol. 48: Geneva 1980	Standardization of albumin, plasma substitutes and plasmapheresis
Vol. 49: Leetown 1981	Fish biologics: Serodiagnostics and vaccines
Vol. 50: Heidelberg 1981	Joint ESACT-IABS Meeting on the use of heteroploid and other cell substrates for the production of biologicals
Vol. 51: Lyon 1981	Immunization of adult birds with inactivated oil adjuvant vaccines
Vol. 52: Lyon 1981	Herpes virus of man and animal: Standardization of immunological procedures
Vol. 53: Dublin 1982	Enteric infections in man and animals: Standardization of immunological procedures

Vol. 54: Athens 1982	Viral hepatitis: Standardization in immunoprophylaxis of infections by hepatitis viruses
Vol. 55: Copenhagen 1982	Fifth General Meeting of European Society of Animal Cell Technology
Vol. 56: Algeria 1983	IIIrd International Symposium on Brucellosis
Vol. 57: Paris 1983	Monoclonal antibodies: Standardization of their characterization and use
Vol. 58: Budapest 1983	BCG vaccines and tuberculins
Vol. 59: Geneva 1983	Standardization and control of biologicals produced by recombinant DNA technology
Vol. 60: Gardone Riviera 1983	Production and exploitation of existing and new animal cell substrates
Vol. 61: Geneva 1984	Proceedings of the Fourth International Symposium on pertussis
Vol. 62: Stockholm 1985	Diagnostics and vaccines for parasitic diseases
Vol. 63: San Francisco 1985	Use and standardization of chemically defined antigens
Vol. 64: London 1985	Reduction of animal usage in the development and control of biological products
Vol. 65: Amsterdam 1985	Use and standardization of combined vaccines
Vol. 66: Baden 1985	Advances in animal cell technology: cell engineering, evaluation and exploitation
Vol. 67: Melbourne 1986	Standardization in blood fractionation including coagulation factors
Vol. 68: Geneva, 1986	Cells – Products – Safety
Vol. 69: London, 1987	Cytokines Laboratory and Clinical Evaluation
Vol. 70:Arlington, VA, 1988	Continuous Cell Lines as Substrates for Biologicals
Vol. 71:Utrecht, 1989	Monoclonal Antibodies for Therapy, Prevention and In vivo Diagnosis of Human Disease
Vol. 72: Annecy, 1989	Progress in Animal Retroviruses
Vol. 73: Shizuoka, 1990	Pertussis: Evaluation and Research on Acellular Pertussis Vaccines
Vol. 74: Bethesda, MD, 1990	Biological Product Freeze-Drying and Formulation
Vol. 75: London, 1990	Virological Aspects of the Safety of Biological Products
Vol. 76: Bethesda, MD, 1991	Continuous Cell Lines - An International Workshop on Current Issues
Vol. 77: Annecy, 1991	Standardization of the Immunopharmacology of Natural and Synthetic Immunomodulators
Vol. 78: Bethesda, MD, 1991	Poliovirus Attenuation: Molecular Mechanisms and Practical Aspects
Vol. 79: Ploufragan, 1992	The First Steps Towards an International Harmonization of Veterinary Biologicals: 1993 and Free Circulation of Vaccines within the EEC
Vol. 80: Heidelberg, 1992	Transmissible Spongiform Encephalopathies - Impact on Animal and Human Health
Vol. 81: Cannes, 1992	Virological Safety Aspects of Plasma Derivatives
Vol. 82: Albany NY, 1993	Recombinant Vectors in Vaccine Development
Vol. 83: Annecy, 1993	Genetic Stability and Recombinant Product Consistency
Vol. 84: Langen, 1993	Non-Target Effects of Live Vaccines
Vol. 85: Santa Fé, NM, 1994	Genetics of Streptococci, Enterococci and Lactococci
Vol. 86: Langen, 1994	Replacement, Reduction and Refinement of Animal Experiments in the Development and Control of Biological Products
Vol. 87: Geneva, 1995	New Approaches to Stabilisation of Vaccines Potency
Vol. 88: Bethesda, MD, 1995	Viral Safety and Evaluation of Viral Clearance from Biopharmaceutical Products
Vol. 89: Rome, 1995	Pertussis Vaccine Trials
Vol. 90: Oslo, 1996	Fish Vaccinology
Vol. 91: San Francisco, CA, 1996	Development of Specifications for Biotechnology Pharmaceuticals Products
Vol. 92: Bergen, 1996	Modulation of the Immune Response to Vaccine Antigens
Vol. 93: Annecy, 1996	Safety of Biological Products Prepared from Mammalian Cell Culture
Vol. 94: Bethesda, MD, 1997	Simian Virus 40 (SV40): A Possible Human Polyomavirus
Vol. 95: Paris, 1997	Preclinical and Clinical Development of New Vaccines
Vol. 96: Washington, DC, 1995	Characterization of Biotechnology Pharmaceutical Products
Vol. 97: London, 1997	Biological Characterization and Assay of Cytokines and Growth Factors

Vol. 98: London, 1997	Inactivated Influenza Vaccines Prepared in Cell Culture
Vol. 99: Strasbourg, 1998	Animal Sera, Animal Sera Derivatives and Substitutes Used in the Manufacture of Pharmaceuticals: Viral Safety and Regulatory Aspects
Vol. 100: Geneva, 1998	A Celebration of 50 Years of Progress in Biological Standardization and Control at WHO
Vol. 101: London, 1998	Alternatives to Animals in the Development and Control of Biological Products for Human and Veterinary Use

Developments in Biologicals

Vol. 102: San Francisco, CA, 1999	Advances in Transfusion Safety
Vol. 103: Annecy, 1999	Physico-Chemical Procedures for the Characterization of Vaccines
Vol. 104: Langen, 1999	Development and Clinical Progress of DNA Vaccines
Vol. 105: Paris, 2000	Progress in Polio Eradication: Vaccine Strategies for the End Game
Vol. 106: Rockville, MD, 2000	Evolving Scientific and Regulatory Perspectives on Cell Substrates for Vaccine Development
Vol. 107: London, 2000	The Design and Analysis of Potency Assays for Biotechnology Products
Vol. 108: Langen, 2001	Advances in Transfusion Safety
Vol. 109: Washington, DC, 2000	Biologics 2000 – Comparability of Biotechnology Products
Vol. 110: Palm Cove, 2001	Orphan Vaccines – Bridging the Gap
Vol. 111: Utrecht, 2001	Advancing Science and Elimination of the Use of Laboratory Animals for Development and Control of Vaccines and Hormones
Vol. 112: Bethesda, MD, 2001	Immunogenicity of Therapeutic Biological Products
Vol. 113: Berlin, 2001	Process Validation for Manufacturing of Biologics and Biotechnology Products
Vol. 114: Ames, IA, 2002	Vaccines for OIE List A and Emerging Animal Diseases
Vol. 115: Bergen, 2002	Laboratory Correlates of Immunity to Influenza – A Reassessment
Vol. 116: Los Angeles, CA, 2003	Development of Therapeutic Cancer Vaccines
Vol. 117: Langen, 2003	Consideration of Alternative Licensing Procedures for Vaccines for Minor Species, Minor Indications and Autogenous/Autologous Products
Vol. 118: Langen, 2003	PDA/EMEA European Virus Safety Forum
Vol. 119: Buenos Aires, 2004	Control of Infectious Animal Diseases by Vaccination
Vol. 120: Bethesda, MD, 2003	Advances in Transfusion Safety
Vol. 121: Bergen, 2003	Progress in Fish Vaccinology
Vol. 122: Bethesda, MD, 2003	State of the Art Analytical Methods for Characterization of Biological Products and Assessment of Comparability
Vol. 123: Rockville, MD, 2004	Vaccine Cell Substrates 2004

IMPRIMERIE MEDECINE HYGIENE GENEVE SUISSE

décembre-2005